Multiple Sclerosis

Editor

DARIN T. OKUDA

NEUROLOGIC CLINICS

www.neurologic.theclinics.com

Consulting Editor
RANDOLPH W. EVANS

February 2018 • Volume 36 • Number 1

ELSEVIER

1600 John F. Kennedy Boulevard • Suite 1800 • Philadelphia, Pennsylvania, 19103-2899

http://www.theclinics.com

NEUROLOGIC CLINICS Volume 36, Number 1
February 2018 ISSN 0733-8619, ISBN-13: 978-0-323-56992-7

Editor: Stacy Eastman
Developmental Editor: Donald Mumford

Neurologic Clinics (ISSN 0733-8619) is published quarterly by Elsevier Inc., 360 Park Avenue South, New York, NY 10010–1710. Months of issue are February, May, August, and November. Periodicals postage paid at New York, NY, and additional mailing offices. Subscription prices are $312.00 per year for US individuals, $631.00 per year for US institutions, $100.00 per year for US students, $390.00 per year for Canadian individuals, $765.00 per year for Canadian institutions, $423.00 per year for international individuals, $765.00 per year for international institutions, and $210.00 for Canadian and foreign students/residents. To receive student/resident rate, orders must be accompanied by name of affiliated institution, date of term, and the *signature* of program/residency coordinator on institution letterhead. Orders will be billed at individual rate until proof of status is received. Foreign air speed delivery is included in all *Clinics* subscription prices. All prices are subject to change without notice. **POSTMASTER:** Send address changes to *Neurologic Clinics*, Elsevier Health Sciences Division, Subscription Customer Service, 3251 Riverport Lane, Maryland Heights, MO 63043. **Customer Service: Telephone: 1-800-654-2452 (U.S. and Canada); 314-447-8871 (outside U.S. and Canada). Fax: 314-447-8029. E-mail: journalscustomerservice-usa@elsevier.com (for print support); journalsonlinesupport-usa@elsevier.com (for online support).**

Reprints. For copies of 100 or more of articles in this publication, please contact the Commercial Reprints Department, Elsevier Inc., 360 Park Avenue South, New York, New York, 10010-1710; Tel.: +1-212-633-3874; Fax: +1-212-633-3820, and E-mail: reprints@elsevier.com.

Neurologic Clinics is also published in Spanish by Nueva Editorial Interamericana S.A., Mexico City, Mexico.

Neurologic Clinics is covered in *Current Contents/Clinical Medicine, MEDLINE/PubMed (Index Medicus), EMBASE/Excerpta Medica, and PsycINFO, and ISI/BIOMED.*

Contributors

CONSULTING EDITOR

RANDOLPH W. EVANS, MD
Clinical Professor, Department of Neurology, Baylor College of Medicine, Houston, Texas, USA

EDITOR

DARIN T. OKUDA, MD, MSc, FAAN, FANA
Professor, Department of Neurology and Neurotherapeutics, The University of Texas Southwestern Medical Center, Clinical Center for Multiple Sclerosis, Director, Neuroinnovation Program, Multiple Sclerosis and Neuroimmunology Imaging Program, Radiologically Isolated Syndrome Consortium, Dallas, Texas, USA

AUTHORS

LILYANA AMEZCUA, MD, MS
Department of Neurology, Keck School of Medicine of USC, Los Angeles, California, USA

CHRISTINA J. AZEVEDO, MD, MPH
Assistant Professor, Department of Neurology, Keck School of Medicine of USC, Los Angeles, California, USA

ELIZABETH CRABTREE-HARTMAN, MD
Associate Professor of Neurology, Medical Director, Tulane Multiple Center, Vice Chair of Clinical Programs, Tulane Center for Clinical Neurosciences, Tulane University School of Medicine, New Orleans, Louisiana, USA

NICOLA DE STEFANO, MD, PhD
Professor of Neurology, Department of Medicine, Surgery and Neuroscience, University of Siena, Siena, Italy

ANTONIO GIORGIO, MD, PhD
Researcher, Department of Medicine, Surgery and Neuroscience, University of Siena, Siena, Italy

JUSTIN D. GLENN, PhD
Department of Neurology, The Johns Hopkins School of Medicine, Baltimore, Maryland, USA

BENJAMIN M. GREENBERG, MD, MHS
Co-Director, Pediatric CONQUER Program, Department of Neurology and Neurotherapeutics, The University of Texas Southwestern Medical Center, Dallas, Texas, USA

MADISON R. HANSEN, BA
Research Assistant, Multiple Sclerosis and Neuroimmunology Imaging Program, Department of Neurology and Neurotherapeutics, The University of Texas Southwestern Medical Center, Clinical Center for Multiple Sclerosis, Dallas, Texas, USA

AMIRHOSSEIN JABERZADEH, PhD
Postdoctoral Scholar, Department of Neurology, Keck School of Medicine of USC, Los Angeles, California, USA

ORHUN H. KANTARCI, MD
Associate Professor, Department of Neurology, Mayo Clinic College of Medicine & Science, Mayo Clinic, Rochester, Minnesota, USA

STEPHEN C. KRIEGER, MD, FAAN
Associate Professor of Neurology, Icahn School of Medicine at Mount Sinai, Corinne Goldsmith Dickinson Center for MS, New York, New York, USA

CHRISTINE LEBRUN, MD, PhD
Service de Neurologie, Centre de Ressources et de Compétences Sclérose en Plaques, Université Nice Sophia Antipolis, Nice, France

HERNAN NICOLAS LEMUS, MD
Department of Neurology, Mayo Clinic, Rochester, Minnesota, USA

ELLEN M. MOWRY, MD, MCR
Department of Neurology, The Johns Hopkins School of Medicine, Baltimore, Maryland, USA

ALEXANDRA MUCCILLI, MD
Division of Neurology, St. Michael's Hospital, University of Toronto, Toronto, Ontario, Canada; Division of Neurology, CHUM Notre-Dame Hospital, University of Montreal, Montreal, Quebec, Canada

JIWON OH, MD, PhD, FRCPC
Division of Neurology, St. Michael's Hospital, University of Toronto, Toronto, Ontario, Canada; Department of Neurology, Johns Hopkins University, Baltimore, Maryland, USA

DARIN T. OKUDA, MD, MSc, FAAN, FANA
Professor, Department of Neurology and Neurotherapeutics, The University of Texas Southwestern Medical Center, Clinical Center for Multiple Sclerosis, Director, Neuroinnovation Program, Multiple Sclerosis and Neuroimmunology Imaging Program, Radiologically Isolated Syndrome Consortium, Dallas, Texas, USA

DANIEL PELLETIER, MD
Vice Chair of Research, Professor, Department of Neurology, Eric and Peggy Lieber Chair in Neurology, Chief, Neuro-immunology Division and USC Multiple Sclerosis Comprehensive Care Center, Keck School of Medicine of USC, Los Angeles, California, USA

ERICA RIVAS-RODRÍGUEZ, MD
Department of Neurology, Keck School of Medicine of USC, Los Angeles, California, USA

MOSES RODRIGUEZ, MD
Departments of Neurology and Immunology, Mayo Clinic, Rochester, Minnesota, USA

ESTELLE SEYMAN, MD
Division of Neurology, St. Michael's Hospital, University of Toronto, Toronto, Ontario, Canada

AKSEL SIVA, MD, FEAN
Professor, Department of Neurology, Istanbul University, Cerrahpaşa School of Medicine, Istanbul, Turkey

JAMES SUMOWSKI, PhD
Associate Professor of Neurology and Psychiatry, Icahn School of Medicine at Mount Sinai, Clinical Neuropsychologist, Corinne Goldsmith Dickinson Center for MS, New York, New York, USA

ANGELA VIDAL-JORDANA, MD, PhD
Department of Neurology-Neuroimmunology, Multiple Sclerosis Centre of Catalonia (Edifici Cemcat), Hospital Universitari Vall d'Hebron, Universitat Autònoma de Barcelona, Barcelona, Spain

CYNTHIA X. WANG, MD
Department of Neurology and Neurotherapeutics, The University of Texas Southwestern Medical Center, Dallas, Texas, USA

ARTHUR E. WARRINGTON, PhD
Department of Neurology, Mayo Clinic, Rochester, Minnesota, USA

BURCU ZEYDAN, MD
Postdoctoral Research Fellow, Departments of Neurology and Radiology, Mayo Clinic, Rochester, Minnesota, USA

Contents

Multiple sclerosis is an inflammatory demyelinating disease of the central nervous system with a variety of presentations and unclear pathogenesis. Multiple sclerosis has been associated with the term *autoimmunity* as a surrogate for pathogenesis. Multiple sclerosis is an organ-specific disease with immune-mediated myelin destruction. Understanding the complex etiology of multiple sclerosis and the importance of axon integrity is critical for clinicians who treat the disease. This article discusses the immune and autoimmune aspects of multiple sclerosis based on the current published data and novel evidence of strategies that promote remyelination and protect axons.

Clinical course in multiple sclerosis (MS) is difficult to predict on group and individual levels. The authors discuss the topographical model of MS as a new approach to characterizing the clinical course, with the potential to personalize disability progression based on each individual patient's pattern of disease burden (eg, lesion location) and reserve. The dynamic clinical threshold depicted in this visual model may help clinicians to educate patients about clinical phenotype and disease burden and foster an understanding of the difference between relapses and pseudoexacerbations. There is an emphasis on building reserve against cognitive and physical decline, encouraging agency among patients.

MRI is the most important tool for diagnosis and management of patients with multiple sclerosis (MS). MRI shows high sensitivity for detection of white matter lesions in the central nervous system and specificity for lesion dissemination in space and time. MRI is also used for tracking disease activity, prognostic evaluation, and monitoring the efficacy and safety of disease-modifying treatments. Nonconventional MRI measures (eg, brain atrophy) and quantitative measures of advanced MRI can capture features of MS beyond white matter lesions but are not currently implemented in clinical practice. Consensus guidelines on standardized MRI acquisition protocol have been recently published.

areas of difficulty: (1) discriminating MS from other diseases when the clinical history and imaging features are atypical or nonspecific and (2) the lack of quantitative imaging metrics with which to follow patients with MS over time in clinical practice. This article highlights promising MRI and postprocessing techniques that have potential applications in these areas. With further study, these tools could be usefully integrated into clinical care.

Pediatric-onset multiple sclerosis (MS) is a rare but increasingly recognized condition that both parallels and diverges from adult-onset MS. Exposure to key risk determinants for MS disease pathogenesis may occur during childhood. The diagnosis of pediatric MS can be challenging because of the potential for atypical presentations and a broad differential diagnosis. MS disease-modifying therapies have not been rigorously studied in children and raise difficult questions on how to manage a chronic inflammatory neurologic disease in a population of patients with developing central nervous and immune systems.

Minorities in the United States such as African Americans and Hispanics may have more severe disease than non-Hispanic whites. Factors contributing to these disparities are reviewed. The variations in disability from non-Hispanic whites may be the result of differences in clinical presentation, genetic underpinnings, and sociocultural factors. Creating awareness and increasing participation in research studies may improve our understanding.

In multiple sclerosis (MS), disease course is defined by a subclinical or clinical relapsing remitting phase, a progressive phase, and the overlapping phase in-between. Each phase can have intermittently active or inactive periods. Subclinical activity in radiologically isolated syndrome evolving to primary-progressive MS is mostly indistinguishable from relapsing-remitting MS evolving to secondary-progressive MS. The onset of progressive-phase MS is age dependent but time and pre-progressive phase agnostic. Pathologic hallmarks of progressive MS onset also appear to be age dependent but pre-progressive phase agnostic. The onset of progressive MS is characterized by a peak in smoldering plaques.

Multiple sclerosis (MS) is a chronic autoimmune disease of the central nervous system in which inflammation, demyelination, and axonal loss occurs from early stages of the disease. It mainly affects people between 20 and 40 years old, with a female predominance. Treatment options have been increasingly growing in the past years, and newer drugs, some with novel mechanisms of action, are being developed for treating patients with MS. There is an increasing interest in developing new drugs that will promote neuroprotection and/or myelin repair through different mechanisms of action that may target the most degenerative component of the disease.

Multiple sclerosis (MS) is a neuroinflammatory autoimmune disease of unknown etiology, although genetic components and environmental triggers are thought to collude to commence pathogenesis. Numerous investigations are now demonstrating the role of the gut microbiota in neuroinflammation and how alterations in its content may be associated with MS disease. This article explores the studies using MS rodent models to determine the roles of gut bacteria in neuroinflammatory disease, evaluate the evidence linking gut bacterial dysbiosis and MS, and give insight into potential MS therapies targeting the gut microbiota currently under investigation.

Meaningful symptom management can have a profound impact on quality of life. It can challenge time parameters during clinic, and therefore thought should be given to strategies that can improve efficiency and thereby make the undertaking more tenable. For any given symptom, the building blocks of care, such as vitamin D status, exercise/physical therapy, nutrition, and stress management, and ensuring disease-modifying therapy coverage, should be maximized. For each symptom, there are pharmacologic and nonpharmacologic interventions. Patient expectations should be queried early in the encounter so that time can be budgeted accordingly.

The average age of onset of multiple sclerosis (MS) is between 20 and 40 years of age. Therefore, most new patients diagnosed with MS within the next 10 to 15 years will be from the millennial generation, representing those born between 1982 and 2000. Certain preferences and trends of this contemporary generation will present new challenges to the MS physician and effective MS care. By first understanding these challenges, relevant and successful solutions can be created to craft a system of care that best benefits the millennial patient with MS.

NEUROLOGIC CLINICS

RELATED INTEREST

Neuroimaging Clinics of North America, May 2017 (Vol. 27, Issue 2)
Advances in Imaging of Multiple Sclerosis
Alex Rovira, *Editor*

THE CLINICS ARE AVAILABLE ONLINE!
Access your subscription at:
www.theclinics.com

Preface
Contemporary Topics in Multiple Sclerosis

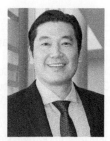

Darin T. Okuda, MD, MSc, FAAN, FANA
Editor

The field of clinical neuroimmunology, focused on the study of multiple sclerosis (MS), is one of the most dynamic subspecialties within neurology given the tremendous advancements made since the last *Neurologic Clinics* report in 2011 dedicated to MS. Not only have there been remarkable developments in our understanding of the origin of disease but also in our ability to detect earlier features supportive of in situ demyelination through enhanced diagnostic metrics and validated criteria. We are also able to offer our patients treatments with mechanisms of action that are greatly different from traditional recommendations. Therapies focused on myelin and axon repair may also be available in the near future! Beyond clinical and radiologic outcomes that may be meaningful to clinicians caring for patients, our management approaches for disabling symptoms associated with MS have also improved considerably along with the generation of strategies in the setting of evolving challenges related to effective care. In this issue of *Neurologic Clinics*, world-class experts from 5 countries share their expertise and knowledge on a variety of contemporary topics in MS including disease in children, disease variability related to ethnic variations, the appreciation of disease prior to first symptom development, the considerations of other diseases that may serve as mimics for central nervous system demyelination, the science of the gut, new brain and spinal cord imaging concepts, the latest in newly emerging treatments for MS and symptom management, and myelin repair, while highlighting the need to adapt our approach to the millennial MS patient given generational differences and the growing use of available technologies when considering the future of MS health care.

This issue aims to provide education by focusing on selected contemporary topics in our field, highlighting key aspects relevant to all health care providers including nurses, advanced practice providers, neurologists with expertise in other fields and those that serve our communities, along with specialists with a focus in MS. A fantastic balance of science along with clinical strategies for direct clinical application is provided. I hope

Neurol Clin 36 (2018) xiii–xiv
https://doi.org/10.1016/j.ncl.2017.10.001
0733-8619/18/© 2017 Published by Elsevier Inc.

neurologic.theclinics.com

that the contents within this issue serve as a catalyst for future innovative scientific efforts and the development of new approaches toward earlier disease recognition and surveillance, improved treatments, and repair of central nervous system injury.

I am deeply grateful to all of the contributors in this issue of *Neurologic Clinics*, all of whom have served as colleagues, mentors, and, most importantly, friends to many of us in the MS community. Please join me in thanking all of the contributors for providing us with their thoughtful contribution to our knowledge so that we may better educate and care for our patients.

Darin T. Okuda, MD, MSc, FAAN, FANA
Department of Neurology & Neurotherapeutics
University of Texas Southwestern Medical Center
Clinical Center for Multiple Sclerosis
5323 Harry Hines Boulevard
Dallas, TX 75390-8806, USA

E-mail address:
darin.okuda@utsouthwestern.edu

Multiple Sclerosis
Mechanisms of Disease and Strategies for Myelin and Axonal Repair

Hernan Nicolas Lemus, MD[a], Arthur E. Warrington, PhD[a,*],
Moses Rodriguez, MD[a,b]

KEYWORDS

- Multiple sclerosis • Autoimmune • Immune • Axon • Remyelination

KEY POINTS

- Multiple sclerosis is an inflammatory demyelinating disease of the central nervous system with a variety of presentations and unclear pathogenesis.
- Multiple sclerosis has been associated with the term *autoimmunity* as a surrogate for pathogenesis.
- Still, multiple sclerosis is an organ-specific disease with immune-mediated myelin destruction.
- Understanding the complex etiology of multiple sclerosis (autoimmune induced, virus induced, or immune mediated) and the importance of axon integrity is critical for clinicians who treat the disease.

INTRODUCTION

Multiple sclerosis (MS) is an inflammatory demyelinating disease of the central nervous system (CNS) with a variety of clinical presentations. The profound heterogeneity of MS is not limited to the symptoms but to neuroradiologic and histologic appearances of lesions and response to therapy.[1] As expected, the pathogenesis of MS is controversial, and there is no effective treatment that halts the neuro-axonal damage

Financial Support: Authors are supported by grants from the Minnesota Partnership Award for Biotechnology and Medical Genomics, Mayo Clinic Center for Multiple Sclerosis and Autoimmune Neurology (CMSAN) through a gift from Dr and Mrs Moon Park.
Competing Interests: Patents for human antibodies that promote remyelination and CNS repair are issued and owned by Mayo Clinic. A.E. Warrington and M. Rodriguez have a potential conflict of interest.
[a] Department of Neurology, Mayo Clinic, 200 First Street Southwest, Rochester, MN 55905, USA; [b] Department of Immunology, Mayo Clinic, 200 First Street Southwest, Rochester, MN 55905, USA
* Corresponding author. Department of Neurology, Mayo Clinic, Guggenheim Building 401, 200 First Street Southwest, Rochester, MN 55905.
E-mail address: Warrington.Arthur@mayo.edu

Neurol Clin 36 (2018) 1–11
https://doi.org/10.1016/j.ncl.2017.08.002
0733-8619/18/© 2017 The Author(s). Published by Elsevier Inc. This is an open access article under the CC BY-NC-ND license (http://creativecommons.org/licenses/by-nc-nd/4.0/).

or promotes remyelination. As a leading cause of disability, MS affects 400,000 people in the United States and 2.5 million of people worldwide.[2]

The demyelinating plaque, the main pathologic hallmark of MS, contains a prominent immunologic response dominated by CD8+ and CD4+ T cells.[1,3] Moreover, the presence of oligoclonal bands in the cerebrospinal fluid of MS patients shows the presence of immunoglobulin-producing B cells suggesting their participation in the pathogenesis of the disease.[4] These findings suggest that MS is an immune-mediated disorder involving multiple antigens of the CNS[5,6] and, further, that MS is an autoimmune disease of the CNS. Understanding the mechanism of MS is essential to elucidate possible strategies to repair myelin and axonal structures.

AUTOIMMUNITY VERSUS IMMUNE-MEDIATED DEMYELINATION

Several criteria have been established to determine whether a disease can be classified as *autoimmune*.[7,8] First, an autoantigen must be present in all patients with a proven immune response directed against it. Second, one must identify autoantibodies within a lesion or serum of patients with a direct correlation to disease activity or observed clinical improvement after immunosuppressive treatment. In systemic lupus erythematous (SLE), a well-characterized autoimmune disorder, the presentation of autoantigens by T cells promotes antibody formation and hence, the clinical manifestations.[9] It is also critical to reproduce the clinical and histopathologic aspects of the human disease after administration of the autoantibody or autoantigen within an animal. For example, when transferring anti-DNA antibodies to naïve recipient mice, there is an immunologic reaction against glomerular antigens leading to nephropathy similar to that seen in SLE.[10] Diseases like SLE have an experimental-based extensive literature that meets all the criteria and proves the role of autoimmunity in the pathophysiology.

MS is also an organ-specific disease (the brain and spinal cord) with immune-mediated myelin destruction. Nevertheless, after extensive research, confirmation of a specific auto-antigen in MS is lacking. The absence/presence of an infectious agent in patients with MS has also not been proven. Other organ-specific immune-mediated diseases such as herpes encephalitis have a persistent exogenous antigen (in this case, the herpes virus) that resides in the CNS and drives the development of acute inflammation and necrotizing lesions.[11] However, the absence of any consistent viral or bacterial antigen in MS patients suggests the presence of an autoantigen that drives this disease. Antibodies directed against CNS myelin proteins, lipids, and carbohydrates (possible candidates as autoantigens) can be identified in the tissue and serum of patients with MS.

Extensive literature is devoted to identifying antibodies against the myelin oligodendrocyte glycoprotein (MOG) in MS patients with inconsistent results. Enzyme-linked immunosorbent assay–based binding studies using a synthetic MOG peptide to identify antibodies found an increase in the frequency of MOG-binding IgGs in patients with MS compared with controls.[12,13] In contrast, other studies using enzyme-linked immunosorbent assay binding to the recombinant human immunoglobulin domain of MOG showed no difference in the levels of bound antibodies in patients with MS or healthy controls.[14] When using other techniques, such as immunoblot to detect antibodies directed against the recombinant human immunoglobulin domain of MOG in patients with MS, the results are inconsistent.[15,16] Antibodies that bind to other antigens such as alpha-B-crystallin, alu repeats, myelin basic protein, and myelin-associated glycoprotein have been reported but not rigorously studied.[17–20] Despite several published attempts to detect and quantify antibodies directed against myelin and nonmyelin antigens in patients with MS, there is no consensus. This lack of a self-directed immune response producing antibodies argues against the hypothesis of MS as an autoimmune disease (**Fig. 1**).

On the other hand, neuromyelitis optica (NMO), an autoimmune astrocytopathy, is a CNS disease driven by the presence of antibodies against aquaporin 4 (AQP4), a plasma membrane–based water-transporting protein (see **Fig. 1**). AQP4 is the most abundant water channel in the brain, expressed primarily in astrocytes and highly involved in neuroexcitation.[21] The discovery of pathogenic immunoglobulin G directed to AQP4 in almost 70% of the patients with NMO was the first evidence that this disease was an inflammatory autoimmune disease of the CNS.[22,23] The pathogenicity of the anti-AQP4 IgG in NMO patients has been reproduced in vivo and their presence confirmed in pathologic lesions.[24,25]

IS MULTIPLE SCLEROSIS AN AUTOIMMUNE DISEASE?

When comparing MS with other autoimmune diseases like neuromyelitis optica, it is clear that MS does not meet the full definition of autoimmune disease (**Table 1**). Although NMO meets 6 of 8 autoimmune disease criteria, MS meets only 2. Although there are some data for several of the other criteria, the evidence is controversial. For example, multiple studies focused on measuring the level of precursor T cells before and then during clinical exacerbations. However, none of these studies found a difference from the prevalence in healthy controls or are not confirmed using other patient populations.[26] It is clear that the data are weak to make a definitive conclusion that MS is an autoimmune disease.

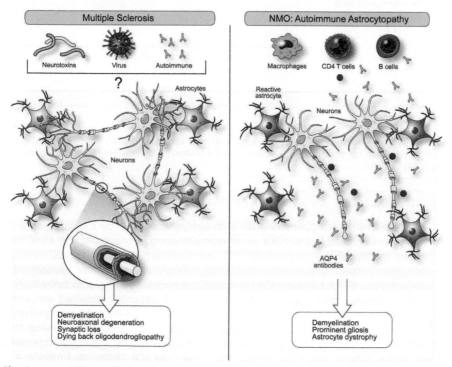

Fig. 1. Autoimmune response hypothesis for MS.

Table 1
Revised criteria for a disease to be considered autoimmune: neuromyelitis optica and multiple sclerosis

Criteria for Autoimmune Disease[7]	NMO	MS
Immune response to a precise autoantigen in all patients	aquaporin 4[22,23]	Multiple antigens have been described, not present in all patients[12,13,17–20]
Lesion reproducibility after administration of autoantibody or T cells	Exacerbation of EAE model after adoptive transfer of neuromyelitis optica Abs[27]	
Animal: induction of lesion by antigen immunization		EAE model: induced by myelin oligodendrocyte glycoprotein, proteolipid protein, myelin basic protein[28] and reactivated CD4+ T cells[29]
Autoantibody or T cell isolation form lesion or serum	aquaporin 4 antibodies[27,30]	
Autoantibody titers or T-cell levels associated with disease activity	Higher antibody titers during relapse than during remission[31]	
Autoimmune disorders or autoantigens associated with the disease	Sjogren syndrome, SLE[32]	No association in population-based cohort studies[33]
Immune absorption with purified autoantigen abrogates pathogenic autoantibody or T cell		
Reduction of autoantibody or T cell associated with clinical improvement	Plasma exchange[34]	Plasma exchange[35,36]

Abbreviations: EAE, experimental autoimmune encephalomyelitis; MBP, myelin basic protein; PLP, proteolipid protein.
Adapted from Paul WE, Schwartz RS, Datta SK. Autoimmunity and autoimmune diseases. In Fundamental immunology. New York: Raven Press; 1989. p. 819-66; and Rodriguez M, Warrington AE, Pease LR. Invited article: human natural autoantibodies in the treatment of neurologic disease. Neurology 2009;72(14):1269–76.

IS MULTIPLE SCLEROSIS A VIRUS-INDUCED DISEASE?

Viral microorganisms are postulated by many investigators to be causal agents of MS. The idea is plausible because other demyelinating diseases of the CNS like progressive multifocal leukoencephalopathy are caused by a virus: the JC virus in immune-compromised individuals.[37] Recently, much attention has focused on Epstein-Barr virus (EBV) because EBV antigens are expressed at significantly higher levels in the cerebrospinal fluid and serum of some MS patients compared with controls.[38] However, studies show an absence of intrathecal anti-EBV antibody synthesis in nearly 93% of patients with MS, which argues against this hypothesis.[39] Hence, the association of EBV with adult MS is not well established, and its role in pathogenesis remains to be determined. Other viral agents like varicella zoster and rubella are considered as possible risk factors but not causal agents.[40,41] Of note, vitamin D deficiency has been linked as a causal agent in relapsing remitting MS. Vitamin D has a role in regulating immune function. Low levels of this vitamin could produce an immune-deficient state against viral agents. Although clinical trials and observational studies using high levels of vitamin D have only shown modest reductions in the levels of interleukin 17, it has not been seen in other inflammatory markers.[42,43] The fact that high dose treatment of vitamin D in MS patients has scant effect on the overall course of the disease does not support this theory.

Demyelinating disease nearly identical to human MS can be consistently established in animals using well-characterized viral agents. Theiler's murine encephalomyelitis virus (TMEV) is a mouse enteric pathogen that belongs to the picornavirus family. It produces a chronic progressive demyelinating condition similar to what it is seen in humans with progressive MS.[44] This model presents with an immune response to virally infected cells and an autoimmune response to CNS antigens.[45] Novel therapies like natural human antibodies that induce either remyelination or neuroprotection have been successfully evaluated in this model of virus-induced demyelination.[46–48] Other virus-induced models with a persistent viral infection without dramatic animal mortality are coronavirus (JHM and MHV-4) and Semliki Forest affecting mice, distemper virus specific for canines, and visna virus in sheep and goats.

MECHANISMS OF MULTIPLE SCLEROSIS: DEMYELINATION VERSUS AXONAL DAMAGE

Demyelination, the major pathologic hallmark of MS, is not sufficient to explain the deficits seen in these patients. In 1969, the first observation of demyelination and complete axonal dysfunction in the CNS was made,[49] and since then, many have considered it as a unique event. Recent studies found that in MS, damage to myelin is not enough to produce the spectrum of symptoms. In humans, levels of demyelination are not strictly correlated to disease stage, neurologic deficits, or lesion pathology.[50–52] Imaging studies in postmortem brains using MRI have shown how axonal injury is the primary event leading to clinical deficits (more than demyelination).[53,54]

On the other hand, murine models of demyelination have also questioned the role of demyelination as the sole event in MS. Despite profound demyelination seen with TMEV murine model, in the absence of major histocompatibility complex (MHC) class I, there is no deficit in motor function.[55] Moreover, there is preservation of axonal transport in these mice despite demyelination.[56] CD8+ T cells direct recognition of MCH class I is a well-known mediator of axonal injury and dropout. In murine models of demyelination and murine culture of neurons, CD8+ T cells injure demyelinated axons selectively.[57,58] CD8+ clones are the dominant cells in active MS lesions[59] and have direct correlation with accumulation of amyloid precursor protein, a marker of acute axonal damage.[60]

Perforin, a critical mediator in cell cytotoxicity and apoptosis, is released by CD8+ T cells after recognition of the MCH class I complex.[61] Once inside the cell, perforin creates a pore in the membrane and delivers granzymes that initiate a cascade of signals causing death of cells.[62] During viral infection with TMEV and in electrically silent neurons in vitro, both have an increased expression of MCH class I complex.[63,64] More importantly, axon injury secondary to demyelination is mediated by inflammatory factors, especially, perforin.[65] Perforin-deficient mice had an increased number of large-diameter axons and better functional motor abilities when compared with perforin-competent controls, despite having the same levels of demyelination.

Sodium channels are also a critical component in demyelinated axons, as changes in their number can influence impulse conduction.[66,67] After an acute injury in peripheral axons, there is a high density of sodium channels.[68] Murine models of demyelination have also shown how formation of nodes of Ranvier (where action potentials are generated) and saltatory conduction precedes remyelination in axons with demyelination.[69] Demyelinated mice with MHC class I deficiency and normal functional status have been previously described.[55] The normal motor function is caused by a preservation of axons and increased intensities of sodium channels suggesting an upregulation or redistribution of these molecules in the axons. Based on these observations, it can be concluded that axonal injury plays a critical role in the neurologic deficits seen in patients with MS and must be taken into account when considering strategies for MS therapies.

MYELIN AND AXONAL REPAIR STRATEGIES

Understanding the complex etiology of MS and the importance of axon integrity is critical for clinicians who expect halting of neuro-axonal damage. When a patient with newly diagnosed MS has the first neurologic symptom, there is already axonal loss. Hence, there is a need to treat early and use multiple strategies that target remyelination and preservation of axons and oligodendrocytes (OL).

The authors' laboratory has done extensive research in natural human recombinant antibodies formerly known as *rHIgM22* and *rHIgM12*. These molecules, part of human innate immunoglobulin repertoire, are able to bind to oligodendrocytes (rHIgM22) and neurons (rHIgM12).[70–72] In TMEV and lysolecithin-induced demyelination, rHIgM22 promotes oligodendrocyte remyelination and protects spinal cord axon number.[47] Currently, this molecule is under a clinical trial to establish its tolerance in MS patients after an acute exacerbation. In addition, rHIgM12 protects against axonal injury in TMEV and amyotrophic lateral sclerosis murine models.[72] It also binds to PSA-NCAM and gangliosides of glia and neurons resulting in neurite extension in vitro and neurite outgrowth.[73] Recently, rHIgM12 showed an immune-modulatory therapeutic effect in an MOG-induced experimental autoimmune encephalomyelitis (EAE).[74]

Inhibition of the leucine rich repeat and immunoglobulinlike domain containing NOGO receptor interacting protein-1 (LINGO-1) increases differentiation of oligodendrocyte progenitor cells into mature oligodendrocytes.[75] In TMEV murine model of demyelination, inhibition of this molecule promoted remyelination leading to the discovery of anti–LINGO-1.[76] This was the first drug entering a clinical trial showing how 41% of patients had improvement of nerve signaling and possibly myelin repair.[77] Despite this, anti–LINGO-1 failed to improve disability and cognitive function after 72 weeks of follow-up.

As explained in the previous section, CD8+ T cells and the upregulation of MHC class I complex are critical in the pathogenesis of MS. Dimethyl fumarate (BG-12 or Tecfidera) is a molecule that showed remarkable efficacy in the treatment of relapsing remitting MS and exposure may result in reductions in CD8+ T-cell populations in certain patients.[78] Fingolimod, the first approved oral therapy for active relapsing remitting MS, modulates T-cell proliferation in vitro as well.[79] Together, these results suggest that an immunotherapy against active CD8+ cells using anti-CD8 antibodies[80] could suppress the immune-mediated reactions in patients with MS.

SUMMARY

MS is an immune-mediated disease that lacks the presence of a specific antigen that drives the inflammatory process. The extensive characterization of MS pathology, immunology, and serology has misled many investigators to conclude that MS is an autoimmune disease. However, there is a lack of scientific evidence supporting the role of active autoantigens and autoantibodies driving the inflammatory and demyelinating cascades seen in patients with MS. Understanding the role of axonal injury and its relationship with clinical deficits is essential for a future drug. Future trials should aim a multifaceted approach with several reagents that target remyelination, protections of axons and oligodendrocyte progenitor cell, and suppressive therapies against active inflammatory cell populations.

ACKNOWLEDGMENTS

The authors acknowledge with many thanks support from the Applebaum, Hilton, Peterson and Sanford Foundations, and the McNeilus family.

REFERENCES

1. Lucchinetti C, Bruck W, Parisi J, et al. Heterogeneity of multiple sclerosis lesions: implications for the pathogenesis of demyelination. Ann Neurol 2000;47(6): 707–17.
2. Pelletier D, Hafler DA. Fingolimod for multiple sclerosis. N Engl J Med 2012; 366(4):339–47.
3. Frohman EM, Racke MK, Raine CS. Multiple sclerosis–the plaque and its pathogenesis. N Engl J Med 2006;354(9):942–55.
4. Qin Y, Duquette P, Zhang Y, et al. Clonal expansion and somatic hypermutation of V(H) genes of B cells from cerebrospinal fluid in multiple sclerosis. J Clin Invest 1998;102(5):1045–50.
5. Ando DG, Clayton J, Kono D, et al. Encephalitogenic T cells in the B10.PL model of experimental allergic encephalomyelitis (EAE) are of the Th-1 lymphokine subtype. Cell Immunol 1989;124(1):132–43.
6. Pettinelli CB, McFarlin DE. Adoptive transfer of experimental allergic encephalomyelitis in SJL/J mice after in vitro activation of lymph node cells by myelin basic protein: requirement for Lyt 1+ 2- T lymphocytes. J Immunol 1981;127(4):1420–3.
7. Paul WE, Schwartz RS, Datta SK. Autoimmunity and autoimmune diseases. In: Fundamental Immunology. New York: Raven Press; 1989. p. 819–66.
8. Rodriguez M, Warrington AE, Pease LR. Invited article: human natural autoantibodies in the treatment of neurologic disease. Neurology 2009;72(14):1269–76.
9. Chan OT, Hannum LG, Haberman AM, et al. A novel mouse with B cells but lacking serum antibody reveals an antibody-independent role for B cells in murine lupus. J Exp Med 1999;189(10):1639–48.
10. Bagavant H, Fu SM. New insights from murine lupus: disassociation of autoimmunity and end organ damage and the role of T cells. Curr Opin Rheumatol 2005; 17(5):523–8.
11. Cinque P, Cleator GM, Weber T, et al. The role of laboratory investigation in the diagnosis and management of patients with suspected herpes simplex encephalitis: a consensus report. J Neurol Neurosurg Psychiatry 1996;61(4):339–45.
12. Kennel De March A, De Bouwerie M, Kolopp-Sarda MN, et al. Anti-myelin oligodendrocyte glycoprotein B-cell responses in multiple sclerosis. J Neuroimmunol 2003;135(1–2):117–25.
13. Khalil M, Reindl M, Lutterotti A, et al. Epitope specificity of serum antibodies directed against the extracellular domain of myelin oligodendrocyte glycoprotein: influence of relapses and immunomodulatory treatments. J Neuroimmunol 2006; 174(1–2):147–56.
14. Karni A, Bakimer-Kleiner R, Abramsky O, et al. Elevated levels of antibody to myelin oligodendrocyte glycoprotein is not specific for patients with multiple sclerosis. Arch Neurol 1999;56(3):311–5.

15. Reindl M, Linington C, Brehm U, et al. Antibodies against the myelin oligodendro-cyte glycoprotein and the myelin basic protein in multiple sclerosis and other neurological diseases: a comparative study. Brain 1999;122(Pt 11):2047–56.
16. Lutterotti A, Reindl M, Gassner C, et al. Antibody response to myelin oligodendro-cyte glycoprotein and myelin basic protein depend on familial background and are partially associated with human leukocyte antigen alleles in multiplex families and sporadic multiple sclerosis. J Neuroimmunol 2002;131(1–2):201–7.
17. Agius MA, Kirvan CA, Schafer AL, et al. High prevalence of anti-alpha-crystallin antibodies in multiple sclerosis: correlation with severity and activity of disease. Acta Neurol Scand 1999;100(3):139–47.
18. Archelos JJ, Trotter J, Previtali S, et al. Isolation and characterization of an oligo-dendrocyte precursor-derived B-cell epitope in multiple sclerosis. Ann Neurol 1998;43(1):15–24.
19. Cruz M, Olsson T, Ernerudh J, et al. Immunoblot detection of oligoclonal anti-myelin basic protein IgG antibodies in cerebrospinal fluid in multiple sclerosis. Neurology 1987;37(9):1515–9.
20. Moller JR, Johnson D, Brady RO, et al. Antibodies to myelin-associated glycopro-tein (MAG) in the cerebrospinal fluid of multiple sclerosis patients. J Neuroimmunol 1989;22(1):55–61.
21. Papadopoulos MC, Verkman AS. Aquaporin water channels in the nervous sys-tem. Nat Rev Neurosci 2013;14(4):265–77.
22. Hinson SR, Pittock SJ, Lucchinetti CF, et al. Pathogenic potential of IgG binding to water channel extracellular domain in neuromyelitis optica. Neurology 2007; 69(24):2221–31.
23. Hinson SR, Roemer SF, Lucchinetti CF, et al. Aquaporin-4-binding autoantibodies in patients with neuromyelitis optica impair glutamate transport by down-regulating EAAT2. J Exp Med 2008;205(11):2473–81.
24. Bennett JL, Lam C, Kalluri SR, et al. Intrathecal pathogenic anti-aquaporin-4 an-tibodies in early neuromyelitis optica. Ann Neurol 2009;66(5):617–29.
25. Lucchinetti CF, Mandler RN, McGavern D, et al. A role for humoral mechanisms in the pathogenesis of Devic's neuromyelitis optica. Brain 2002;125(Pt 7):1450–61.
26. Steinman L. Immunology of relapse and remission in multiple sclerosis. Annu Rev Immunol 2014;32:257–81.
27. Bradl M, Misu T, Takahashi T, et al. Neuromyelitis optica: pathogenicity of patient immunoglobulin in vivo. Ann Neurol 2009;66(5):630–43.
28. Olitsky PK, Yager RH. Experimental disseminated encephalomyelitis in white mice. J Exp Med 1949;90(3):213–24.
29. Swanborg RH. Experimental autoimmune encephalomyelitis in the rat: lessons in T-cell immunology and autoreactivity. Immunol Rev 2001;184:129–35.
30. Lennon VA, Kryzer TJ, Pittock SJ, et al. IgG marker of optic-spinal multiple scle-rosis binds to the aquaporin-4 water channel. J Exp Med 2005;202(4):473–7.
31. Jarius S, Wildemann B. AQP4 antibodies in neuromyelitis optica: diagnostic and pathogenetic relevance. Nat Rev Neurol 2010;6(7):383–92.
32. Pittock SJ, Lennon VA, de Seze J, et al. Neuromyelitis optica and non organ-specific autoimmunity. Arch Neurol 2008;65(1):78–83.
33. Wynn DR, Rodriguez M, O'Fallon WM, et al. A reappraisal of the epidemiology of multiple sclerosis in Olmsted County, Minnesota. Neurology 1990;40(5):780–6.
34. Bonnan M, Valentino R, Olindo S, et al. Plasma exchange in severe spinal attacks associated with neuromyelitis optica spectrum disorder. Mult Scler 2009;15(4): 487–92.

35. Rodriguez M, Karnes WE, Bartleson JD, et al. Plasmapheresis in acute episodes of fulminant CNS inflammatory demyelination. Neurology 1993;43(6):1100–4.
36. Magana SM, Keegan BM, Weinshenker BG, et al. Beneficial plasma exchange response in central nervous system inflammatory demyelination. Arch Neurol 2011;68(7):870–8.
37. SantaCruz KS, Roy G, Spigel J, et al. Neuropathology of JC virus infection in progressive multifocal leukoencephalopathy in remission. World J Virol 2016;5(1):31–7.
38. Cepok S, Zhou D, Srivastava R, et al. Identification of Epstein-Barr virus proteins as putative targets of the immune response in multiple sclerosis. J Clin Invest 2005;115(5):1352–60.
39. Villegas E, Santiago O, Carrillo JA, et al. Low intrathecal immune response of anti-EBNA-1 antibodies and EBV DNA from multiple sclerosis patients. Diagn Microbiol Infect Dis 2011;70(1):85–90.
40. Eftekharian MM, Ghannad MS, Taheri M, et al. Frequency of viral infections and environmental factors in multiple sclerosis. Hum Antibodies 2016;24(1–2):17–23.
41. Shaygannejad V, Rezaie N, Paknahad Z, et al. The environmental risk factors in multiple sclerosis susceptibility: a case-control study. Adv Biomed Res 2016;5:98.
42. Toghianifar N, Ashtari F, Zarkesh-Esfahani SH, et al. Effect of high dose vitamin D intake on interleukin-17 levels in multiple sclerosis: a randomized, double-blind, placebo-controlled clinical trial. J Neuroimmunol 2015;285:125–8.
43. Golan D, Halhal B, Glass-Marmor L, et al. Vitamin D supplementation for patients with multiple sclerosis treated with interferon-beta: a randomized controlled trial assessing the effect on flu-like symptoms and immunomodulatory properties. BMC Neurol 2013;13:60.
44. Theiler M. Spontaneous encephalomyelitis of mice–a new virus disease. Science 1934;80(2066):122.
45. dal Canto MC, Lipton HL. A new model of persistent viral infection with primary demyelination. Neurol Neurocir Psiquiatr 1977;18(2–3 Suppl):455–67.
46. Warrington AE, Bieber AJ, Ciric B, Pease LR, et al. A recombinant human IgM promotes myelin repair after a single, very low dose. J Neurosci Res 2007;85(5):967–76.
47. Wootla B, Denic A, Watzlawik JO, et al. Antibody-mediated oligodendrocyte remyelination promotes axon health in progressive demyelinating disease. Mol Neurobiol 2016;53(8):5217–28.
48. Wootla B, Denic A, Warrington AE, et al. A monoclonal natural human IgM protects axons in the absence of remyelination. J Neuroinflammation 2016;13(1):94.
49. McDonald WI, Sears TA. Effect of demyelination on conduction in the central nervous system. Nature 1969;221(5176):182–3.
50. Stevens JC, Farlow MR, Edwards MK, et al. Magnetic resonance imaging. Clinical correlation in 64 patients with multiple sclerosis. Arch Neurol 1986;43(11):1145–8.
51. Bruck W, Bitsch A, Kolenda H, et al. Inflammatory central nervous system demyelination: correlation of magnetic resonance imaging findings with lesion pathology. Ann Neurol 1997;42(5):783–93.
52. Mews I, Bergmann M, Bunkowski S, et al. Oligodendrocyte and axon pathology in clinically silent multiple sclerosis lesions. Mult Scler 1998;4(2):55–62.
53. van Waesberghe JH, Kamphorst W, De Groot CJ, et al. Axonal loss in multiple sclerosis lesions: magnetic resonance imaging insights into substrates of disability. Ann Neurol 1999;46(5):747–54.

54. Fisher E, Chang A, Fox RJ, et al. Imaging correlates of axonal swelling in chronic multiple sclerosis brains. Ann Neurol 2007;62(3):219–28.
55. Rivera-Quinones C, McGavern D, Schmelzer JD, et al. Absence of neurological deficits following extensive demyelination in a class I-deficient murine model of multiple sclerosis. Nat Med 1998;4(2):187–93.
56. Ure DR, Rodriguez M. Preservation of neurologic function during inflammatory demyelination correlates with axon sparing in a mouse model of multiple sclerosis. Neuroscience 2002;111(2):399–411.
57. Medana I, Martinic MA, Wekerle H, et al. Transection of major histocompatibility complex class I-induced neurites by cytotoxic T lymphocytes. Am J Pathol 2001;159(3):809–15.
58. Johnson AJ, Upshaw J, Pavelko KD, et al. Preservation of motor function by inhibition of CD8+ virus peptide-specific T cells in Theiler's virus infection. FASEB J 2001;15(14):2760–2.
59. Babbe H, Roers A, Waisman A, et al. Clonal expansions of CD8(+) T cells dominate the T cell infiltrate in active multiple sclerosis lesions as shown by micromanipulation and single cell polymerase chain reaction. J Exp Med 2000;192(3): 393–404.
60. Bitsch A, Schuchardt J, Bunkowski S, et al. Acute axonal injury in multiple sclerosis. Correlation with demyelination and inflammation. Brain 2000;123(Pt 6): 1174–83.
61. Lieberman J. The ABCs of granule-mediated cytotoxicity: new weapons in the arsenal. Nat Rev Immunol 2003;3(5):361–70.
62. Metkar SS, Wang B, Aguilar-Santelises M, et al. Cytotoxic cell granule-mediated apoptosis: perforin delivers granzyme B-serglycin complexes into target cells without plasma membrane pore formation. Immunity 2002;16(3):417–28.
63. Lindsley MD, Patick AK, Prayoonwiwat N, et al. Coexpression of class I major histocompatibility antigen and viral RNA in central nervous system of mice infected with Theiler's virus: a model for multiple sclerosis. Mayo Clin Proc 1992;67(9): 829–38.
64. Neumann H, Cavalie A, Jenne DE, et al. Induction of MHC class I genes in neurons. Science 1995;269(5223):549–52.
65. Howe CL, Adelson JD, Rodriguez M. Absence of perforin expression confers axonal protection despite demyelination. Neurobiol Dis 2007;25(2):354–9.
66. Waxman SG, Black JA, Kocsis JD, et al. Low density of sodium channels supports action potential conduction in axons of neonatal rat optic nerve. Proc Natl Acad Sci U S A 1989;86(4):1406–10.
67. Johnston WL, Dyer JR, Castellucci VF, et al. Clustered voltage-gated Na+ channels in Aplysia axons. J Neurosci 1996;16(5):1730–9.
68. Foster RE, Whalen CC, Waxman SG. Reorganization of the axon membrane in demyelinated peripheral nerve fibers: morphological evidence. Science 1980; 210(4470):661–3.
69. Smith KJ, Bostock H, Hall SM. Saltatory conduction precedes remyelination in axons demyelinated with lysophosphatidyl choline. J Neurol Sci 1982;54(1): 13–31.
70. Avrameas S. Natural autoantibodies: from 'horror autotoxicus' to 'gnothi seauton'. Immunol Today 1991;12(5):154–9.
71. Watzlawik J, Holicky E, Edberg DD, et al. Human remyelination promoting antibody inhibits apoptotic signaling and differentiation through Lyn kinase in primary rat oligodendrocytes. Glia 2010;58(15):1782–93.

72. Xu X, Denic A, Jordan LR, et al. A natural human IgM that binds to gangliosides is therapeutic in murine models of amyotrophic lateral sclerosis. Dis Model Mech 2015;8(8):831–42.
73. Watzlawik J, Kahoud RJ, Ng S, et al. Polysialic acid as an antigen for monoclonal antibody HIgM12 to treat multiple sclerosis and other neurodegenerative disorders. J Neurochem 2015;134(5):865–78.
74. Lemus HN, Warrington AE, Denic A, et al. Treatment with a recombinant human IgM that recognizes PSA-NCAM preserves brain pathology in MOG-induced experimental autoimmune encephalomyelitis. Hum Antibodies 2017;25(3–4): 121–9.
75. Mi S, Miller RH, Lee X, et al. LINGO-1 negatively regulates myelination by oligodendrocytes. Nat Neurosci 2005;8(6):745–51.
76. Mi S, Miller RH, Tang W, et al. Promotion of central nervous system remyelination by induced differentiation of oligodendrocyte precursor cells. Ann Neurol 2009; 65(3):304–15.
77. MS Society 2016. 2016. Available at: https://www.mssociety.org.uk/node/690821. Accessed September 26, 2017.
78. Wu Q, Wang Q, Mao G, et al. Dimethyl fumarate selectively reduces memory T cells and shifts the balance between Th1/Th17 and Th2 in multiple sclerosis patients. J Immunol 2017;198(8):3069–80.
79. Thomas K, Sehr T, Proschmann U, et al. Fingolimod additionally acts as immunomodulator focused on the innate immune system beyond its prominent effects on lymphocyte recirculation. J Neuroinflammation 2017;14(1):41.
80. Clement M, Pearson JA, Gras S, et al. Targeted suppression of autoreactive CD8+ T-cell activation using blocking anti-CD8 antibodies. Sci Rep 2016;6: 35332.

New Insights into Multiple Sclerosis Clinical Course from the Topographical Model and Functional Reserve

CrossMark

Stephen C. Krieger, MD*, James Sumowski, PhD

KEYWORDS

- Multiple sclerosis • Clinical course • Prognosis • Topographical model • Reserve

KEY POINTS

- The topographical model of multiple sclerosis (MS) visually represents the dynamic nature of lesion patterns, functional reserve, and transient fluctuations owing to physiologic stressors, in the evolution of MS clinical course.
- The topographical model of MS may be used as a clinical tool for educating patients about the clinical expression of MS disease, and may aid in predicting future disability.
- An emphasis on reserve in the model encourages future research on sources of reserve against disability, and motivates patients to engage in lifestyle choices that may build reserve.

INTRODUCTION

Multiple sclerosis (MS) is distinct among neurologic diseases in that it is characterized by both acute relapses and incremental progression of disability. This Is but one source of heterogeneity across people with MS, because the disease varies considerably in symptoms, severity, and course, and is notoriously difficult to prognosticate at the individual patient level. The topographical model of MS[1] was proposed as a clinical framework through which both archetypal features of the clinical course of MS, as well as essential factors driving interpersonal variability, can be visualized. This model reflects the growing recognition of the way that functional reserve influences MS phenotype and prognosis, and also acknowledges the need for inclusion of

Disclosures: S.C. Krieger has received compensation for consulting and advisory board work with Acorda Therapeutics, Bayer HealthCare, Biogen Idec, EMD Serono, Genentech, Genzyme, Mallinckrodt, Novartis, Teva, and TG Therapeutics, and has given non-promotional lectures with Biogen Idec and Genzyme. J. Sumowski has no disclosures to report.
Icahn School of Medicine at Mount Sinai, Corinne Goldsmith Dickinson Center for MS, 5 East 98th Street, Box 1138, New York, NY 10029, USA
* Corresponding author.
E-mail address: stephen.krieger@mssm.edu

MS-related cognitive dysfunction in representations of the disease course. Indeed, this insidious but pervasive symptom has not been fully incorporated into longstanding approaches to disability assessment or conceptualizations of MS phenotypes. This paper reviews important concepts in the clinical course of MS, the novel contributions of the topographical model, and the crucial role of functional reserve in MS prognosis and outcomes.

BACKGROUND

Approximately 80% to 90% of MS cases begin as a relapsing disease characterized by acute neurologic events caused by focal inflammatory lesions.[2] Characteristic neurologic symptoms indicative of relapse—principally optic neuritis, partial myelitis, and brainstem syndromes—are essential to the international panel diagnostic criteria for MS.[3] The accepted clinical course phenotypes initially published in the 1990s divide MS into relapsing remitting MS, secondary progressive MS (SPMS), and primary progressive MS (PPMS) forms of the disease (**Fig. 1**). The updated phenotype descriptions include an emphasis on close observation for evidence of ongoing inflammatory relapsing disease activity, and the presence or absence of insidious worsening of neurologic function in the absence of relapses referred to as disease progression.[4] MS has thus often been conceptualized as a "2-phase" disease,[5] with the early inflammatory relapsing phase followed by progression characterized by neurodegeneration.

Although acute relapse is the diagnostic and phenotypic hallmark of MS, and approved disease-modifying therapies for MS have demonstrated their efficacy fundamentally through prevention of relapses, the long-term impact of relapses on the clinical course and the accumulation of disability continues to be a matter of debate.[6,7] Numerous studies have demonstrated that a substantial portion of relapses do not result in a full recovery; therefore, residual neurologic dysfunction may be observed.[8] An increased frequency and severity of relapses early in disease course may also confer an unfavorable prognosis and rapid development of disability.[9] In contrast, older studies of long-term outcomes in MS had identified a very limited impact of early relapses to the development of disability once the progressive phase of MS has become apparent.[10]

Recent work characterizing relapse symptomatology more precisely has shown that motor system relapses and those with incomplete recovery measured at several time points exert a more significant prognostic impact on disability accumulation.[11,12] These data provide an argument that the localization of relapse-causative lesions, their severity, and their degree of recovery are important drivers of subsequent disability. Acute lesions seen on MRI are strongly associated with the occurrence of clinical relapse, and serve as a surrogate marker for inflammatory disease activity.[13] Furthermore, MRI lesions accumulated early in disease course have been shown to be a strong predictor of disability accumulated 20 years later.[14] That the MRI burden of disease often seems to be more substantial than clinical symptoms apparent early in disease has been referred to as the "clinical–radiologic paradox," although the concept of reserve in the topographical model of MS may help to make this less paradoxical.

In addition to early clinical and MRI prognostic factors, the role of advancing age as a significant contributor to the clinical course of MS has more recently come into focus.[15] The likelihood of developing progressive disease increases with age, with more than one-half of the MS population older than 65 having a progressive course.[16] Those diagnosed at an older age are at higher risk of manifesting a PPMS course or

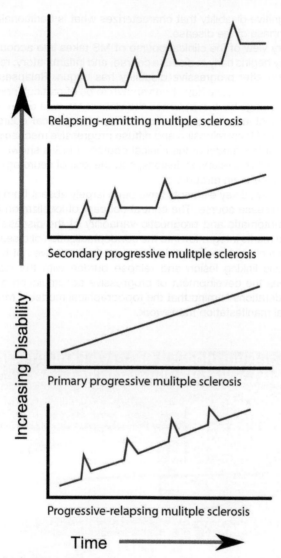

Increasing Disability

Relapsing-remitting multiple sclerosis

Secondary progressive mulitple sclerosis

Primary progressive mulitple sclerosis

Progressive-relapsing mulitple sclerosis

Time

Fig. 1. The 4 classic disease course phenotypes in multiple sclerosis. (*Adapted from* Lublin FD, Reingold SC. Defining the clinical course of multiple sclerosis: results of an international survey. Neurology 1996;46:907–11.)

developing SPMS after a short interval from diagnosis. Two possible age-related explanations for this phenomenon are that patients with older-onset disease may have had longstanding unrecognized and untreated disease with progressive late-in-life manifestations, or that compensatory mechanisms may not be as robust in the older-onset MS population.[17] Indeed, these explanations are not mutually exclusive, noting that the effect of age on the clinical course of MS can be attributed in large measure to the role of brain atrophy in MS, which proceeds at a rate several fold higher than in the general population.[18] It is hypothesized that the accelerated loss of brain volume is attended by a loss of the compensatory mechanisms that constitute neurologic reserve. The decline of functional reserve yields the insidious accumulation of physical and cognitive disability that characterizes what is traditionally thought of as the progressive phase of the disease.

A contemporary view of the clinical course of MS takes into account that accelerated brain atrophy begins early in disease course, and inflammatory, relapsing disease may continue long after progressive disability has begun. Relapses occurring in a context of progressive disease have been shown to be of particular prognostic significance.[19] These findings have supplanted the view of MS as a distinctly 2-phase disease, advancing instead a conceptualization that the clinical course of MS is an evolving admixture of focal relapsing and diffuse progressive mechanisms. A comprehensive example of this model of the clinical course of MS is shown in **Fig. 2**, which depicts the role of clinical relapses, lesions, and the loss of neurologic reserve in tandem with accelerated brain atrophy.

In the authors' view, 2 key elements have been largely absent from prior conceptualizations of MS disease course. The central concept of localization in MS underlies much of the symptomatic and prognostic variability of the disease[20–22] and, thus, lesion localization merits integration into the conceptualization of disease course. Second, prior work on clinical course and prognostic factors have not been based on a unifying hypothesis linking lesion and relapse burden with the loss of functional reserve that drives the development of progressive accumulation of disability. It is with these considerations in mind that the topographical model of MS was proposed as a novel clinical manifestation framework.

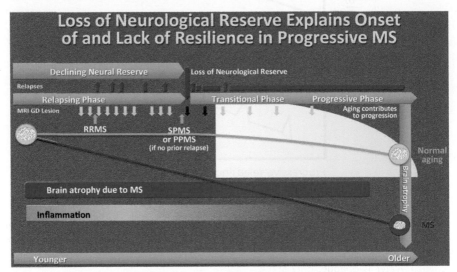

Fig. 2. Archetypal clinical course for multiple sclerosis (MS) incorporating clinical relapses, lesions, and the loss of neurologic reserve in tandem with accelerated brain atrophy. PPMS, primary progressive multiple sclerosis; SPMS, secondary progressive multiple sclerosis. (*Courtesy of* Dr Tim Vollmer, Aurora, CO; with permission.)

THE TOPOGRAPHICAL MODEL OVERVIEW

The topographical model of MS provides a unified depiction of the clinical course of MS across the spectrum of relapsing and progressive forms of the disease.[1] Like other conceptual depictions of a clinical course of disease, it remains agnostic to pathophysiologic and cellular mechanisms of the disease; however, the topographical model intends to encapsulate the specific clinical paradigm through which the clinical course of MS manifests. In the topographical model the central nervous system is visualized as a pool with increasing levels of depth, with the spinal cord and optic nerves at the shallow end, the brainstem and cerebellum with intermediate depth, and the cerebral hemispheres comprising the deep end. The depth of the water in this visual model corresponds with the degree of functional reserve intrinsic to these different regions of the central nervous system. Thus, the spinal cord and optic nerves—the simplest, most linear structures commonly affected by MS—have the least redundancy and capacity for organizational plasticity and rewiring, whereas the cerebral hemispheres possess the greatest such structural and functional resilience.

DISEASE ACTIVITY IN THE TOPOGRAPHICAL MODEL

In the topographical model, lesions rise as focal peaks emerging from the base of the pool; those that cross the surface of the water—the clinical threshold—cause demonstrable signs and symptoms of an MS relapse. Those that remain below the threshold are clinically silent lesions seen on MRI. Disease activity in the spinal cord and optic nerves is predisposed to causing the hallmark clinical relapses of MS: symptoms referable to partial myelitis and optic neuritis. The phenomenon of the "clinical–radiologic paradox" in MS is immediately apparent in the model, insofar as symptomatic relapses occur less frequently than the development of new lesions, the majority of lesions are initially below the clinical threshold, and a patient's clinical picture lags behind the extent of disease burden revealed on MRI (**Fig. 3**). That the emergence of new lesions and the occurrence of relapses are both depicted as topographical peaks is fundamentally congruent with the work Sormani and associates[13] have done, showing that new MRI lesions are an excellent surrogate marker for relapse, and both are manifestations of inflammatory disease activity.

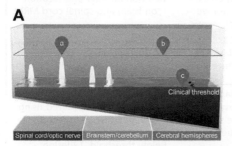 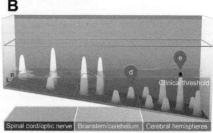

Fig. 3. The topographical model of multiple sclerosis (MS), clinical (*A*) and subclinical (*B*) views. (*A*) Water is opaque, only above-threshold peaks are visible. (*a*) Above-threshold topographical peaks depict relapses and quantified Expanded Disability Status Scale (EDSS)/functional system disability measures. Each peak yields localizable clinical findings; the topographical distribution defines the clinical picture for an individual patient. (*b*) Water level at outset reflects baseline functional capacity and may be estimated by baseline brain volume. (*c*) Water level decrease reflects loss of functional reserve and may be estimated by metrics of annualized brain atrophy. (*B*) Subclinical view. The water is translucent, both clinical signs and subthreshold lesions are visible. (*d*) Subthreshold topographical peaks depict T2 lesion number and volume. (*e*) The tallest peaks (ie, the most destructive) in the cerebral hemispheres are shown capped in black as T1 black holes. (*Data from* Krieger SC, Cook K, De Nino S, et al. The topographical model of multiple sclerosis: a dynamic visualization of disease course. Neurol Neuroimmunol Neuroinflamm 2016;3:e279.)

Drawing on the work of Scott and colleagues,[9,11] defining the prognostic importance of relapse symptomatology, severity, and degree of recovery, the topographical model of MS incorporates these variable factors to depict a wide range of the clinical course of MS phenotypes (**Table 1**). In the model, lesion or relapse severity is indicated by the height of a topographical peak and the degree of recovery is depicted as the extent to which the peak settles back down toward the base of the pool, further below the clinical threshold. Lesion localization defines the particular clinical symptoms invoked and functional systems affected—those in the spinal cord yield pyramidal, sensory, and bowel and bladder symptoms; those in the brainstem and cerebellum cause diplopia, vertigo, ataxia, and imbalance; and those in the hemispheres yield cerebral signs, most notably cognitive dysfunction. In this way, the model can be individualized to encapsulate a particular patient's "disease topography"—the regions of multifocal central nervous system damage that characterizes their individual lesion pattern and severity of disease. The concept and impact of lesion topography is an area of current investigation,[23] and similarly lesion morphology is becoming increasingly well-characterized.[24] Spinal cord lesions, in particular, occupying the shallow end of the pool, have been shown to confer a worse prognosis.[25]

The topographical model operates not solely as a visual depiction, but rather posits that there is a distinct relationship between lesion topography and the loss of functional reserve that drives the clinical course of MS. The model depicts that as time passes and functional reserve (the water level) declines, progression clinically recapitulates a patient's prior relapse symptoms and unmasks previously clinically silent lesions, incrementally manifesting above the clinical threshold a patient's underlying disease topography.[1] This *recapitulation hypothesis* is based on the observation

Table 1
Variable factors in the topographical model of multiple sclerosis

Factor	Depiction in Model	Clinical/Imaging Correlate
Localization	Topographical distribution of relapses and their causative lesions in referable anatomic regions	T2 lesion number and location on brain and spinal cord MRI
Relapse frequency	Rate of occurrence of lesions crossing the clinical threshold as relapses	Annualized relapse rate
Relapse severity	Height of each topographical peak; the tallest, most destructive peaks are shown capped in black to indicate T1 black holes	Above threshold: relapse symptoms, as measured using Expanded Disability Status Scale functional systems Below threshold: T2 lesion volume, and metrics of lesion destructiveness, including T1 black holes
Relapse recovery	Recovery capacity: the degree to which each topographical peak recedes below the clinical threshold	Relapse residua or complete recovery back to prerelapse baseline
Baseline volume and progression rate	Initial starting volume in the pool, and the rate at which water level declines	Estimated baseline brain volume and metrics of annualized brain volume loss

Adapted from Krieger SC, Cook K, De Nino S, et al. The topographical model of multiple sclerosis: a dynamic visualization of disease course. Neurol Neuroimmunol Neuroinflamm 2016;3:e279.

that the clinical signs and symptoms of a particular patient's progression manifest as a permanent, incremental recapitulation of prior relapse symptoms and a cumulative unmasking of previously clinically silent lesions. Although it is in some respects a relapse-centric model, progressive MS without relapses (PPMS) can also be depicted in the topographical model, whereby at the time of formation, inflammatory MS lesions did not cross the clinical threshold to yield relapses; however once the threshold has sufficiently declined, the multifocal signs and symptoms of MS referable to these lesions emerges gradually (**Fig. 4**). The loss of reserve, and neuroimaging correlates of this process, will be discussed in detail in a subsequent section.

There are several potential implications of this model on the understanding of MS disease course. The topographical model blurs the distinctions between phenotypic categories and animates dynamic periods of transition across them, taking into account that in practice there can be a long period of diagnostic uncertainty as patients transition from relapsing remitting MS to SPMS,[26] and a precise moment of "conversion to SPMS" can rarely be identified. The concept that the loss of reserve may yield progressive worsening through a loss of compensation for lesion burden helps to explain why high lesion burden early in the course of disease—even if the lesions are initially asymptomatic—is a poor prognostic factor for disability accrued many years later[14]: once compensatory reserve declines, those sub-clinical lesions are no longer sub-threshold. The model depicts the loss of reserve as beginning at the outset of disease,[27] congruent with findings at CIS and RIS supporting the concept that early treatment to prevent disease activity[28]—keeping the disease topography flat—may forestall the development of progressive disability later in the disease course.

The recapitulation hypothesis central to this clinical framework may allow clinicians to identify evidence of progression more precisely in individual patients, because familiarity with the topography of a given patient's disease may speak to the form their progression will take.[29] Identifying a leading indicator of evidence of progression in an individual patient could allow for earlier identification of a progressive phenotype, and may have implications for prognosis and treatment.

The topographical model is further congruent with findings that progressive accumulation of disability– be it in a context of SPMS or PPMS—is an age-related phenomenon. In the model, it takes years for reserve to be lost and for the clinical threshold to

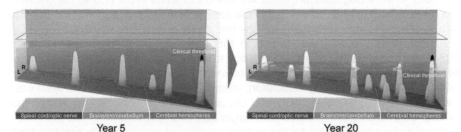

Year 5   Year 20

Fig. 4. Representative disease course archetype at 5 and 20 of years disease duration. The model conceptualizes relapsing and progressive contributions to disease course along a continuum: an individual's disease course can be driven predominantly by relapses, or predominantly by progression, and those with very mild or stable disease may demonstrate neither. This archetypal disease course is shown at years 5 and 20. In progressive multiple sclerosis, several subthreshold lesions denote underlying early disease activity, which cross the clinical threshold as functional reserve declines yielding gradual accumulation of disability. (*Data from* Krieger SC, Cook K, De Nino S, et al. The topographical model of multiple sclerosis: a dynamic visualization of disease course. Neurol Neuroimmunol Neuroinflamm 2016;3:e279.)

decline sufficiently for the progressive unmasking of disease topography to begin. In this way, the model does not distinguish between the clinical manifestation framework of PPMS and SPMS, which is consistent with the lack of categorical differences in the genetics or pathophysiology between these progressive phenotypes.[30] The model does, however, prioritize the loss of reserve—the declining threshold—as the crucial driver of disability in progressive disease.

DECLINE OF RESERVE IN THE TOPOGRAPHICAL MODEL

The concept of reserve against disability emerged from the aforementioned clinical–radiologic paradox: the observation that some persons are better able to withstand neurologic disease without or before suffering disability. Research on reserve began with the finding that many persons who die without dementia nevertheless met neuro-pathologic criteria for Alzheimer's disease on autopsy.[31] Similarly, many persons with MS can withstand considerable lesion burden with minimal to no cognitive or physical disability. Reserve is, in essence, the difference between the actual and expected disability for a given level of disease burden. One goal of research on reserve is to identify and maximize the protective factors underlying reserve, and to minimize risk factors associated with depletion of reserve. In the topographical model, reserve is represented as the water in the pool.

Research on cognitive and physical disability in aging and dementia (for review, see Stern[32]), and MS[33–35] has shown that premorbid maximal lifetime brain size is a largely heritable source of reserve. That is, persons with greater brain volume are better able to withstand MS lesion burden without cognitive impairment[33,34] or physical disability progression.[35] This advantage may be realized through more robust neural networks resistant to disease-related disruption, and/or greater capacity or degrees of freedom to compensate for disease. Importantly, although maximal lifetime brain growth is heritable, one's level of reserve and brain volume is dynamic across the lifespan. Aging and MS disease are steadily depleting this reserve; however, there is increasing evidence for modifiable factors to maintain as much reserve as possible (ie, "brain maintenance"[36]), including disease-modifying treatments[37] and lifestyle factors such as diet, physical exercise, and other health factors (eg, managing blood sugar, sleep apnea, etc). In the topographical model, the amount of water in the pool at the outset of the disease, and the rate at which it declines, are both variable factors, and the fluid nature of reserve inherently opens up the possibility of its replenishment.

Almost all of the work on reserve in MS has focused on cognitive outcomes (eg, memory, processing speed). In addition to maximal lifetime brain size as a source of reserve, several studies have linked estimates of lifetime intellectual enrichment with preserved cognition (eg, education, vocabulary knowledge, cognitive leisure activities; for review, see Sumowski and Leavitt[38]). More recently, it was shown that greater cognitive leisure is linked with larger hippocampal volume in MS patients,[39] which may be a neural basis for the protective effect of enrichment on memory function. The link between environment, brain structure, and functional outcomes may also extend to noncognitive domains, such as balance. Indeed, balance training has been linked to improved stability function in MS patients (eg, Prosperini and associates[40]), which provides a proof of concept that lifestyle choices and interventions may help to build reserve in noncognitive domains. This is an area for future research.

Personality may also relate to reserve, because high neuroticism and low openness to new experiences are linked to worse memory in MS patients.[41] These 2 personality traits may have different mechanisms of action. Persons who are open to new experiences are likely the same persons engaging in enriching activities, which we know are beneficial. In contrast, persons with high neuroticism may be prone to the negative effects of stress and stress hormones on the brain. Although stress is not good for anyone, there is a specific link between stress and disease activity in persons with MS,[42] which may be mitigated through stress reduction interventions.[43] Proactive and effective treatment of anxiety and depression may also have beneficial effects on brain structure and function.

USE OF THE TOPOGRAPHICAL MODEL IN CLINICAL CARE AND EDUCATION

The concept of reserve and the topographical model of MS can facilitate communication about the clinical course of MS with people with MS, particularly around 3 key issues: understanding disease phenotypes and the role of reserve, the importance of asymptomatic lesions seen on MRI, and distinguishing a true relapse from a pseudoexacerbation.

In the authors' experience, well-informed people with MS are often intent on knowing "which type of MS" they have, which can be difficult to answer methodically, particularly if there is uncertainty about the onset of progressive disease. Using the principles of the updated clinical course phenotypes as depicted in the topographical model, we discuss our remaining vigilant both for evidence of disease activity and for evidence of insidious progression, because these processes may coexist in parallel. In the parlance of the topographical model, the goals of care in MS include both preventing new disease topography, as well as maximizing reserve and "keeping the tank full" to augment a person's capacity to keep the disease submerged.

The concept of brain reserve has traditionally focused on individual differences in maximal lifetime brain size (estimated with intracranial volume[44]), and the link between larger size and protection from disability. More recently, there has been an appropriate focus on brain maintenance—the observation that brain-healthy modifiable lifestyle factors (eg, diet, exercise) can help to preserve remaining brain volume, which is a source of reserve. Persons with MS can be educated about various brain-healthy lifestyle choices that may help to preserve the water level and keep the lesions under the surface. These examples of intellectual enrichment, cognitive leisure, and stress reduction interventions demonstrate how lifestyle choices can contribute to reserve. Many of these factors can be addressed by the patients themselves, thereby affording patients control over reserve maintenance. In addition to protecting against disability, the goal of "keeping the tank full" provides a psychologically healthy agency for persons who may otherwise feel helpless in the face of an unpredictable illness. The topographical model and the concept of reserve can thus help clinicians to convey a more inclusive, optimistic, and personalized description of MS disease course to our patients. Framing disease course in such a way helps to steer people with MS away from the consideration of progressive MS as a categorical distinction and indicative of certain decline, and mitigates the sense of futility that being classified in such a way has historically conferred.

Second, it can be challenging to explain how an MRI can reveal new lesions even if patients feel clinically stable and are experiencing no new symptoms. The need for surveillance MRIs, even in periods of clinical quiescence, and clinicians' emphasis on preventing the formation of new lesions, may seem to some patients to be incongruous or even superfluous. The water level depiction of the clinical threshold in the topographical model can help clinicians to convey that new lesions on MRI may indicate areas of damage existing "beneath the surface." This concept can allow people with MS to visualize how new lesions and new clinical relapses are both manifestations of MS disease activity, and that an MRI allows us to see disease activity that does not cross the threshold to cause symptoms. The authors have found success using the model to allow people with MS to envision the goal of disease modifying therapy for relapsing MS fundamentally as keeping the topography flat, preventing new lesions from emerging and relapses from crossing the threshold.

Finally, the topographical model can help people with MS to distinguish between a pseudoexacerbation and an MS relapse. Water is used to depict reserve in the model in part to capture the dynamic, day-to-day physiologic fluctuations in compensatory ability that people with MS often experience. The model can be used to show that, when someone with MS is overheated, the pool drains transiently, and the clinical threshold temporarily declines. Preexisting, subthreshold disease topography reemerges above the threshold, and a recrudescence of prior symptoms occurs. When the fever, heat, or other physiologic stressor is removed, these symptoms recede again below the clinical threshold as the person feels repleted and the pool refills. In the authors' experience, this visualization allows for a clear distinction between a true relapse—the emergence of a new topographical peak, which may require treatment with steroids—from a pseudoexacerbation, or fluctuation in reserve, which does not.

WHAT EMPIRICAL QUESTIONS REMAIN TO BE ANSWERED?

As clinicians and scientists, we must identify the most impactful and clinically useful sources of reserve, so that we may counsel our patients appropriately. There are several remaining questions about the origins of reserve, including the neurophysiologic basis of preserved function in the face of disease. For instance, is it simply that some persons have greater brain volume, or is there a more dynamic aspect of reserve instantiated in active recovery (eg, remyelination, synaptogenesis)? Is reserve afforded through more robust networks as a product of development, or greater capacity for compensatory rewiring? Such questions may ultimately have implications for rehabilitation. In the context of the topographical model, however, one goal is to measure a person's reserve in an attempt to accurately predict outcomes. Toward this end, one important unanswered question is whether reserve is best estimated with global measures (eg, total gray matter volume), or whether estimates of reserve need to be more specific to a function (eg, cortical thickness in primary sensorimotor areas, fractional anisotropy within the corticospinal tract). Although the topographical model depicts a single clinical threshold and reserve declining globally, this can be further refined as data are acquired on regionally and functionally specific changes. The ultimate goal is the development of an empirically validated model of disease course and phenotype that can be used for individual prognostication and as a therapeutic guide.

ACKNOWLEDGMENTS

The authors thank Karin Cook, Madhuri Fletcher, John Panagis, Erik Gorka, and Scott De Nino for their work in developing the topographical model and contributing to the images, figures, and ideas in this article.

REFERENCES

1. Krieger SC, Cook K, De Nino S, et al. The topographical model of multiple sclerosis: a dynamic visualization of disease course. Neurol Neuroimmunol Neuroinflamm 2016;3:e279.
2. Compston A, Coles A. Multiple sclerosis. Lancet 2008;372:1502–17.

3. Polman CH, Reingold SC, Banwell B, et al. Diagnostic criteria for multiple sclerosis: 2010 revisions to the McDonald criteria. Ann Neurol 2011;69:292–302.
4. Lublin FD, Reingold SC, Cohen JA, et al. Defining the clinical course of multiple sclerosis: the 2013 revisions. Neurology 2014;83:278–86.
5. Leray E, Yaouanq J, Le Page E, et al. Evidence for a two-stage disability progression in multiple sclerosis. Brain 2010;133:1900–13.
6. Lublin FD. Relapses do not matter in relation to long-term disability: no (they do). Mult Scler 2011;17:1415–6.
7. Casserly C, Ebers GC. Relapses do not matter in relation to long-term disability: yes. Mult Scler 2011;17(12):1412–4.
8. Lublin FD, Baier M, Cutter G. Effect of relapses on development of residual deficit in multiple sclerosis. Neurology 2003;61:1528–32.
9. Scott TF, Schramke CJ. Poor recovery after the first two attacks of multiple sclerosis is associated with poor outcome five years later. J Neurol Sci 2010;292:52–6.
10. Confavreux C, Vukusic S, Moreau T, et al. Relapses and progression of disability in multiple sclerosis. N Engl J Med 2000;343:1430–8.
11. Scott TF, Gettings EJ, Hackett CT, et al. Specific clinical phenotypes in relapsing multiple sclerosis: the impact of relapses on long-term outcomes. Mult Scler Relat Disord 2016;5:1–6.
12. Novotna M, Paz Soldan MM, Abou Zeid N, et al. Poor early relapse recovery affects onset of progressive disease course in multiple sclerosis. Neurology 2015;85:722–9.
13. Sormani MP, Li DK, Bruzzi P, et al. Combined MRI lesions and relapses as a surrogate for disability in multiple sclerosis. Neurology 2011;77:1684–90.
14. Fisniku LK, Brex PA, Altmann DR, et al. Disability and T2 MRI lesions: a 20-year follow-up of patients with relapse onset of multiple sclerosis. Brain 2008;131:808–17.
15. Sanai SA, Saini V, Benedict RH, et al. Aging and multiple sclerosis. Mult Scler 2016;22:717–25.
16. Minden SL, Frankel D, Hadden LS, et al. Disability in elderly people with multiple sclerosis: an analysis of baseline data from the Sonya Slifka Longitudinal Multiple Sclerosis Study. NeuroRehabilitation 2004;19:55–67.
17. Scalfari A, Neuhaus A, Daumer M, et al. Age and disability accumulation in multiple sclerosis. Neurology 2011;77:1246–52.
18. De Stefano N, Stromillo ML, Giorgio A, et al. Establishing pathological cut-offs of brain atrophy rates in multiple sclerosis. J Neurol Neurosurg Psychiatry 2016;87:93–9.
19. Paz Soldan MM, Novotna M, Abou Zeid N, et al. Relapses and disability accumulation in progressive multiple sclerosis. Neurology 2015;84:81–8.
20. Sastre-Garriga J, Tintore M. Multiple sclerosis: lesion location may predict disability in multiple sclerosis. Nat Rev Neurol 2010;6:648–9.
21. Kincses ZT, Ropele S, Jenkinson M, et al. Lesion probability mapping to explain clinical deficits and cognitive performance in multiple sclerosis. Mult Scler 2011;17:681–9.
22. Dalton CM, Bodini B, Samson RS, et al. Brain lesion location and clinical status 20 years after a diagnosis of clinically isolated syndrome suggestive of multiple sclerosis. Mult Scler 2012;18:322–8.
23. Tintore M, Otero-Romero S, Rio J, et al. Contribution of the symptomatic lesion in establishing MS diagnosis and prognosis. Neurology 2016;87:1368–74.

24. Newton BD, Wright K, Winkler MD, et al. 3-dimensional shape and surface characteristics differentiate multiple sclerosis lesions from other etiologies. Annual Meeting of the European Congress on Treatment and Rehabilitation in Multiple Sclerosis (ECTRIMS). London (United Kingdom), 14-17 September, 2016.
25. Arrambide G, Rovira A, Sastre-Garriga J, et al. Spinal cord lesions: a modest contributor to diagnosis in clinically isolated syndromes but a relevant prognostic factor. Mult Scler 2017. [Epub ahead of print].
26. Katz Sand I, Krieger S, Farrell C, et al. Diagnostic uncertainty during the transition to secondary progressive multiple sclerosis. Mult Scler 2014;20:1654–7.
27. De Stefano N, Giorgio A, Battaglini M, et al. Assessing brain atrophy rates in a large population of untreated multiple sclerosis subtypes. Neurology 2010;74: 1868–76.
28. Giovannoni G, Butzkueven H, Dhib-Jalbut S, et al. Brain health: time matters in multiple sclerosis. Mult Scler Relat Disord 2016;9(Suppl 1):S5–48.
29. Laitman BM, Cook K, Fletcher M, et al. The topographical model of multiple sclerosis: first empirical test of the recapitulation hypothesis. Poster presented at the Annual Meeting of the American Academy of Neurology. Boston (MA), 22-28 April, 2017.
30. Lassmann H, van Horssen J, Mahad D. Progressive multiple sclerosis: pathology and pathogenesis. Nat Rev Neurol 2012;8:647–56.
31. Katzman R, Terry R, DeTeresa R, et al. Clinical, pathological, and neurochemical changes in dementia: a subgroup with preserved mental status and numerous neocortical plaques. Ann Neurol 1988;23:138–44.
32. Stern Y. Cognitive reserve in ageing and Alzheimer's disease. Lancet Neurol 2012;11:1006–12.
33. Sumowski JF, Rocca MA, Leavitt VM, et al. Brain reserve and cognitive reserve in multiple sclerosis: what you've got and how you use it. Neurology 2013;80: 2186–93.
34. Sumowski JF, Rocca MA, Leavitt VM, et al. Brain reserve and cognitive reserve protect against cognitive decline over 4.5 years in MS. Neurology 2014;82: 1776–83.
35. Sumowski JF, Rocca MA, Leavitt VM, et al. Brain reserve against physical disability progression over 5 years in multiple sclerosis. Neurology 2016;86: 2006–9.
36. Nyberg L, Lovden M, Riklund K, et al. Memory aging and brain maintenance. Trends Cogn Sci 2012;16:292–305.
37. Sormani MP, Arnold DL, De Stefano N. Treatment effect on brain atrophy correlates with treatment effect on disability in multiple sclerosis. Ann Neurol 2014; 75:43–9.
38. Sumowski JF, Leavitt VM. Cognitive reserve in multiple sclerosis. Mult Scler 2013; 19:1122–7.
39. Sumowski JF, Rocca MA, Leavitt VM, et al. Reading, writing, and reserve: literacy activities are linked to hippocampal volume and memory in multiple sclerosis. Mult Scler 2016;22(12):1621–5.
40. Prosperini L, Fortuna D, Gianni C, et al. Home-based balance training using the Wii balance board: a randomized, crossover pilot study in multiple sclerosis. Neurorehabil Neural Repair 2013;27:516–25.
41. Leavitt VM, Buyukturkoglu K, Inglese M, et al. Protective personality traits: high openness and low neuroticism linked to better memory in multiple sclerosis. Mult Scler 2017. [Epub ahead of print].

42. Mohr DC, Hart SL, Julian L, et al. Association between stressful life events and exacerbation in multiple sclerosis: a meta-analysis. BMJ 2004;328:731.
43. Mohr DC, Lovera J, Brown T, et al. A randomized trial of stress management for the prevention of new brain lesions in MS. Neurology 2012;79:412–9.
44. Courchesne E, Chisum HJ, Townsend J, et al. Normal brain development and aging: quantitative analysis at in vivo MR imaging in healthy volunteers. Radiology 2000;216:672–82.

Effective Utilization of MRI in the Diagnosis and Management of Multiple Sclerosis

Antonio Giorgio, MD, PhD, Nicola De Stefano, MD, PhD*

KEYWORDS

- MRI • Multiple sclerosis • Disease-modifying treatment • Diagnosis • Management
- Lesions • Atrophy • Standardized MRI protocol

KEY POINTS

- MRI is the most important tool for diagnosis and management of patients with multiple sclerosis (MS).
- MRI is able to detect white matter (WM) lesions in the central nervous system and their dissemination in space and time.
- MRI is used for tracking disease activity and for prognostic evaluation, as well for monitoring treatment efficacy and safety.
- Nonconventional and quantitative MRI measures can capture features of MS histopathologic findings beyond WM lesions but, for various reasons, are not currently implemented in clinical practice.
- Consensus guidelines on standardized MRI acquisition protocol have been recently published.

INTRODUCTION

Multiple sclerosis (MS) is an autoimmune, inflammatory, demyelinating and degenerative disease of the central nervous system (CNS), leading to a wide range of disability. The diagnosis of MS relies on the McDonald criteria, revised in 2010,[1] which is based on the evaluation of clinical symptoms (at presentation with clinically isolated syndrome [CIS] and/or in the history) and MRI of the CNS. The relevance of MRI as a noninvasive tool for the initial investigation of suspected MS and for disease monitoring over time has constantly grown due to the widespread availability of magnetic resonance (MR) scanners, advances in computational technology, and a plethora of scientific studies.

Department of Medicine, Surgery and Neuroscience, University of Siena, Viale Bracci 2, Siena 53100, Italy
* Corresponding author.
E-mail address: destefano@unisi.it

Neurol Clin 36 (2018) 27–34
https://doi.org/10.1016/j.ncl.2017.08.013
0733-8619/18/© 2017 Elsevier Inc. All rights reserved.

In recent years, several disease-modifying treatments (DMTs), acting with different mechanisms, have become available for MS. In particular, DMTs can decrease the focal inflammatory activity; the rate of brain atrophy; and, ultimately, the accrual of disability. It is important to choose for each patient the most adequate DMT and to monitor its efficacy and possible adverse effects over time.

USE OF MRI IN THE DIAGNOSIS OF MULTIPLE SCLEROSIS

Over the past 20 years, the neurologic community has adopted for MS various diagnostic criteria, which have been regularly modified as new lines of evidence and expert recommendations have emerged. The latest criteria were established in 2010 by an international panel and consist of a revision of the classic McDonald criteria.[1] The diagnostic criteria for MS have shown their validity and reliability when applied to patients younger than age 50 years with a typical clinical syndrome consistent with demyelination of the CNS (ie, CIS), such as optic neuritis, transverse myelitis, and brainstem syndromes, and after exclusion of alternative conditions mimicking MS.

MRI is currently the most relevant tool for MS diagnosis and is formally included in the diagnostic workup of patients with CIS suggestive of MS. Indeed, it shows high sensitivity for detection of focal white matter (WM) lesions in the CNS and specificity for lesion dissemination in space (DIS) and dissemination in time (DIT). In particular, DIS is fulfilled by the presence of 1 or more lesions in 2 of 4 characteristic anatomic locations (periventricular, juxtacortical, infratentorial, or spinal cord). DIT is demonstrated by simultaneous presence of gadolinium (Gd)-enhancing and Gd-nonenhancing lesions, thus indicating at least 2 demyelinating events, or by new T2 and/or Gd-enhancing lesion at follow-up MR examination. For the first time, the latest criteria allow an MS diagnosis based on a single MRI scan showing both DIS and DIT.

Sizes, shapes, and locations of MS lesions are variable. However, typically, they have an ovoid shape, a diameter greater than or equal to 3 mm, and cluster close to the ventricles and in the corpus callosum, although juxtacortical and infratentorial regions are other common sites of involvement. On sagittal images, lesions can appear as "fingers" stemming from the ventricular borders and reaching the corona radiata. A well-defined nodular enhancement usually occurs in acute small lesions, whereas a ring-like appearance may be present in subacute large lesions, which have a higher level of tissue destruction and, therefore, tend to resolve more slowly.

Importantly, the diagnostic work-up may be inconclusive in early MS, thus clinical and MRI follow-up may be needed to confirm the diagnosis. A 3 to 6 month interval between the baseline and follow-up MR examination has been recommended and, in the case in which no DIT occurs at that time, a further scan is recommended 6 to 12 months later.[2] If the brain MRI is normal over time, the diagnosis of MS appears less likely.

MRI is also able to detect incidental lesions suggestive of MS histopathologic findings in the brain and spinal cord of subjects without past or current neurologic symptoms. This condition has been termed radiologically isolated syndrome.[3] A new consensus article by the Magnetic Resonance Imaging in Multiple Sclerosis (MAG-NIMS) network provides recommendations useful for a proper stratification and management of these patients, which distinguishes between those at high risk for developing MS and those who have a low risk and thus are improperly exposed to unnecessary medical testing and treatment.[4]

The 2010 revisions of the McDonald criteria have received some criticism regarding their leniency, possibly leading to false-positive diagnosis, and the lack of consideration of MS pathologic findings beyond WM lesions. Against this background, there is a need for additional MRI measures to help differentiate among lesions of different pathogenesis. The demonstration of the "central vein sign", based on the perivascular location of MS lesions, and increased iron deposition help differentiate MS lesions from lesions of ischemic small vessel disease or neuromyelitis optica. These findings are particularly visible at high MR field strengths ($\geq$3.0 T) and when using specific sequences, such as susceptibility-weighted imaging and a special type of fluid attenuated inversion recovery (FLAIR*).[5,6]

Pathologic gray matter (GM) is present in MS brain and has a clear-cut clinical relevance, especially for cognitive impairment.[7] Indeed, cortical lesions (CLs) turn out to be rather specific for MS and their incorporation into diagnostic criteria would further increase their specificity.[8] Relatively novel MR sequences, such as double inversion recovery and phase-sensitive inversion recovery, have increased the detection rate of CLs and the sensitivity can be even further improved by using high MR field strengths.[9,10] Despite these advantages, CLs have not yet been incorporated into the McDonald diagnostic criteria and are not used as an imaging endpoint for treatment trials. Indeed, there is currently a lack of standardized image acquisition and analysis for CLs and, even using a dedicated protocol, the MRI sensitivity is much lower than histopathology.[11]

USE OF MRI IN THE MANAGEMENT OF MULTIPLE SCLEROSIS

Alongside its fundamental role for MS diagnosis, MRI is used for tracking subclinical disease activity, for prognostic evaluation, and for monitoring treatment effect, thus providing important pieces of information for ongoing patient management.

MRI for Monitoring Disease Activity

A high WM lesion load or the occurrence of lesions in a particular location (eg, brainstem) at the time of MS diagnosis predicts the development of future clinical disability in the medium to long term.[12,13] Although a cutoff for lesion count is debatable, patients with CIS showing greater than 10 T2 lesions have a significantly higher risk for long-term (eg, 20 years) disability progression compared with those patients having less than 4 T2 lesions.[14] It is well known that disease activity as measured by MRI is more sensitive than the frequency of clinical relapses. For this reason, serial MRI examinations are a reliable tool for detection and tracking subclinical disease activity. The occurrence of new lesions during the first 5 years of disease is associated with worse long-term (ie, 20 years) prognosis, even in presence of low lesion count.[14]

The most commonly used MRI measures of disease activity in clinical practice are the active lesions, characterized by Gd-enhancing T1 lesions, new or enlarging T2 lesions in serial MR scans, and the disease burden, which is based on the total T2 lesion volume. Although Gd-enhancing lesions are a reliable measure of acute inflammation with blood-brain barrier breakdown, their enhancement is transient, typically lasting about 6 to 8 weeks, thus monitoring disease activity by this method would require MRI acquisitions more frequently than is normally feasible in clinical practice (eg, monthly rather than annually or semiannually). For this reason, monitoring changes of T2 lesion number and volume currently remains the most practical measure of disease activity over time.

Another lesional MRI measure is characterized by hypointense T1 lesions (so-called "black holes"), which reflect old and inactive lesions associated with severe tissue damage (demyelination and, especially, axonal loss). Their count may be low in the early disease course and they are not suitable for monitoring disease activity.

Moreover, they showed no independent role for predicting conversion of CIS to clinically definite MS.[15]

MRI for Treatment Response

Lesion measures

As for any chronic disease, monitoring treatment in MS is necessary to achieve favorable long-term outcomes. The aims of DMTs in MS are reduction of disease activity, in terms of relapse frequency and new MRI lesions, and prevention of disability worsening over time. Clinical trials investigating the efficacy of DMTs in MS include standard MRI measures, such as active MRI lesions as secondary outcome measure. A recent meta-analysis has demonstrated that treatment effect on relapses until 2 years is predicted by the effect on active MS lesions within 6 to 9 months.[16]

It is common in clinical practice to start a DMT and then monitor its efficacy using follow-up MRI examinations. Indeed, MRI activity occurs with a frequency 5 to 10 times higher than clinical activity in relapsing-remitting MS (RRMS), thus providing a sensitive measure of disease activity and treatment efficacy. Several studies have evaluated the role of lesional MRI measures obtained early in the course of a DMT, such as interferon (IFN) β, and risk for disease worsening in the long term. The most predictive measures in this context include 2 to 5 new T2 lesions in the first 1 to 2 years of treatment.[17] Detection or absence of disease activity by MRI in a patient receiving a DMT represents a measure of treatment response. This implies that before the initiation or the switch of a treatment, a baseline and a follow-up MRI examination are needed. However, due to different mechanisms of action and time to treatment response of the various DMTs in MS, some investigators suggested that the reference scan should be obtained 3 to 6 months after treatment initiation or switch. Further MRI scans useful to monitor subclinical MS activity in RRMS should be obtained at intervals of 6 to 12 months, depending on the level of disease activity. A less frequent monitoring would be more suitable for patients who have been clinically stable for several years or who have a progressive disease without evidence of disease activity on previous assessments.

The evaluation of longitudinal MR examinations in clinical practice can be difficult because images are acquired with different scanners and acquisition parameters. In this context, detection of Gd lesions is a simple task for clinicians, whereas help from MRI experts is warranted for detection of new or enlarging T2 lesions.

Studies from other chronic autoimmune diseases (eg, rheumatologic) suggest that defining an explicit treatment target for close disease monitoring may have significant benefit on long-term outcome.[18] In the context of MS, it was recently proposed to use the so-called no evidence of disease activity (NEDA), which is conventionally defined as no relapses, no active MRI lesions (new T2 or Gd lesions), and no new disability accumulation, typically measured using the Expanded Disability Status Scale.[19] Based on this definition, assessment of NEDA status relies heavily on MRI monitoring. Recent studies on real-world cohorts of RRMS patients showed that NEDA can be found in the long term (7–10 years) in a minimal proportion of cases (8%–9%) and is even more difficult to sustain when a potential marker of neurodegeneration, such as brain atrophy, is included in the definition.[20,21] It is currently unknown whether the NEDA concept can be extended to treatments different from IFN.

Nonconventional measures

In clinical practice, widespread changes (ie, neurodegeneration or possible remyelination) in the normal-appearing WM and GM beyond WM lesions cannot be assessed adequately by conventional MRI (eg, T2-weighted and post-Gd T1 sequences) but need the application of nonconventional MRI measures and techniques.

Brain atrophy In the last decade or so, several studies have demonstrated that brain volume reduction (atrophy), which is a measure of neurodegeneration, occurs even in the earliest MS stages. The clinical relevance of brain atrophy, especially of the GM, stems from a better association, compared with WM lesion measures, with clinical progression, in terms of both disability and cognitive impairment.[22] Both GM compartments, the cortex and deep GM (especially thalamus), are affected.

Pathogenesis of brain atrophy in MS is complex and not completely clear.[7] It is mostly driven by GM atrophy, which may be a primary process[23] or may be secondary to axonal transection by WM lesions.[24,25] However, recent studies showed that the relationship of GM atrophy with WM focal pathologic findings may depend on the anatomic region considered (eg, motor cortex thinning related to corticospinal tract damage)[26] and on the disease course, with cortical atrophy more related to normal-appearing WM in longstanding RRMS.[27]

Being a measure of neurodegeneration, preventing brain atrophy will surely lead to relevant clinical benefit. MRI brain volume measures have been used in several clinical trials as outcome measure to assess the effect of DMT. A recent meta-analysis performed at the trial level demonstrated that treatment effect on brain atrophy correlates with treatment effect on disability.[28] Against this background, brain atrophy should ideally become a primary outcome measure in clinical trials. However, it should be taken into account that during the first 6 months to 1 year of DMT use, brain volume may decrease due to the treatment-related resolution of ongoing WM inflammation and edema ("pseudoatrophy").[29]

Although proposed by different groups, no standardized protocol for atrophy measurement is available and, for this reason, this measure is not currently implemented in clinical practice for routine assessment of single MS patients.

Remyelination Several remyelinating treatments are currently under investigation in phase 1 and 2 clinical trials.[30,31] Conventional MRI measures are of limited value in monitoring remyelination, although a recent randomized trial with IFN β-1b in CIS demonstrated a reduction of black holes.[32] Various advanced MRI techniques exist for a more specific in vivo assessment of the myelin content, including magnetization transfer (MT) imaging and diffusion tensor imaging, which would be the most feasible techniques in a clinical setting, and positron emission tomography. In particular, significant changes in MT ratio, consistent with demyelination and remyelination, and following different temporal evolution, were found in different regions of MS lesions for at least 3 years after formation.[33] Although the use of quantitative MRI measures for the assessment of remyelination has some potential, clinicians should consider that effective utilization of these measures in clinical practice and in multicenter studies is prevented with respect to conventional MRI by various factors, including longer scan time, complex postprocessing analyses, and lack of standardization.

Monitoring treatment adverse effects
Since the approval of the novel and potent DMT for MS, the need for monitoring potential adverse effects has increased.[34] In particular, brain MRI has been used for monitoring MS patients treated with natalizumab (NTZ), a recombinant humanized monoclonal antibody.[35] Progressive multifocal leukoencephalopathy (PML) is a relatively rare but serious opportunistic infection caused by reactivation of the John Cunningham (JC) virus during NTZ treatment; brain MRI represents the most valuable

screening tool for its early detection, even at asymptomatic stage.[36] Guidelines for MRI screening in NTZ-treated patients have been recently published.[2] Brain MRI, including FLAIR, T2-weighted, and diffusion-weighted imaging sequences, is recommended every 3 to 4 months in patients at high risk (ie, JC virus seropositive, treatment duration $\geq$18 months) and once a year in patients at low risk of PML (ie, JC virus seronegative). However, clinicians should consider that MRI-based monitoring for early PML detection is not limited only to patients treated with NTZ, but it should be extended to patients treated with other DMTs, such as alemtuzumab, rituximab, or dimethylfumarate.[34]

STANDARDIZED MRI PROTOCOL

Despite the routine use of MRI in the diagnosis and management of MS patients, there is currently no evidence defining its optimal use. It is well known that several MRI acquisition parameters (eg, field strength, sequence, spatial resolution, coil type) can influence the detection of focal MS histopathologic findings, especially in a multicenter setting. Thus, it is widely accepted that standardized MRI protocols are urgently needed. However, even in the 2010 revision of the McDonald criteria, specific suggestions for MRI acquisition are lacking. In this respect, the MAGNIMS network has recently published European consensus guidelines.[2,37]

Brain MRI should be performed at least on a 1.5-T scanner but a 3 T scanner is recommended for the better sensitivity to MS lesions due to improved image resolution and signal-to-noise ratio, although this does not seem to allow an earlier MS diagnosis.[38] The spatial resolution should be 1×1 mm in-plane and 3-mm slice thickness (voxel size: 1×1×3 mm). Proton-density (PD) and T2-weighted sequences are considered the reference for detection of hyperintense (ie, bright) WM lesions. FLAIR sequence is useful for excluding cerebrospinal fluid (CSF)-filled enlarged Virchow–Robin spaces and it shows a higher sensitivity for juxtacortical and periventricular lesions but lower sensitivity for those lesions in the infratentorial area. High-resolution (3-dimensional, voxel size: 1 mm^3) FLAIR is ideally preferred due to higher contrast-to-noise ratio, availability of multiplanar reconstructions, and registration of longitudinal images.

A standard T1-weighted spin echo sequence can show chronic T1 hypointense lesions ("black holes"), reflecting irreversible tissue damage, and macroscopic atrophy. Gd should be administered before the acquisition of PD, T2 or FLAIR sequences to allow longer circulation time and better detection of acute lesions.

Spinal cord MRI is relevant for MS diagnosis, but it may be less sensitive for assessing subclinical disease activity and thus for disease management. It is more demanding than brain MRI due to small tissue volume, occurrence of various artifacts (eg, CSF flow and blood vessel pulsations), harder detection of MS lesions, and prolonged scan time. Spinal MRI images should be acquired on a scanner with at least 1.5-T field strength and, unlike brain MRI, no evidence exists that 3 T scanners have higher sensitivity for lesion detection. For spinal cord, the standard sequence for MS is considered dual-echo (PD and T2-weighted) with at least 1×1×3 mm spatial resolution and sagittal orientation. Indeed, in this case, FLAIR lacks sensitivity for spinal lesions. Alternatively, short-tau inversion recovery T2-weighted sequence may be used in presence of flow-related artifacts, which may lead to false-positive results. The role of Gd administration in spinal cord MRI is still unclear because, compared with brain lesions, only a small proportion of spinal lesions show enhancement and, when it occurs, it is commonly associated with neurologic symptoms.[39]

REFERENCES

1. Polman CH, Reingold SC, Banwell B, et al. Diagnostic criteria for multiple sclerosis: 2010 revisions to the McDonald criteria. Ann Neurol 2011;69(2):292–302.
2. Wattjes MP, Rovira A, Miller D, et al. Evidence-based guidelines: MAGNIMS consensus guidelines on the use of MRI in multiple sclerosis-establishing disease prognosis and monitoring patients. Nat Rev Neurol 2015;11(10):597–606.
3. Okuda DT, Mowry EM, Beheshtian A, et al. Incidental MRI anomalies suggestive of multiple sclerosis: the radiologically isolated syndrome. Neurology 2009;72(9): 800–5.
4. De Stefano N, Giorgio A, Tintore M, et al. Radiologically isolated syndrome or subclinical multiple sclerosis: MAGNIMS consensus recommendations. Mult Scler 2017. in press.
5. Haacke EM, Makki M, Ge Y, et al. Characterizing iron deposition in multiple sclerosis lesions using susceptibility weighted imaging. J Magn Reson Imaging 2009; 29(3):537–44.
6. Sati P, George IC, Shea CD, et al. FLAIR*: a combined MR contrast technique for visualizing white matter lesions and parenchymal veins. Radiology 2012;265(3): 926–32.
7. Geurts JJ, Calabrese M, Fisher E, et al. Measurement and clinical effect of grey matter pathology in multiple sclerosis. Lancet Neurol 2012;11(12):1082–92.
8. Filippi M, Rocca MA, Calabrese M, et al. Intracortical lesions: relevance for new MRI diagnostic criteria for multiple sclerosis. Neurology 2010;75(22):1988–94.
9. Simon B, Schmidt S, Lukas C, et al. Improved in vivo detection of cortical lesions in multiple sclerosis using double inversion recovery MR imaging at 3 Tesla. Eur Radiol 2010;20(7):1675–83.
10. de Graaf WL, Kilsdonk ID, Lopez-Soriano A, et al. Clinical application of multi-contrast 7-T MR imaging in multiple sclerosis: increased lesion detection compared to 3 T confined to grey matter. Eur Radiol 2013;23(2):528–40.
11. Seewann A, Kooi EJ, Roosendaal SD, et al. Postmortem verification of MS cortical lesion detection with 3D DIR. Neurology 2012;78(5):302–8.
12. Fisniku LK, Chard DT, Jackson JS, et al. Gray matter atrophy is related to long-term disability in multiple sclerosis. Ann Neurol 2008;64(3):247–54.
13. Tintore M, Rovira A, Arrambide G, et al. Brainstem lesions in clinically isolated syndromes. Neurology 2010;75(21):1933–8.
14. Fisniku LK, Brex PA, Altmann DR, et al. Disability and T2 MRI lesions: a 20-year follow-up of patients with relapse onset of multiple sclerosis. Brain 2008;131(Pt 3):808–17.
15. Mitjana R, Tintore M, Rocca MA, et al. Diagnostic value of brain chronic black holes on T1-weighted MR images in clinically isolated syndromes. Mult Scler 2014;20(11):1471–7.
16. Sormani MP, Bruzzi P. MRI lesions as a surrogate for relapses in multiple sclerosis: a meta-analysis of randomised trials. Lancet Neurol 2013;12(7):669–76.
17. Sormani MP, De Stefano N. Defining and scoring response to IFN-beta in multiple sclerosis. Nat Rev Neurol 2013;9(9):504–12.
18. Grigor C, Capell H, Stirling A, et al. Effect of a treatment strategy of tight control for rheumatoid arthritis (the TICORA study): a single-blind randomised controlled trial. Lancet 2004;364(9430):263–9.
19. Havrdova E, Galetta S, Stefoski D, et al. Freedom from disease activity in multiple sclerosis. Neurology 2010;74(Suppl 3):S3–7.

20. Rotstein DL, Healy BC, Malik MT, et al. Evaluation of no evidence of disease activity in a 7-year longitudinal multiple sclerosis cohort. JAMA Neurol 2015;72(2): 152–8.
21. De Stefano N, Stromillo ML, Giorgio A, et al. Long-term assessment of no evidence of disease activity in relapsing-remitting MS. Neurology 2015;85(19): 1722–3.
22. De Stefano N, Airas L, Grigoriadis N, et al. Clinical relevance of brain volume measures in multiple sclerosis. CNS Drugs 2014;28(2):147–56.
23. Popescu V, Klaver R, Voorn P, et al. What drives MRI-measured cortical atrophy in multiple sclerosis? Mult Scler 2015;21(10):1280–90.
24. Charil A, Dagher A, Lerch JP, et al. Focal cortical atrophy in multiple sclerosis: relation to lesion load and disability. Neuroimage 2007;34(2):509–17.
25. Battaglini M, Giorgio A, Stromillo ML, et al. Voxel-wise assessment of progression of regional brain atrophy in relapsing-remitting multiple sclerosis. J Neurol Sci 2009;282(1–2):55–60.
26. Bergsland N, Lagana MM, Tavazzi E, et al. Corticospinal tract integrity is related to primary motor cortex thinning in relapsing-remitting multiple sclerosis. Mult Scler 2015;21(14):1771–80.
27. Steenwijk MD, Daams M, Pouwels PJ, et al. What explains gray matter atrophy in long-standing multiple sclerosis? Radiology 2014;272(3):832–42.
28. Sormani MP, Arnold DL, De Stefano N. Treatment effect on brain atrophy correlates with treatment effect on disability in multiple sclerosis. Ann Neurol 2014; 75(1):43–9.
29. De Stefano N, Arnold DL. Towards a better understanding of pseudoatrophy in the brain of multiple sclerosis patients. Mult Scler 2015;21(6):675–6.
30. Kremer D, Kury P, Dutta R. Promoting remyelination in multiple sclerosis: current drugs and future prospects. Mult Scler 2015;21(5):541–9.
31. Rottlaender A, Kuerten S. Stepchild or prodigy? Neuroprotection in multiple sclerosis (MS) Research. Int J Mol Sci 2015;16(7):14850–65.
32. Nagtegaal GJ, Pohl C, Wattjes MP, et al. Interferon beta-1b reduces black holes in a randomised trial of clinically isolated syndrome. Mult Scler 2014;20(2): 234–42.
33. Chen JT, Collins DL, Atkins HL, et al. Magnetization transfer ratio evolution with demyelination and remyelination in multiple sclerosis lesions. Ann Neurol 2008; 63(2):254–62.
34. Soelberg Sorensen P. Safety concerns and risk management of multiple sclerosis therapies. Acta Neurol Scand 2016;136(3):168–86.
35. Gupta S, Weinstock-Guttman B. Natalizumab for multiple sclerosis: appraising risk versus benefit, a seemingly demanding tango. Expert Opin Biol Ther 2014; 14(1):115–26.
36. Wattjes MP, Wijburg MT, Vennegoor A, et al. Diagnostic performance of brain MRI in pharmacovigilance of natalizumab-treated MS patients. Mult Scler 2016;22(9): 1174–83.
37. Rovira A, Wattjes MP, Tintore M, et al. Evidence-based guidelines: MAGNIMS consensus guidelines on the use of MRI in multiple sclerosis-clinical implementation in the diagnostic process. Nat Rev Neurol 2015;11(8):471–82.
38. Wattjes MP, Harzheim M, Lutterbey GG, et al. Does high field MRI allow an earlier diagnosis of multiple sclerosis? J Neurol 2008;255(8):1159–63.
39. Gass A, Rocca MA, Agosta F, et al. MRI monitoring of pathological changes in the spinal cord in patients with multiple sclerosis. Lancet Neurol 2015;14(4):443–54.

Spinal Cord MRI in Multiple Sclerosis

Alexandra Muccilli, MD[a,b], Estelle Seyman, MD[a], Jiwon Oh, MD, PhD, FRCPC[a,c,*]

KEYWORDS

- Spinal cord • MRI • Multiple sclerosis • Clinical usefulness • Prediction
- Quantitative techniques

KEY POINTS

- The spinal cord (SC) is an important structure to image for clinical and research purposes in MS.
- Conventional MRI techniques are useful in detecting lesions in the SC, and a variety of sequences can be used for this purpose.
- Conventional MRI techniques have diagnostic and prognostic usefulness in the clinical management of patients with MS, clinically isolated syndrome, and radiologically isolated syndrome.
- A number of advanced, quantitative SC measures have demonstrated usefulness in investigational settings.
- Among quantitative SC MRI measures, SC atrophy and magnetization transfer imaging have been most extensively studied; with further validation, these quantitative techniques may become useful clinically.

INTRODUCTION

The last few decades have seen extraordinary advances in the field of multiple sclerosis (MS), with notable developments in neuroimaging. The increased availability of MRI and continuous advances in MRI techniques have enabled earlier diagnosis of MS and the routine use of MRI in clinical practice to monitor MS disease activity. Moreover, advanced MRI techniques have been an important contributor to our evolving understanding of the complex inflammatory and neurodegenerative processes involved in MS disease mechanisms.

Although the brain has long been the focus of MRI use in clinical practice and research in MS, in recent years, the importance of assessing the spinal cord (SC) has become apparent. This article outlines the usefulness of assessing the SC using

[a] Division of Neurology, St. Michael's Hospital, University of Toronto, 30 Bond Street, Toronto, Ontario, M5B 1W8, Canada; [b] Division of Neurology, Centre Hospitalier de L'Université de Montréal, Université de Montréal, 1058 Saint-Denis Street, Montreal, Quebec H2X 3J4, Canada; [c] Department of Neurology, Johns Hopkins University, Baltimore, MD, USA
* Corresponding author. Division of Neurology, St. Michael's Hospital, University of Toronto, 30 Bond Street, Toronto, Ontario, M5B 1W8, Canada.
E-mail address: ohjiw@smh.ca

Neurol Clin 36 (2018) 35–57
https://doi.org/10.1016/j.ncl.2017.08.009
0733-8619/18/© 2017 Elsevier Inc. All rights reserved.

neurologic.theclinics.com

both conventional and advanced MRI techniques as a promising tool with clinical diagnostic and predictive usefulness, to gain insight into MS disease pathogenesis, and as a potential outcome measure in clinical trial settings.

SPINAL CORD MRI IN MULTIPLE SCLEROSIS: CONSIDERATIONS

The SC is a compact tubular structure with tightly packed and highly organized functional columns of gray and white matter. Its small size and precise organization of motor and sensory tracts make the SC an ideal target to study the structural and functional impact of the pathology of MS.

Imaging the SC using MRI can be challenging owing to significant technical limitations. The SC is susceptible to artifacts from partial volume averaging owing to the surrounding cerebrospinal fluid (CSF), bone, and epidural fat. In addition, owing to the proximity of the SC to other vital organs in the thoracic cavity, motion-induced artifacts resulting from respiration, heartbeat, CSF flow, and swallowing can contribute to diminished signal-to-noise ratio.[1]

Efforts have been made in the last decade to optimize the signal-to-noise ratio, thus improving image quality and minimizing unwanted interference. Improved coil technology, higher field strengths, image acquisition with cardiac and respiratory "gating," as well as newer sequences that better delineate intrinsic SC anatomy and MS lesions, are among the technical developments that have led to improved detection of demyelinating and degenerative changes in the SC.

CONVENTIONAL SPINAL CORD MRI: LESION DETECTION
T2-Weighted Sequences for Spinal Cord Lesion Detection

T2-weighted sequences of the SC are relatively sensitive in detecting MS-related disease activity. In the brain, MRI has been shown to identify new lesions up to 10 times more frequently than clinical relapses occur.[2–5] T2-hyperintense lesions on MRI, however, are not specific for acute demyelination and can represent a variety of heterogeneous histopathologic changes.[6–9]

Initially, focal T2-hyperintense lesions in the brain and SC were visualized on sagittal dual spin echo sequences.[10] The advent of fluid attenuated inversion recovery (FLAIR) sequences, which are T2-weighted images with CSF suppression and consequent reduction in CSF-related artifacts, led to improved sensitivity in detecting MS lesions in the brain.[11,12] Unfortunately, FLAIR sequences in the SC were found to be insensitive at detecting MS lesions.[13,14] Further technical advances led to the development of fast spin echo (FSE) sequences with improved resolution and signal-to-noise ratio in comparison with FLAIR and dual spin echo sequences.[15,16] The increased sensitivity and shorter acquisition time of FSE in comparison with FLAIR and dual spin echo sequences, respectively, has made this sequence the current reference standard to image SC lesions in MS (**Fig. 1**).[13,15–18]

Additional MRI Sequences for Spinal Cord Lesion Detection

Several modified T1- and T2-weighted sequences have been evaluated as complementary additions to standard T2-weighted FSE sequences with the goal of improving SC lesion detection. Short tau inversion recovery (STIR) is a fat suppression technique that has demonstrated usefulness in detecting SC lesions in MS.[15,19] Several studies have compared cervical SC imaging with STIR and FSE, and observed improved signal-to-noise ratio and increased sensitivity to SC lesions with STIR over FSE sequences.[15,20–22] In contrast, contradictory results were observed in a few studies, where an increase in signal artifact, lower image quality, and more interobserver

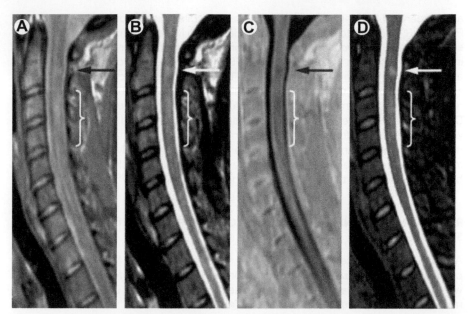

Fig. 1. Visualization of cervical spinal cord (SC) lesions in multiple sclerosis (MS) using various MRI sequences. Cervical SC lesions in MS visualized on a 3T MRI using different MRI sequences. (A) Proton density-weighted images demonstrate both focal and diffuse lesions, but diffuse lesions are better visualized in comparison with other sequences. (B) T2-weighted, (C) phase sensitive inversion recovery, and (D) short tau inversion recovery images demonstrate focal lesions clearly. (*From* Kearney H, Miller DH, Ciccarelli O. Spinal cord MRI in multiple sclerosis–diagnostic, prognostic and clinical value. Nat Rev Neurol 2015;11(6):327–38; with permission from "Nature Publishing group".)

differences were demonstrated with STIR versus FSE, despite the increased sensitivity of STIR to SC lesion detection.[19,23] Based on the observed advantages and drawbacks of STIR, this sequence is typically suggested as an adjunct to conventional sagittal FSE sequences for SC lesion detection. Similarly, double inversion recovery, which suppresses signals from both the CSF and white matter, has shown increased sensitivity with regard to SC lesion detection, but also significant issues with artifact, thus limiting its use.[24,25]

Gradient echo (GRE) sequences are another possible complementary sequence to core T2-weighted, FSE sequences. Axial GRE sequences have demonstrated increased sensitivity to SC lesions in MS in comparison with T2-weighted FSE.[26,27] Multiple echo recombinant GRE is a newer GRE sequence that provides increased signal-to-noise ratio in comparison with conventional T2-FSE sequences, thus resulting in exceptional gray–white matter resolution and enhanced conspicuity of cervical SC lesions.[28,29] One study comparing multiple echo recombinant GRE with T2-weighted FSE in detecting cervical SC lesions demonstrated superior sensitivity with multiple echo recombinant GRE, but better specificity with standard axial T2-weighted FSE.[28]

There has been increasing enthusiasm over the ability of phase-sensitive inversion recovery (PSTI-IR or PSIR), a T1-weighted inversion recovery sequence, to detect cervical SC lesions. PSIR was initially developed and used in visualizing white and gray matter MS lesions in the brain and has since been used in a number of studies to assess cervical SC lesions.[30–32] Poonawalla and colleagues[33] compared the ability of PSIR, STIR, and FSE to detect cervical SC lesions in MS and found that PSIR enabled superior lesion demarcation and localization. These findings were recently confirmed in a number of studies that demonstrated PSIR's superior lesion detection capabilities and interobserver reliability over STIR and T2W-FSE imaging.[34,35] Similarly, magnetization prepared rapid GRE, another promising T1-weighted sequence, exhibits superior lesion detection and improved correlations between lesion volume and Expanded Disability Status Scale (EDSS) in comparison with T2-weighted FSE, STIR, and T1-weighted GRE.[36] Unfortunately, PSIR and magnetization prepared rapid GRE are not widely available and thus have not been implemented widely in MS imaging protocols. However, based on accumulating evidence, this will likely change as centers become more comfortable using these sequences (see **Fig. 1**).[18]

RECOMMENDED STANDARDIZED SPINAL CORD MRI PROTOCOL IN MULTIPLE SCLEROSIS

A group of experienced neurologists and neuroradiologists in MS imaging recently proposed a standardized MRI protocol for the diagnosis and follow-up of patients with MS, which included a dedicated segment on SC imaging.[37] Details of the recommended SC MRI protocol are outlined in **Table 1**.

To summarize, sagittal and axial T2-weighted images are recommended with T2-weighted axial slices at the level of the identified lesions. In addition, STIR or PSIR sequences are suggested in addition to T2-weighted sequences to detect more subtle or discreet lesions. A cervical SC MRI is recommended in patients suspected of having MS, both with and without symptoms referable to the SC. For follow-up imaging, SC

Table 1 Recommended SC MRI protocol in MS	
Parameter	Description and Important Instructions
Core sequences	• Sagittal T2 • Sagittal proton attenuation, STIR, or PST1-IR • Axial T2 that covers lesions
Optional sequences	• Axial T2 through complete SC • Sagittal T1 • Postgadolinium sagittal T1-weighted with a minimum of a 5-minute delay before obtaining the postgadolinium scan, additional contrast material is not required for SC MRI if follows a contrast brain MRI study.
Coverage	• Cervical cord coverage • Thoracic and conus medullaris coverage is recommended only if localizing symptoms are present.
Acquisition parameters	• Scans should be in good quality, with adequate SNR • In section pixel resolution (<1 × 1 mm) • Closed magnets preferred (large bore for patients with claustrophobia) • Slice thickness in sagittal scans <3 mm, axial scans <5 mm • No gaps

Abbreviations: PST1-IR, phase-sensitive T1 inversion recovery; SC, spinal cord; SNR, signal to noise ratio; STIR, short tau inversion recovery.

Adapted from Traboulsee A, Simon JH, Stone L, et al. Revised recommendations of the consortium of MS Centers Task Force for a standardized MRI protocol and clinical guidelines for the diagnosis and follow-up of multiple sclerosis. AJNR Am J Neuroradiol 2016;37(3):395; with permission.

MRI may be indicated in specific situations, which are outlined in elsewhere in this article.

CLINICAL USEFULNESS OF SPINAL CORD MRI IN MULTIPLE SCLEROSIS: DIAGNOSIS AND PREDICTION
Diagnosis

The SC is a common site of lesions in MS, making it an important region to image to ascertain the extent of MS disease processes in the central nervous system. A number of imaging studies have noted that upwards of 70% to 80% of patients with relapsing remitting MS (RRMS) have focal SC lesions, even within a few years of diagnosis. Patients with progressive variants of MS also frequently have SC lesions, which can appear both focal and diffuse on MRI.[10,38–40] Focal SC lesions in MS are frequently located in the dorsal white matter tracts, but are also frequently observed in the lateral corticospinal tracts, and usually involve both gray and white matter (**Fig. 2**).[10,18,39–41] Typically, SC lesions in MS do not span more than 1 to 2 vertebral segments.

In MS, the cervical portion of the SC is the most commonly lesioned region. One large retrospective cohort analysis (n = 202) found that the cervical SC was involved in 59% of MS cases, but only 16% had lesions exclusive to this region, with the lower

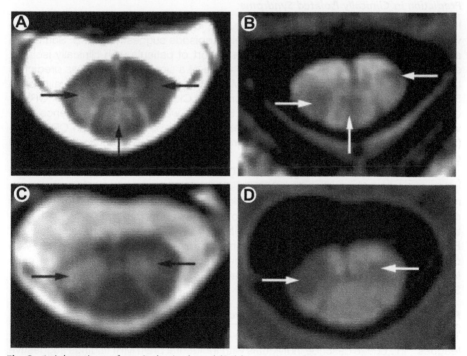

Fig. 2. Axial sections of cervical spinal cord (SC) lesions in multiple sclerosis. (*A*) Hyperintense signal abnormalities on axial fast field echo (FFE) sequences demonstrate lesions in the lateral and posterior columns. (*B*) Hypointense signal abnormalities seen on phase sensitive inversion recovery (PSIR) sequence imaging indicate lesions in the lateral and posterior columns. (*C, D*) Lateral column lesions extending from the SC white matter into the gray matter are seen on (*C*) FFE sequence and (*D*) PSIR sequence. All images were acquired at the C2 to C3 intervertebral disc level, on a 3T MRI. (*From* Kearney H, Miller DH, Ciccarelli O. Spinal cord MRI in multiple sclerosis–diagnostic, prognostic and clinical value. Nat Rev Neurol 2015;11(6):327–38; with permission from "Nature Publishing group".)

thoracic SC segments also frequently demonstrating focal SC lesions (20%).[40] Another study demonstrated that the number of cervical SC lesions predicted the presence of thoracic SC lesions, independent of brain MRI findings.[42]

Given how common SC lesions are in MS, they naturally have a role in an MS diagnosis. Initial MRI diagnostic criteria did not include SC lesions.[43–45] They were, however, incorporated in the original edition of the McDonald Criteria (2001), but their role in diagnosis was not detailed.[46] In the next iteration of the McDonald criteria, SC lesions were deemed equivalent to infratentorial lesions in demonstrating dissemination in space (DIS).[47] The most recent version of the McDonald criteria (2010) clearly designates the SC as 1 of the 4 anatomic sites constituting DIS.[48] This is likely owing to the recognition that inclusion of an SC lesion results in a much higher percentage of patients meeting the diagnostic criteria for MS compared with using brain MRI alone (84.6% of newly diagnosed patients with MS meeting criteria for DIS when including the SC as a distinct anatomic site for DIS, compared with only 66.3% with brain MRI alone).[38] Moreover, lesions in the SC provide an additional element of specificity when diagnosing MS, because cerebral white matter disease lesions can often be seen incidentally in older subjects, in other inflammatory conditions, and in patients with migraines and microvascular ischemic disease, and this is not the case in the SC.

Prediction in Clinically Isolated Syndrome

In addition to their central diagnostic role, SC lesions have a significant predictive value in patients presenting with a first clinical episode suggestive of MS. Sombekke and colleagues[49] prospectively followed a cohort of patients with clinically isolated syndrome (CIS) and observed that the presence of a single SC lesion was predictive of conversion to clinically definite MS (CDMS). Interestingly, the predictive value of an SC lesion was stronger in patients with nonspinal CIS, where the odds ratio (OR) for conversion to CDMS in the presence of an SC lesion was 6.48 (95% confidence interval [CI], 2.34–17.95) over an average 5-year follow-up period versus an OR of 1.24 (95% CI, 0.35–4.44) in the spinal CIS subgroup. This finding was confirmed in several other studies.[50–52]

Furthermore, recent data suggest that SC involvement in CIS is associated with an increased risk of future disability. One prospective cohort study of 131 patients with nonspinal CIS followed patients with serial imaging of the neuroaxis for a 5-year period. During the follow-up period, 71% of patients converted to CDMS. Of the patients who did not convert to MS, none had SC lesions at baseline or follow-up. Furthermore, SC lesion number was the only baseline MRI measure associated with disability (EDSS) at follow-up.[50] Given the predictive value of SC lesions in early MS, recent expert consensus guidelines have suggested the incorporation of cervical SC imaging in initial investigations.[37]

Prediction in Radiologically Isolated Syndrome

The term radiologically isolated syndrome (RIS) was first coined by Okuda and colleagues[53] in 2009 to describe individuals with incidental brain MRI findings suggestive of MS in the absence of any current or prior signs and symptoms. A subsequent retrospective study of 71 subjects with RIS identified cervical spine lesions in 25 subjects (35%), of which clinical progression to CIS or primary progressive multiple sclerosis (PPMS) was noted in 21 patients (84%) over a 1.6-year median time period. Of note, in the multivariate logistic regression model, the presence of a typical MS cervical SC lesion increased the risk of conversion to CIS or CDMS by 128-fold (OR, 128.0; 95% CI, 13.0–1256.5; $P<.0001$) versus only by 9 times with brainstem or posterior fossa involvement (OR, 9.2; 95% CI, 1.1–75.2; $P = .04$).[54]

Recently, a large retrospective cohort of 456 RIS subjects from 5 countries identified a number of risk factors predicting a first demyelinating episode, which include younger age (≤37 years), male sex, and the presence of a cervical or thoracic SC lesion. Interestingly, in the multivariate regression analysis, the presence of a cervical or thoracic spine lesion was identified as the strongest predictor of future clinical events (hazard ratio, 3.08; 95% CI, 2.06–4.62; $P<.001$).[55]

Based on these studies, it is evident that the presence of SC lesions has clinical usefulness with regard to prediction in early stages of MS (CIS and RIS).

Prediction in Established Multiple Sclerosis

Although lesions of the SC are often symptomatic, given its compact arrangement of eloquent white matter tracks, accumulating evidence confirms the prevalence of asymptomatic SC lesions in both early and established MS.[38,49,50,56,57] Unfortunately, despite the relative frequency of known clinically silent SC lesions, the latter is rarely imaged outside of suspected SC relapses in routine clinical practice. Thus, there is limited information on the predictive value of SC lesions on future disease course.

New lesions on brain MRI are strongly correlated with relapse and disability progression. Thus, MRI activity in the brain is used as a surrogate marker of disease activity in MS.[58,59] Studies of a much smaller magnitude have demonstrated an association between SC lesions and clinical disability.[60,61] Coret and colleagues[60] retrospectively reviewed prospectively collected data of 25 with RRMS over a minimum 10-year follow-up period who had a cervical SC MRI during the first 3 years of symptom onset. The authors demonstrated that diffuse SC lesions (poorly defined areas of high T2-weighted signal) predicted greater disability (EDSS ≥4) than a nodular pattern (≥1 focal lesions; hazard ratio, 7.2; 95% CI, 1.4–36.4) and patients attained a predefined endpoint of an EDSS of 4 more quickly in the former (mean of 7 years vs 11 years; log-rank 10.3; $P = .01$). Moreover, in a longitudinal study of 52 patients with MS presenting with a first episode of acute partial transverse myelitis, a high number of SC lesions at baseline predicted a greater number of relapses ($P = .04$).[62]

More recently, Kearney and colleagues[56] demonstrated that SC lesion load was associated independently with EDSS, independent of brain or SC atrophy. The authors acquired conventional and advanced quantitative SC MRI on 92 patients with MS and 28 healthy controls. They demonstrated that SC lesion load was significantly higher in progressive forms of MS (secondary progressive MS [SPMS] $P = .008$ and PPMS $P = .02$) versus RRMS. Moreover, in the multivariate regression model, SC lesion load was associated independently with EDSS ($P<.001$).[56] Furthermore, Brownlee and colleagues[50] showed an independent association between baseline SC lesion count, change in SC lesion number, as well as cervical SC cross-sectional area and disability level (based on the EDSS).

THE CLINICORADIOLOGIC PARADOX

Despite accumulating evidence from these relatively small studies that lesions in the SC in MS are relevant to clinical disability, using conventional MRI techniques to image the SC, a phenomenon known as the clinicoradiologic paradox, limits observed correlations between SC lesions and clinical measures.[63]

The clinicoradiologic paradox has been well-described in the brain and refers to the observation that lesion-based measures (lesion count and volume) often have limited correlations with measures of clinical disability in patients with MS. This "paradox" is also observed in the SC, with a number of studies demonstrating that a lack of association between SC lesion load and disability.[10,39]

There are many reasons underlying the clinicoradiologic paradox, including the fact that conventional MRI techniques (T2-weighted sequences) lack sensitivity and specificity to underlying tissue microstructural changes that are relevant to MS disease processes.[64–67] In addition, the limited methods with which we quantify neurologic dysfunction in MS contribute to this phenomenon.[68] With the SC, specifically, owing to additional technical challenges, the clinicoradiologic paradox can be more accentuated.[63,69]

Advanced quantitative MRI measures, which are more sensitive and specific to MS-related structural changes in brain and SC tissue, allow for many of the limitations of conventional MRI to be addressed.

ADVANCED QUANTITATIVE SPINAL CORD MRI TECHNIQUES: STRUCTURAL TECHNIQUES

A variety of advanced quantitative SC MRI techniques have been developed that have the ability to assess the SC beyond simply identifying lesions. Quantitative techniques can be largely divided into those that assess the structural and functional integrity, because both aspects are impacted by disease states such as MS. These sections summarize a number of quantitative MRI techniques that assess the structural integrity of SC tissue in MS.

Spinal Cord Atrophy

Given the previously described limitations in the evaluation of SC lesions, alternative methods that have the ability to quantify MS-related SC damage beyond lesion detection are being developed. One of the most commonly used quantitative measures of disease-related change in MS is SC atrophy. Measures of SC atrophy (SC volume and SC cross-sectional area) have been shown to occur across all stages of MS and consistently demonstrate strong correlations with clinical disability.[70–73]

Methods to measure SC atrophy have evolved substantially over the past few decades. Early studies relied on manual delineation, but this method is impractical because it is labor intensive, time consuming, and has poor reproducibility.[74] Subsequently, Losseff and colleagues[75] developed a more refined and reproducible threshold-based method that exploited the contrast in signal intensity between CSF and the SC, and a used a semiautomated measurement of area at the C2/C3 level. This technique was widely used in atrophy imaging protocols, but still had ,limitations including being time consuming. Subsequently, a rapid, semiautomatic SC segmentation technique was developed by Horsfield and colleagues[76] in 2010 that improved reproducibility and time requirements. Various other groups have subsequently developed and used automated and semiautomated methods with different strengths and weaknesses.[77–79] Recently, a voxel-based statistical analysis of 3-dimensional cervical SC images has enabled the evaluation of regional patterns of atrophy in particular MS phenotypes.[80]

Generally, SC atrophy in MS has been measured by assessing SC volume or cross-sectional area (**Fig. 3**). Recent studies that have assessed various normalization factors of SCV have demonstrated that SC cross-sectional area (which is SC volume normalized by SC length) may be the most robust measure of SC atrophy, in that it consistently has the strongest correlations with clinical disability, and is able to detect differences between MS and healthy subjects, and between MS subtypes.[81,82]

Several studies in patients with long-standing MS (>10 years since symptom onset) demonstrated that SC atrophy, as measured by the upper cervical cross-sectional area on MRI, is associated with clinical disability, independent of various other MRI

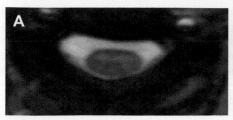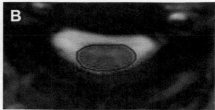

Fig. 3. Automated segmentation of spinal cord (SC) cross-sectional area. (*A*) Axial section of cervical SC (*B*) with superimposed region of interest encompassing the SC cross-sectional area. (*From* Oh J, Sotirchos ES, Saidha S, et al. Relationships between quantitative spinal cord MRI and retinal layers in multiple sclerosis. Neurology 2015;84:723; with permission from "Wolters Kluwer Inc" publishing house.)

metrics including T2-weighted lesion load and brain atrophy.[71,83] Moreover, Biber-acher and colleagues[70] went on to demonstrate atrophy in patients with early MS (CIS). Cervical SC atrophy seems to be more significant in patients with progressive disease, independent of disease duration.[82,84,85] A recent study found that both SC and retinal layer atrophy exhibited independent associations with clinical dysfunction beyond measuring brain atrophy, highlighting the importance of including assessments of small compartments such as the SC and optic nerve when attempting to understand disease mechanism relevant to disability in MS.[86]

Lukas and colleagues[73] sought to quantify the rate of volume loss in a longitudinal diverse cohort of patients with MS. The median decrease in SC area was 1.5% per year across all subgroups, but was notably highest in patients with SPMS (−2.2% per year) and significantly greater in those with disease progression versus stable disease. Remarkably, rates of brain atrophy did not differ between subtypes or between progressive and stable patients. A recent systematic review and metaanalysis confirmed that SC atrophy occurs in both relapsing and progressive MS, and the pooled rate of SC atrophy was 1.8% per year, which is substantially larger in magnitude than what is reported for brain atrophy in MS (0.5%–1.0% per year).[87] Thus, these studies suggest that, given the magnitude of SC atrophy on an annual basis, this may be a viable biomarker of disease progression in MS.

There have been conflicting data regarding SC atrophy in early MS, namely, CIS.[88–90] One study with a phenotypically diverse cohort of patients (CIS, RRMS, SPMS, and PPMS) revealed cervical SC atrophy in those with progressive disease and its absence CIS and patients with RRMS.[90] Biberacher and colleagues,[70] however, demonstrated atrophy early on in the disease course, including in CIS. Interestingly, this study also highlighted the possible contribution of increased SC structural variability on disability status, because the data suggests a positive association between the two.

The regional distribution of SC atrophy seems to vary by MS disease subtype. Those with RRMS display clusters of atrophy primarily localized to the posterior SC, whereas patients with progressive MS seemed to have more generalized volume loss, but atrophy is most significant in the posterior and lateral columns.[80,84]

Spinal Cord Atrophy: Gray Matter

Although MS has traditionally been thought to be a disease of the white matter, a wealth of evidence has demonstrated that MS-related pathologic processes affect both the white and gray matter in the brain and SC, and that gray matter pathology is highly relevant to clinical disability.[91–95]

In the SC specifically, Schlaeger and colleagues[95] observed evidence of gray matter atrophy in with RRMS versus healthy controls and that patients with progressive MS subtypes had significantly more gray matter atrophy than those with RRMS. In multivariate models of clinical disability where a spectrum of MRI measures were included (SC lesion count, SC gray matter atrophy, SC white matter atrophy, brain T2-weighted lesion load, brain T1-weighted lesion load), SC gray matter atrophy was the most significant correlate of clinical disability (**Fig. 4**).

Magnetization Transfer Imaging

Among quantitative MRI techniques, magnetization transfer imaging (MTI) has been one of the most extensively studied over the last 2 decades and has been used

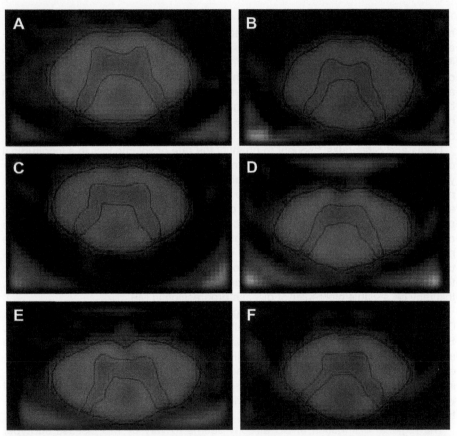

Fig. 4. Axial 2-dimensional phase sensitive inversion images at the C2/C3 disc level in patients with multiple sclerosis (MS) with gray matter (GM) and white matter (WM) segmented. (*A, C, E*) A patient with relapsing remitting MS (RRMS) and mild disability. (*B*) A patient with primary progressive MS and moderate disability. (*D, F*) A patient with secondary progressive MS and severe disability. There is selective atrophy of the spinal cord GM in the patient with primary progressive MS and moderate disability (*B*) and both WM and GM atrophy in severely disabled secondary progressive MS of long disease duration (*F*). (*From* Schlaeger R, Papinutto N, Panara V, et al. Spinal cord gray matter atrophy correlates with multiple sclerosis disability. Ann Neurol 2014;76(4):568–80; with permission from "John Wiley and sons" publishing house.)

frequently to assess microstructural changes in the brain and SC of patients with MS. MTI is sensitive to the myelin content of underlying tissue being imaged, and quantifies this by measuring magnetization transfer between macromolecule-bound protons that consist of predominately myelin in the central nervous system, and those in free water. The magnetization transfer ratio (MTR) is the most commonly used MTI-derived index, and is reduced with myelin and axonal loss.[96,97] MRI–histopathologic correlational studies have shown that reduced MTR values in both demyelinating lesions as well as normal appearing white matter strongly correlate with post mortem demyelination and axonal degeneration.[97,98]

MTI has been applied in the SC in MS by a number of groups. Early reports demonstrated decreased MTR in SC lesions as well as in normal-appearing white matter in patients with progressive MS.[99,100] Another study by Rovaris and colleagues[101] revealed significantly reduced cervical SC MTI indices in SPMS and PPMS, whereas no MTR abnormalities were observed in healthy controls. More recently, a study that assessed a variety of quantitative SC MRI metrics found differences between cervical SC MTR measures in patients with low cervical SC lesion count but substantially different disability levels. In those with high SC lesion counts, however, there was no difference in the MTR, even when disability levels differed significantly.[102] The authors postulate that this finding might be the result of the propensity of MTR to reflect demyelination more than axonal degeneration, the latter being the more likely culprit of significant disability in patients with heavy lesion burdens.

The role of meningeal inflammatory pathology is of increasing interest in MS, and a number of studies have evaluated this phenomenon in the brain.[103–107] Recently, Kearney and colleagues[108] attempted to evaluate pial inflammation in the SC using MTI metrics and found isolated reduction of MTR in the subpial region of the SC (outer region), suggestive of pial inflammation and/or subpial demyelination in patients with CIS and RRMS. In addition, there was a significant association of reduced subpial MTR with SC atrophy in progressive MS. The authors concluded that subpial MTR might be useful in detecting early meningeal inflammatory abnormalities in the SC in MS.

MTI has also been applied in specific SC regions. Zackowski and colleagues[109] found that MT-CSF (an MTI-derived metric)[110] in the dorsal and lateral columns of the cervical SC in patients with MS correlated with vibration sensation threshold and motor strength, respectively.

Finally, recent work by Lema and colleagues[111] used a novel approach of quantitative MT saturation to enhance the precision of standard MTI, theoretically resulting in increased sensitivity to microstructural changes in the underlying tissue. The authors demonstrated that, although cervical SC MTR did not correlate with EDSS or 25-foot timed walk, an association between MT saturation and both of these disability measures was present, suggesting the improved sensitivity of MT saturation over conventional MTI.

Diffusion Tensor Imaging

Diffusion tensor imaging (DTI) is another quantitative MRI technique that addresses some of the limitations of conventional MRI to study MS. DTI permits a quantitative evaluation of tissue architecture by evaluating the motion of water molecules.[112–114] The magnitude and direction of water diffusion in 3-dimensional space are reflected in the various DTI indices. The most commonly used DTI indices are mean diffusivity and fractional anisotropy (FA)[115–117] (**Fig. 5**).

In MS-mediated damage to the central nervous system, the typical physiologic barriers to diffusion are impaired, resulting in altered DTI indices, not only in lesions, but

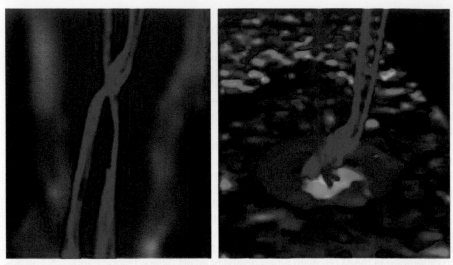

Fig. 5. Axial view of the fractional anisotropy color map of the spinal cord (SC). The figure is color coded with the direction of the principal eigenvector of the diffusion tensor. The right and left corticospinal tracts are shown in red and blue, exiting the SC and crossing. (*From* Wheeler-Kingshott CA, Stroman PW, Schwan JM, et al. The current state-of-the-art of spinal cord imaging: applications. NeuroImage 2014;84:1082–93; with permission from "Elsevier" publishing house.)

also in normal-appearing white and gray matter.[118–120] Post mortem histopathologic studies have correlated these changes in DTI indices with pathologic demyelination and axonal injury.[97,121–123]

Although a wealth of literature exists on DTI use in the brain of patients with MS, DTI studies in the SC are much more limited, likely owing to technical limitations. A number of groups have demonstrated that the cervical SC has an increased mean diffusivity and a decreased FA in patients with MS versus healthy control subjects, in both lesioned tissue and normal-appearing tissue.[124–128] A recent cross-sectional multi-parametric MRI study examined relationships between DTI indices and various measures of clinical disability in a heterogeneous group of patients with MS. The authors found significant independent correlations in multivariate models despite the inclusion of measures of SC and brain atrophy.[129] Likewise, patients with PPMS display similar abnormalities in cervical SC DTI indices.[130]

There have been few longitudinal studies assessing SC DTI measures in MS. One study found that future disability correlated with cervical SC FA at baseline, but there were no observed correlations between DTI index change and clinical disability progression over a mean follow-up period of 2.4 years.[124] Other small studies evaluated DTI indices and disability status at baseline and at several time points over 6 months in patients with MS presenting with cervical myelitis. Overall, the results demonstrated that lower radial diffusivity (RD) at baseline, and a significant reduction in RD over the follow-up period correlated with a better functional outcome.[131–133]

Like MTI, DTI has also been applied in regional assessments of the SC in MS. Naismith and colleagues[134] evaluated column-specific DTI indices in MS, and found correlations between dorsal column FA and RD and vibration thresholds. Moreover, EDSS was significantly correlated with FA and RD in both dorsolateral and corticospinal tracts. Finally, DTI indices (RD, FA, and mean diffusivity) have also been found to be abnormal in the gray matter of patients with MS and correlate strongly with disability.[94]

Ultra–High-Field MRI

Ultra–high-field (UHF) MRI enables a more detailed characterization of structural change in underlying tissue by enabling improved signal-to-noise ratio, greater chemical shift dispersion, and improved contrast owing to magnetic susceptibility variations, which can lead to increased sensitivity to underlying tissue changes. At present, UHF MRI is mainly used in investigational settings.[135] In the brain, the application of UHF MRI in MS has enabled enhanced characterization of white matter lesions, improved visualization of gray matter lesions and their exact location, and the quantification of "novel" metabolites, which may be markers of axonal degeneration.[135–137]

Studies assessing UHF MRI in the SC have been limited. In a pilot study that imaged the cervical SC at 7T in 10 healthy subjects, clear gray/white matter differentiation and improved visualization of smaller peripheral structures (pia mater, dura mater, denticulate ligaments, nerve roots, rostral–caudal blood vessels) that typically are not visualized on 3T MRI was observed.[138]

In the SC in MS, 7T MRI has only been recently reported by Dula and colleagues,[139] who evaluated 15 patients with MS. In comparison with SC MRI at 3T, 7T MRI demonstrated improved lesion detection (lesion counts increased by 52% vs 3T MRI) and enhanced demarcation of gray and white matter. In addition, nerve roots were clearly visualized. The authors concluded that there were clear advantages of using UHF MRI in the SC over conventional techniques.

ADVANCED QUANTITATIVE MRI: FUNCTIONAL IMAGING

The preceding sections summarized quantitative MRI techniques that assess SC tissue structural integrity. Another important factor when considering tissue aberrations in diseased states is the functional integrity of the underlying tissue. The following sections summarize emerging functional techniques in the SC in MS.

Functional MRI

Functional MRI (fMRI) analyzes changes in the pattern of regional blood flow corresponding to specific neurologic stimuli. This technique relies on the neurovascular coupling theory, and uses the blood oxygen level–dependent effect as the contrast method to measure metabolic activity in underlying tissue, which corresponds with tissue activation.[140]

To date, most fMRI studies in MS have focused on cortical functional changes, and applying fMRI to the SC has required adaptation from the well-established methods in the brain.[141–143] Although sparse, a number of studies have demonstrated in healthy controls and in different neurologic disease states that fMRI in the SC is feasible, and can capture particular areas of SC neuronal activity that correspond to specific stimuli.[117,144,145]

In MS, the few fMRI studies that have been reported have demonstrated increased activation of the cervical SC in response to specific stimuli in all of the major MS clinical phenotypes. The magnitude of increased activation was correlated with the severity of clinical disability and the extent of structural tissue damage.[146–148] These early studies are intriguing, and warrant further investigation in larger cohorts of patients.

Magnetic Resonance Spectroscopy

Proton MR spectroscopy provides information on the metabolic and biochemical status of underlying tissue by quantifying the concentrations of specific metabolites that act as markers for underlying pathologic processes. *N*-acetylaspartate (NAA) is the most widely studied metabolite in the SC in patients with MS to date, and is considered to be a specific in vivo marker for neuronal number, health, and viability.[149]

MR spectroscopy studies assessing metabolite concentrations in MS in the cervical SC have been performed in cross-sectional and longitudinal settings. Patients with MS with a cervical SC relapse were shown to have reduced NAA concentration and lower structural connectivity in the corticospinal and posterior tracts.[127] Significant associations between reduced NAA in the cervical SC and acute and chronic disability have also been described.[127] Interestingly, SC NAA levels partially increased over time after an acute relapse, especially in patients who improved clinically, suggesting that SC NAA may reflect clinically relevant changes in axonal integrity.[150]

CONCLUSIONS AND FUTURE DIRECTIONS

Imaging the SC in MS has significant value, both in clinical and investigational settings. Conventional MRI techniques have been used predominately to evaluate SC lesions, and newer sequences have improved the ability to detect SC lesions. Conventional MRI of the SC is routinely used in clinical practice, because it has both diagnostic and prognostic usefulness.

A number of advanced quantitative SC MRI measures that assess both the structural and functional integrity of the SC have been evaluated in investigational settings. These techniques include measures of SC atrophy, DTI, MTI, UHF MRI, fMRI, and MR spectroscopy. These techniques have collectively demonstrated significant usefulness in improving our understanding of microstructural and functional changes relevant to disability in MS, and have contributed to our understanding of MS and the role the SC plays in MS disease mechanisms. However, these quantitative techniques cannot yet be applied in clinical settings in individual patients because variability and complex postprocessing algorithms prohibit their routine use. Future studies are necessary to establish whether these quantitative measures may be useful as biomarkers of neurodegeneration and neuroprotection in clinical trial settings and in day-to-day clinical practice, particularly in progressive MS. Finally, novel functional techniques and UHF MRI hold promise in providing needed insights into the underlying mechanisms of disease in MS. Such knowledge will enable a more comprehensive understanding of the complex disease mechanisms underlying MS, which will lay the foundation for the development of superior treatments that will improve the lives of people living with MS.

REFERENCES

1. Taber KH, Herrick RC, Weathers SW, et al. Pitfalls and artifacts encountered in clinical MR imaging of the spine. Radiographics 1998;18(6):1499–521.
2. Cadavid D, Wolansky LJ, Skurnick J, et al. Efficacy of treatment of MS with IFNbeta-1b or glatiramer acetate by monthly brain MRI in the BECOME study. Neurology 2009;72(23):1976–83.
3. McFarland HF, Frank JA, Albert PS, et al. Using gadolinium-enhanced magnetic resonance imaging lesions to monitor disease activity in multiple sclerosis. Ann Neurol 1992;32(6):758–66.

4. Tortorella C, Codella M, Rocca MA, et al. Disease activity in multiple sclerosis studied by weekly triple-dose magnetic resonance imaging. J Neurol 1999; 246(8):689–92.

5. Willoughby EW, Grochowski E, Li DK, et al. Serial magnetic resonance scanning in multiple sclerosis: a second prospective study in relapsing patients. Ann Neurol 1989;25(1):43–9.

6. Bekiesinska-Figatowska M. T2-hyperintense foci on brain MR imaging. Med Sci Monit 2004;10(Suppl 3):80–7.

7. Haller S, Kövari E, Herrmann FR, et al. Do brain T2/FLAIR white matter hyperintensities correspond to myelin loss in normal aging? A radiologic-neuropathologic correlation study. Acta Neuropathol Commun 2013;1:14.

8. Nesbit GM, Forbes GS, Scheithauer BW, et al. Multiple sclerosis: histopathologic and MR and/or CT correlation in 37 cases at biopsy and three cases at autopsy. Radiology 1991;180(2):467–74.

9. Nijeholt GJ, Bergers E, Kamphorst W, et al. Post-mortem high-resolution MRI of the spinal cord in multiple sclerosis: a correlative study with conventional MRI, histopathology and clinical phenotype. Brain 2001;124(Pt 1):154–66.

10. Kidd D, Thorpe JW, Thompson AJ, et al. Spinal cord MRI using multi-array coils and fast spin echo. II. Findings in multiple sclerosis. Neurology 1993;43(12): 2632–7.

11. Thomas DJ, Pennock JM, Hajnal JV, et al. Magnetic resonance imaging of spinal cord in multiple sclerosis by fluid-attenuated inversion recovery. Lancet 1993; 341(8845):593–4.

12. White SJ, Hajnal JV, Young IR, et al. Use of fluid-attenuated inversion-recovery pulse sequences for imaging the spinal cord. Magn Reson Med 1992;28(1): 153–62.

13. Filippi M, Yousry TA, Alkadhi H, et al. Spinal cord MRI in multiple sclerosis with multicoil arrays: a comparison between fast spin echo and fast FLAIR. J Neurol Neurosurg Psychiatry 1996;61(6):632–5.

14. Keiper MD, Grossman RI, Brunson JC, et al. The low sensitivity of fluid-attenuated inversion-recovery MR in the detection of multiple sclerosis of the spinal cord. AJNR Am J Neuroradiol 1997;18(6):1035–9.

15. Hittmair K, Mallek R, Prayer D, et al. Spinal cord lesions in patients with multiple sclerosis: comparison of MR pulse sequences. AJNR Am J Neuroradiol 1996; 17(8):1555–65.

16. Stevenson VL, Gawne-Cain ML, Barker GJ, et al. Imaging of the spinal cord and brain in multiple sclerosis: a comparative study between fast FLAIR and fast spin echo. J Neurol 1997;244(2):119–24.

17. Thorpe JW, Kidd D, Kendall BE, et al. Spinal cord MRI using multi-array coils and fast spin echo. I. Technical aspects and findings in healthy adults. Neurology 1993;43(12):2625–31.

18. Kearney H, Miller DH, Ciccarelli O. Spinal cord MRI in multiple sclerosis–diagnostic, prognostic and clinical value. Nat Rev Neurol 2015;11(6):327–38.

19. Bot JC, Barkhof F, Lycklama A, et al. Comparison of a conventional cardiac-triggered dual spin-echo and a fast STIR sequence in detection of spinal cord lesions in multiple sclerosis. Eur Radiol 2000;10(5):753–8.

20. Campi A, Pontesilli S, Gerevini S, et al. Comparison of MRI pulse sequences for investigation of lesions of the cervical spinal cord. Neuroradiology 2000;42(9): 669–75.

21. Nayak NB, Salah R, Huang JC, et al. A comparison of sagittal short T1 inversion recovery and T2-weighted FSE sequences for detection of multiple sclerosis spinal cord lesions. Acta Neurol Scand 2014;129(3):198–203.

22. Ross JS. Newer sequences for spinal MR imaging: smorgasbord or succotash of acronyms? AJNR Am J Neuroradiol 1999;20(3):361–73.

23. Thorpe JW, MacManus DG, Kendall BE, et al. Short tau inversion recovery fast spin-echo (fast STIR) imaging of the spinal cord in multiple sclerosis. Magn Reson Imaging 1994;12(7):983–9.

24. Redpath TW, Smith FW. Technical note: use of a double inversion recovery pulse sequence to image selectively grey or white brain matter. Br J Radiol 1994;67(804):1258–63.

25. Riederer I, Karampinos DC, Settles M, et al. Double inversion recovery sequence of the cervical spinal cord in multiple sclerosis and related inflammatory diseases. AJNR Am J Neuroradiol 2015;36(1):219–25.

26. Finelli DA, Hurst GC, Karaman BA, et al. Use of magnetization transfer for improved contrast on gradient-echo MR images of the cervical spine. Radiology 1994;193(1):165–71.

27. Ozturk A, Aygun N, Smith SA, et al. Axial 3D gradient-echo imaging for improved multiple sclerosis lesion detection in the cervical spinal cord at 3T. Neuroradiology 2013;55(4):431–9.

28. Martin N, Malfair D, Zhao Y, et al. Comparison of MERGE and axial T2-weighted fast spin-echo sequences for detection of multiple sclerosis lesions in the cervical spinal cord. AJR Am J Roentgenol 2012;199(1):157–62.

29. White ML, Zhang Y, Healey K. Cervical spinal cord multiple sclerosis: evaluation with 2D multi-echo recombined gradient echo MR imaging. J Spinal Cord Med 2011;34(1):93–8.

30. Harel A, Ceccarelli A, Farrell C, et al. Phase-Sensitive Inversion-Recovery MRI Improves Longitudinal Cortical Lesion Detection in Progressive MS. PLoS One 2016;11(3):e0152180.

31. Hou P, Hasan KM, Sitton CW, et al. Phase-sensitive T1 inversion recovery imaging: a time-efficient interleaved technique for improved tissue contrast in neuroimaging. AJNR Am J Neuroradiol 2005;26(6):1432–8.

32. Sethi V, Yousry TA, Muhlert N, et al. Improved detection of cortical MS lesions with phase-sensitive inversion recovery MRI. J Neurol Neurosurg Psychiatry 2012;83(9):877–82.

33. Poonawalla AH, Hou P, Nelson FA, et al. Cervical spinal cord lesions in multiple sclerosis: T1-weighted inversion-recovery MR imaging with phase-sensitive reconstruction. Radiology 2008;246(1):258–64.

34. Alcaide-Leon P, Pauranik A, Alshafai L, et al. Comparison of sagittal FSE T2, STIR, and T1-weighted phase-sensitive inversion recovery in the detection of spinal cord lesions in MS at 3T. AJNR Am J Neuroradiol 2016;37(5):970–5.

35. Sundarakumar DK, Smith CM, Hwang WD, et al. Evaluation of focal cervical spinal cord lesions in multiple sclerosis: comparison of white matter-suppressed t1 inversion recovery sequence versus conventional STIR and proton density-weighted turbo spin-echo sequences. AJNR Am J Neuroradiol 2016;37(8):1561–6.

36. Nair G, Absinta M, Reich DS. Optimized T1-MPRAGE sequence for better visualization of spinal cord multiple sclerosis lesions at 3T. AJNR Am J Neuroradiol 2013;34(11):2215–22.

37. Traboulsee A, Simon JH, Stone L, et al. Revised recommendations of the consortium of MS Centers Task Force for a standardized MRI protocol and clinical

guidelines for the diagnosis and follow-up of multiple sclerosis. AJNR Am J Neuroradiol 2016;37(3):394–401.
38. Bot JC, Barkhof F, Polman CH, et al. Spinal cord abnormalities in recently diagnosed MS patients: added value of spinal MRI examination. Neurology 2004; 62(2):226–33.
39. Lycklama A, Nijeholt GJ, Castelijns JA, et al. Sagittal MR of multiple sclerosis in the spinal cord: fast versus conventional spin-echo imaging. AJNR Am J Neuroradiol 1998;19(2):355–60.
40. Weier K, Mazraeh J, Naegelin Y, et al. Biplanar MRI for the assessment of the spinal cord in multiple sclerosis. Mult Scler 2012;18(11):1560–9.
41. Bot JC, Barkhof F. Spinal-cord MRI in multiple sclerosis: conventional and nonconventional MR techniques. Neuroimaging Clin N Am 2009;19(1):81–99.
42. Hua LH, Donlon SL, Sobhanian MJ, et al. Thoracic spinal cord lesions are influenced by the degree of cervical spine involvement in multiple sclerosis. Spinal Cord 2015;53(7):520–5.
43. Barkhof F, Filippi M, Miller DH, et al. Comparison of MRI criteria at first presentation to predict conversion to clinically definite multiple sclerosis. Brain 1997; 120(Pt 11):2059–69.
44. Fazekas F, Barkhof F, Filippi M. Unenhanced and enhanced magnetic resonance imaging in the diagnosis of multiple sclerosis. J Neurol Neurosurg Psychiatry 1998;64(Suppl 1):S2–5.
45. Paty DW, Oger JJ, Kastrukoff LF, et al. MRI in the diagnosis of MS: a prospective study with comparison of clinical evaluation, evoked potentials, oligoclonal banding, and CT. Neurology 1988;38(2):180–5.
46. McDonald WI, Compston A, Edan G, et al. Recommended diagnostic criteria for multiple sclerosis: guidelines from the International Panel on the diagnosis of multiple sclerosis. Ann Neurol 2001;50(1):121–7.
47. Polman CH, Reingold SC, Edan G, et al. Diagnostic criteria for multiple sclerosis: 2005 revisions to the "McDonald Criteria". Ann Neurol 2005;58(6):840–6.
48. Polman CH, Reingold SC, Banwell B, et al. Diagnostic criteria for multiple sclerosis: 2010 Revisions to the McDonald criteria. Ann Neurol 2011;69(2):292–302.
49. Sombekke MH, Wattjes MP, Balk LJ, et al. Spinal cord lesions in patients with clinically isolated syndrome: a powerful tool in diagnosis and prognosis. Neurology 2013;80(1):69–75.
50. Brownlee WJ, Altmann DR, Alves Da Mota P, et al. Association of asymptomatic spinal cord lesions and atrophy with disability 5 years after a clinically isolated syndrome. Mult Scler 2017;23(5):665–74.
51. O'Riordan JI, Thompson AJ, Kingsley DP, et al. The prognostic value of brain MRI in clinically isolated syndromes of the CNS. A 10-year follow-up. Brain 1998;121(Pt 3):495–503.
52. Patrucco L, Rojas JI, Cristiano E. Assessing the value of spinal cord lesions in predicting development of multiple sclerosis in patients with clinically isolated syndromes. J Neurol 2012;259(7):1317–20.
53. Okuda DT, Mowry EM, Beheshtian A, et al. Incidental MRI anomalies suggestive of multiple sclerosis: the radiologically isolated syndrome. Neurology 2009; 73(20):1714.
54. Okuda DT, Mowry EM, Cree BA, et al. Asymptomatic spinal cord lesions predict disease progression in radiologically isolated syndrome. Neurology 2011;76(8): 686–92.
55. Okuda DT, Siva A, Kantarci O, et al. Radiologically isolated syndrome: 5-year risk for an initial clinical event. PLoS One 2014;9(3):e90509.

56. Kearney H, Altmann DR, Samson RS, et al. Cervical cord lesion load is associated with disability independently from atrophy in MS. Neurology 2015;84(4): 367–73.
57. Nijeholt GJ, van Walderveen MA, Castelijns JA, et al. Brain and spinal cord abnormalities in multiple sclerosis. Correlation between MRI parameters, clinical subtypes and symptoms. Brain 1998;121(Pt 4):687–97.
58. Sormani MP, Arnold DL, De Stefano N. Treatment effect on brain atrophy correlates with treatment effect on disability in multiple sclerosis. Ann Neurol 2014; 75(1):43–9.
59. Sormani MP, Bruzzi P. MRI lesions as a surrogate for relapses in multiple sclerosis: a meta-analysis of randomised trials. Lancet Neurol 2013;12(7):669–76.
60. Coret F, Bosca I, Landete L, et al. Early diffuse demyelinating lesion in the cervical spinal cord predicts a worse prognosis in relapsing-remitting multiple sclerosis. Mult Scler 2010;16(8):935–41.
61. Trop I, Bourgouin PM, Lapierre Y, et al. Multiple sclerosis of the spinal cord: diagnosis and follow-up with contrast-enhanced MR and correlation with clinical activity. AJNR Am J Neuroradiol 1998;19(6):1025–33.
62. Cordonnier C, de Seze J, Breteau G, et al. Prospective study of patients presenting with acute partial transverse myelopathy. J Neurol 2003;250(12): 1447–52.
63. Barkhof F. The clinico-radiological paradox in multiple sclerosis revisited. Curr Opin Neurol 2002;15(3):239–45.
64. Bergers E, Bot JC, De Groot CJ, et al. Axonal damage in the spinal cord of MS patients occurs largely independent of T2 MRI lesions. Neurology 2002;59(11): 1766–71.
65. Bergers E, Bot JC, van der Valk P, et al. Diffuse signal abnormalities in the spinal cord in multiple sclerosis: direct postmortem in situ magnetic resonance imaging correlated with in vitro high-resolution magnetic resonance imaging and histopathology. Ann Neurol 2002;51(5):652–6.
66. Bitsch A, Kuhlmann T, Stadelmann C, et al. A longitudinal MRI study of histopathologically defined hypointense multiple sclerosis lesions. Ann Neurol 2001;49(6):793–6.
67. Stankiewicz J, Neema M, Alsop D, et al. Spinal cord lesions and clinical status in multiple sclerosis: a 1.5T and 3T MRI study. J Neurol Sci 2009;279(1–2):99–105.
68. Kalkers NF, Bergers L, de Groot V, et al. Concurrent validity of the MS functional composite using MRI as a biological disease marker. Neurology 2001;56(2): 215–9.
69. Filippi M, Agosta F. Imaging biomarkers in multiple sclerosis. J Magn Reson Imaging 2010;31(4):770–88.
70. Biberacher V, Boucard CC, Schmidt P, et al. Atrophy and structural variability of the upper cervical cord in early multiple sclerosis. Mult Scler 2015;21(7):875–84.
71. Daams M, Weiler F, Steenwijk MD, et al. Mean upper cervical cord area (MUCCA) measurement in long-standing multiple sclerosis: relation to brain findings and clinical disability. Mult Scler 2014;20(14):1860–5.
72. Kearney H, Yiannakas MC, Abdel-Aziz K, et al. Improved MRI quantification of spinal cord atrophy in multiple sclerosis. J Magn Reson Imaging 2014;39(3): 617–23.
73. Lukas C, Knol DL, Sombekke MH, et al. Cervical spinal cord volume loss is related to clinical disability progression in multiple sclerosis. J Neurol Neurosurg Psychiatry 2015;86(4):410–8.

74. Kidd D, Thorpe JW, Kendall BE, et al. MRI dynamics of brain and spinal cord in progressive multiple sclerosis. J Neurol Neurosurg Psychiatry 1996;60(1):15–9.

75. Losseff NA, Webb SL, O'Riordan JI, et al. Spinal cord atrophy and disability in multiple sclerosis. A new reproducible and sensitive MRI method with potential to monitor disease progression. Brain 1996;119(Pt 3):701–8.

76. Horsfield MA, Sala S, Neema M, et al. Rapid semi-automatic segmentation of the spinal cord from magnetic resonance images: application in multiple sclerosis. Neuroimage 2010;50(2):446–55.

77. Hickman SJ, Coulon O, Parker GJ, et al. Application of a B-spline active surface technique to the measurement of cervical cord volume in multiple sclerosis from three-dimensional MR images. J Magn Reson Imaging 2003;18(3):368–71.

78. Liu C, Edwards S, Gong Q, et al. Three dimensional MRI estimates of brain and spinal cord atrophy in multiple sclerosis. J Neurol Neurosurg Psychiatry 1999; 66(3):323–30.

79. Vaithianathar L, Tench CR, Morgan PS, et al. Magnetic resonance imaging of the cervical spinal cord in multiple sclerosis–a quantitative T1 relaxation time mapping approach. J Neurol 2003;250(3):307–15.

80. Valsasina P, Rocca MA, Horsfield MA, et al. Regional cervical cord atrophy and disability in multiple sclerosis: a voxel-based analysis. Radiology 2013;266(3): 853–61.

81. Healy BC, Arora A, Hayden DL, et al. Approaches to normalization of spinal cord volume: application to multiple sclerosis. J Neuroimaging 2012;22(3):e12–9.

82. Oh J, Seigo M, Saidha S, et al. Spinal cord normalization in multiple sclerosis. J Neuroimaging 2014;24(6):577–84.

83. Kearney H, Rocca MA, Valsasina P, et al. Magnetic resonance imaging correlates of physical disability in relapse onset multiple sclerosis of long disease duration. Mult Scler 2014;20(1):72–80.

84. Rocca MA, Valsasina P, Damjanovic D, et al. Voxel-wise mapping of cervical cord damage in multiple sclerosis patients with different clinical phenotypes. J Neurol Neurosurg Psychiatry 2013;84(1):35–41.

85. Lukas C, Sombekke MH, Bellenberg B, et al. Relevance of spinal cord abnormalities to clinical disability in multiple sclerosis: MR imaging findings in a large cohort of patients. Radiology 2013;269(2):542–52.

86. Oh J, Sotirchos ES, Saidha S, et al. Relationships between quantitative spinal cord MRI and retinal layers in multiple sclerosis. Neurology 2015;84(7):720–8.

87. Casserly C, Baral S, Oh J. MRI quantification of spinal cord atrophy in multiple sclerosis: a systematic review and meta-analysis. Neurology 2016;86 (P3.016). Available at: http://www.neurology.org/content/86/16_Supplement/P3.016.

88. Brex PA, Leary SM, O'Riordan JI, et al. Measurement of spinal cord area in clinically isolated syndromes suggestive of multiple sclerosis. J Neurol Neurosurg Psychiatry 2001;70(4):544–7.

89. Rashid W, Davies GR, Chard DT, et al. Increasing cord atrophy in early relapsing-remitting multiple sclerosis: a 3 year study. J Neurol Neurosurg Psychiatry 2006;77(1):51–5.

90. Rocca MA, Horsfield MA, Sala S, et al. A multicenter assessment of cervical cord atrophy among MS clinical phenotypes. Neurology 2011;76(24):2096–102.

91. Fisniku LK, Brex PA, Altmann DR, et al. Disability and T2 MRI lesions: a 20-year follow-up of patients with relapse onset of multiple sclerosis. Brain 2008; 131(Pt 3):808–17.

92. Gilmore CP, Geurts JJ, Evangelou N, et al. Spinal cord grey matter lesions in multiple sclerosis detected by post-mortem high field MR imaging. Mult Scler 2009;15(2):180–8.

93. Kearney H, Miszkiel KA, Yiannakas MC, et al. Grey matter involvement by focal cervical spinal cord lesions is associated with progressive multiple sclerosis. Mult Scler 2016;22(7):910–20.

94. Kearney H, Schneider T, Yiannakas MC, et al. Spinal cord grey matter abnormalities are associated with secondary progression and physical disability in multiple sclerosis. J Neurol Neurosurg Psychiatry 2015;86(6):608–14.

95. Schlaeger R, Papinutto N, Panara V, et al. Spinal cord gray matter atrophy correlates with multiple sclerosis disability. Ann Neurol 2014;76(4):568–80.

96. Bot JC, Blezer EL, Kamphorst W, et al. The spinal cord in multiple sclerosis: relationship of high-spatial-resolution quantitative MR imaging findings to histopathologic results. Radiology 2004;233(2):531–40.

97. Mottershead JP, Schmierer K, Clemence M, et al. High field MRI correlates of myelin content and axonal density in multiple sclerosis–a post-mortem study of the spinal cord. J Neurol 2003;250(11):1293–301.

98. van Waesberghe JH, Kamphorst W, De Groot CJ, et al. Axonal loss in multiple sclerosis lesions: magnetic resonance imaging insights into substrates of disability. Ann Neurol 1999;46(5):747–54.

99. Filippi M. The role of magnetization transfer and diffusion-weighted MRI in the understanding of multiple sclerosis evolution. Neurol Sci 2000;21(4 Suppl 2): S877–81.

100. Gass A, Davie CA, Barker GJ, et al. Demonstration of plaque development in multiple sclerosis using magnetisation transfer ratio images and protein spectroscopy with short echo time. Nervenarzt 1997;68(12):996–1001 [in German].

101. Rovaris M, Bozzali M, Santuccio G, et al. In vivo assessment of the brain and cervical cord pathology of patients with primary progressive multiple sclerosis. Brain 2001;124(Pt 12):2540–9.

102. Oh J, Saidha S, Chen M, et al. Spinal cord quantitative MRI discriminates between disability levels in multiple sclerosis. Neurology 2013;80(6):540–7.

103. Absinta M, Vuolo L, Rao A, et al. Gadolinium-based MRI characterization of leptomeningeal inflammation in multiple sclerosis. Neurology 2015;85(1):18–28.

104. Howell OW, Reeves CA, Nicholas R, et al. Meningeal inflammation is widespread and linked to cortical pathology in multiple sclerosis. Brain 2011; 134(Pt 9):2755–71.

105. Magliozzi R, Howell OW, Reeves C, et al. A Gradient of neuronal loss and meningeal inflammation in multiple sclerosis. Ann Neurol 2010;68(4):477–93.

106. Serafini B, Rosicarelli B, Magliozzi R, et al. Detection of ectopic B-cell follicles with germinal centers in the meninges of patients with secondary progressive multiple sclerosis. Brain Pathol 2004;14(2):164–74.

107. Zurawski J, Lassmann H, Bakshi R. Use of magnetic resonance imaging to visualize leptomeningeal inflammation in patients with multiple sclerosis: a review. JAMA Neurol 2017;74(1):100–9.

108. Kearney H, Yiannakas MC, Samson RS, et al. Investigation of magnetization transfer ratio-derived pial and subpial abnormalities in the multiple sclerosis spinal cord. Brain 2014;137(Pt 9):2456–68.

109. Zackowski KM, Smith SA, Reich DS, et al. Sensorimotor dysfunction in multiple sclerosis and column-specific magnetization transfer-imaging abnormalities in the spinal cord. Brain 2009;132(Pt 5):1200–9.

110. Smith SA, Golay X, Fatemi A, et al. Magnetization transfer weighted imaging in the upper cervical spinal cord using cerebrospinal fluid as intersubject normalization reference (MTCSF imaging). Magn Reson Med 2005;54(1):201–6.

111. Lema A, Bishop C, Malik O, et al. A comparison of magnetization transfer methods to assess brain and cervical cord microstructure in multiple sclerosis. J Neuroimaging 2017;27(2):221–6.

112. Chenevert TL, Brunberg JA, Pipe JG. Anisotropic diffusion in human white matter: demonstration with MR techniques in vivo. Radiology 1990;177(2):401–5.

113. Beaulieu C. The basis of anisotropic water diffusion in the nervous system - a technical review. NMR Biomed 2002;15(7–8):435–55.

114. Moseley ME, Cohen Y, Kucharczyk J, et al. Diffusion-weighted MR imaging of anisotropic water diffusion in cat central nervous system. Radiology 1990; 176(2):439–45.

115. Fox RJ, Beall E, Bhattacharyya P, et al. Advanced MRI in multiple sclerosis: current status and future challenges. Neurol Clin 2011;29(2):357–80.

116. Basser PJ. Inferring microstructural features and the physiological state of tissues from diffusion-weighted images. NMR Biomed 1995;8(7–8):333–44.

117. Wheeler-Kingshott CA, Stroman PW, Schwab JM, et al. The current state-of-the-art of spinal cord imaging: applications. Neuroimage 2014;84:1082–93.

118. Cruz LC Jr, Domingues RC, Gasparetto EL. Diffusion tensor imaging of the cervical spinal cord of patients with relapsing-remising multiple sclerosis: a study of 41 cases. Arq Neuropsiquiatr 2009;67(2B):391–5.

119. Hesseltine SM, Law M, Babb J, et al. Diffusion tensor imaging in multiple sclerosis: assessment of regional differences in the axial plane within normal-appearing cervical spinal cord. AJNR Am J Neuroradiol 2006;27(6):1189–93.

120. Ohgiya Y, Oka M, Hiwatashi A, et al. Diffusion tensor MR imaging of the cervical spinal cord in patients with multiple sclerosis. Eur Radiol 2007;17(10):2499–504.

121. Klawiter EC, Schmidt RE, Trinkaus K, et al. Radial diffusivity predicts demyelination in ex vivo multiple sclerosis spinal cords. Neuroimage 2011;55(4): 1454–60.

122. Schmierer K, Wheeler-Kingshott CA, Boulby PA, et al. Diffusion tensor imaging of post mortem multiple sclerosis brain. Neuroimage 2007;35(2):467–77.

123. Zollinger LV, Kim TH, Hill K, et al. Using diffusion tensor imaging and immunofluorescent assay to evaluate the pathology of multiple sclerosis. J Magn Reson Imaging 2011;33(3):557–64.

124. Agosta F, Absinta M, Sormani MP, et al. In vivo assessment of cervical cord damage in MS patients: a longitudinal diffusion tensor MRI study. Brain 2007; 130(Pt 8):2211–9.

125. Benedetti B, Rocca MA, Rovaris M, et al. A diffusion tensor MRI study of cervical cord damage in benign and secondary progressive multiple sclerosis patients. J Neurol Neurosurg Psychiatry 2010;81(1):26–30.

126. Cercignani M, Horsfield MA, Agosta F, et al. Sensitivity-encoded diffusion tensor MR imaging of the cervical cord. AJNR Am J Neuroradiol 2003;24(6):1254–6.

127. Ciccarelli O, Wheeler-Kingshott CA, McLean MA, et al. Spinal cord spectroscopy and diffusion-based tractography to assess acute disability in multiple sclerosis. Brain 2007;130(Pt 8):2220–31.

128. Valsasina P, Rocca MA, Agosta F, et al. Mean diffusivity and fractional anisotropy histogram analysis of the cervical cord in MS patients. Neuroimage 2005;26(3): 822–8.

129. Oh J, Zackowski K, Chen M, et al. Multiparametric MRI correlates of sensori-motor function in the spinal cord in multiple sclerosis. Mult Scler 2013;19(4):427–35.

130. Agosta F, Benedetti B, Rocca MA, et al. Quantification of cervical cord pathology in primary progressive MS using diffusion tensor MRI. Neurology 2005;64(4):631–5.

131. Freund P, Wheeler-Kingshott C, Jackson J, et al. Recovery after spinal cord relapse in multiple sclerosis is predicted by radial diffusivity. Mult Scler 2010;16(10):1193–202.

132. Theaudin M, Saliou G, Ducot B, et al. Short-term evolution of spinal cord damage in multiple sclerosis: a diffusion tensor MRI study. Neuroradiology 2012;54(10):1171–8.

133. Toosy AT, Kou N, Altmann D, et al. Voxel-based cervical spinal cord mapping of diffusion abnormalities in MS-related myelitis. Neurology 2014;83(15):1321–5.

134. Naismith RT, Xu J, Klawiter EC, et al. Spinal cord tract diffusion tensor imaging reveals disability substrate in demyelinating disease. Neurology 2013;80(24):2201–9.

135. Absinta M, Sati P, Gaitan MI, et al. Seven-tesla phase imaging of acute multiple sclerosis lesions: a new window into the inflammatory process. Ann Neurol 2013;74(5):669–78.

136. Gaitan MI, Shea CD, Evangelou IE, et al. Evolution of the blood-brain barrier in newly forming multiple sclerosis lesions. Ann Neurol 2011;70(1):22–9.

137. Harrison DM, Oh J, Roy S, et al. Thalamic lesions in multiple sclerosis by 7T MRI: clinical implications and relationship to cortical pathology. Mult Scler 2015;21(9):1139–50.

138. Sigmund EE, Suero GA, Hu C, et al. High-resolution human cervical spinal cord imaging at 7 T. NMR Biomed 2012;25(7):891–9.

139. Dula AN, Pawate S, Dethrage LM, et al. Chemical exchange saturation transfer of the cervical spinal cord at 7 T. NMR Biomed 2016;29(9):1249–57.

140. Ogawa S, Lee TM, Kay AR, et al. Brain magnetic resonance imaging with contrast dependent on blood oxygenation. Proc Natl Acad Sci U S A 1990;87(24):9868–72.

141. Filippi M, Rocca MA, Colombo B, et al. Functional magnetic resonance imaging correlates of fatigue in multiple sclerosis. Neuroimage 2002;15(3):559–67.

142. Filippi M, Rocca MA, Mezzapesa DM, et al. Simple and complex movement-associated functional MRI changes in patients at presentation with clinically isolated syndromes suggestive of multiple sclerosis. Hum Brain Mapp 2004;21(2):108–17.

143. Rocca MA, Gavazzi C, Mezzapesa DM, et al. A functional magnetic resonance imaging study of patients with secondary progressive multiple sclerosis. Neuroimage 2003;19(4):1770–7.

144. Madi S, Flanders AE, Vinitski S, et al. Functional MR imaging of the human cervical spinal cord. AJNR Am J Neuroradiol 2001;22(9):1768–74.

145. Stroman PW, Tomanek B, Krause V, et al. Mapping of neuronal function in the healthy and injured human spinal cord with spinal fMRI. Neuroimage 2002;17(4):1854–60.

146. Agosta F, Valsasina P, Absinta M, et al. Primary progressive multiple sclerosis: tactile-associated functional MR activity in the cervical spinal cord. Radiology 2009;253(1):209–15.

147. Agosta F, Valsasina P, Rocca MA, et al. Evidence for enhanced functional activity of cervical cord in relapsing multiple sclerosis. Magn Reson Med 2008;59(5): 1035–42.
148. Valsasina P, Agosta F, Absinta M, et al. Cervical cord functional MRI changes in relapse-onset MS patients. J Neurol Neurosurg Psychiatry 2010;81(4):405–8.
149. Moffett JR, Ross B, Arun P, et al. N-Acetylaspartate in the CNS: from neurodiagnostics to neurobiology. Prog Neurobiol 2007;81(2):89–131.
150. Ciccarelli O, Altmann DR, McLean MA, et al. Spinal cord repair in MS: does mitochondrial metabolism play a role? Neurology 2010;74(9):721–7.

Anomalies Characteristic of Central Nervous System Demyelination

Radiologically Isolated Syndrome

Christine Lebrun, MD, PhD[a],*, Orhun H. Kantarci, MD[b],
Aksel Siva, MD, FEAN[c], Daniel Pelletier, MD[d],
Darin T. Okuda, MD, MSc[e], on behalf RISConsortium

KEYWORDS

- MRI • Multiple sclerosis • Radiologically isolated syndrome
- Clinically isolated syndrome • Incidental findings

KEY POINTS

- The widespread use of MRI has increased the incidence of incidentalomas, and to date, there is no consensus of what physicians should advise their patients. The risk of progression to multiple sclerosis should be discussed with the patient.
- When incidental T2 hyperintensities are suggestive of multiple sclerosis according to 2005 dissemination in space criteria for MS, it is defined as radiologically isolated syndrome (RIS).
- Spinal cord lesions, male gender, and age less than 35 years are pejorative factors for clinical conversion.
- As one-third of patients will present a clinical event within the 5 years following the first MRI, clinical and radiological follow-up of these patients is recommended.
- Individual initiatives with off-label use of disease-modifying treatments are not validated in any group of RIS patients.

Disclosures: None for this article.
[a] Service de Neurologie, Centre de Ressources et de Compétences Sclérose en Plaques, Université Nice Sophia Antipolis, Hôpital Pasteur 2, 30 voie romaine, Nice Cedex 06002, France;
[b] Department of Neurology, Mayo Clinic College of Medicine, 200 1st Street SW, Rochester, MN 55902, USA; [c] Department of Neurology, University of Istanbul, Cerrahpasa School of Medicine, Beyazıt, Fatih/Istanbul 34452, Turkey; [d] Department of Neuroradiology, University Southern California, 1520 San Pablo Street, Los Angeles, CA 90032, USA; [e] Department of Neurology, University of Texas Southwestern Medical Center, 5959 Harry Hines Boulevard, Dallas, TX 75390, USA
* Corresponding author.
E-mail address: lebrun.c@chu-nice.fr

Neurol Clin 36 (2018) 59–68
https://doi.org/10.1016/j.ncl.2017.08.004
0733-8619/18/© 2017 Elsevier Inc. All rights reserved.

neurologic.theclinics.com

CASE REPORT

The patient is a 35-year-old woman who developed recurrent headaches. She had no neurologic history. On physical examination, she has no abnormality. Brain MRI shows T2 hyperintense lesions suggestive of a demyelinating disease. One lesion is enhancing on T1-weighted with contrast images and spinal cord MRI, demonstrating a cervical cord lesion hyperintense on T2-weighted images (**Fig. 1**). Blood tests were negative for infectious or systemic inflammatory disease, and cerebrospinal fluid (CSF) was positive for oligoclonal bands.

INTRODUCTION

With the widespread use of MRI, it is not uncommon that healthy individuals who do not exhibit signs of neurologic dysfunction have a brain MRI that reveals unexpected white matter T2 lesions.[1] Nevertheless, only a few patients presenting with T2 abnormalities that are highly suggestive of demyelinating plaques given their size, location, and morphology, will fulfill dissemination in space criteria.[2–4] These healthy subjects lack a history or symptomatology suggestive of multiple sclerosis (MS), and, although fulfilling dissemination in space (DIS) MRI criteria, are now diagnosed with radiologically isolated syndrome (RIS).[5]

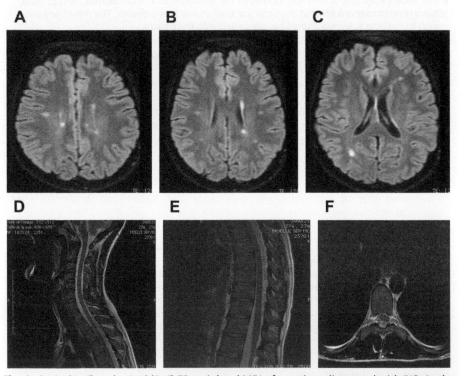

Fig. 1. Brain (*A–C*) and spinal (*D–F*) T2-weighted MRI of a patient diagnosed with RIS. As the patient complained of headache, it is important to strictly apply Barkhof and Tintore criteria and to check for the lack of a neurologic history or symptoms. As spinal cord lesions, either cervical or thoracic, are a pejorative marker for clinical conversion, paraclinical screening including blood tests and CSF analysis can be proposed.

THE SIGNIFICANCE OF INCIDENTALOMAS

Incidental MS findings were described as of the late 20th century in autopsy-based studies and indicated a frequency of unexpected postmortem MS in the range 0.08% to 0.2%.[6–9] A Canadian series of general autopsy of nearly 2500 individuals demonstrated changes compatible with MS in 5 patients (0.2%). Data from autopsy-based studies cannot determine the proportion of patients with a pathologically isolated syndrome, but all have described it as occurring in the range of 0.1% to 0.2%. In the spirit of describing the frequency of unexpected imaging findings on MRI, or incidentalomas, a meta-analysis of 16 studies including 15,559 healthy control participants reported 9 cases of definite demyelination and 4 cases of possible demyelination, yielding a frequency of 0.06% and 0.03%, respectively.[9,10] The incidence and prevalence of newly defined RIS is currently unknown, but Swedish studies have provided evidence for an estimate of 0.1%. These data were generated following a systematic review of MRI scans from a tertiary MS center in a region of high prevalence in Sweden.[11] Among 2105 individuals with a median age of 48 years, only 1 patient was identified with RIS, yielding a prevalence of 0.05% in the studied population, or 0.15% among patients aged 15 to 40 years. A second study has confirmed the same cumulative incidence of 0.1%.[12] These data imply that prevalence of RIS may not be far from the mean prevalence of MS around the world.

A NEW SYNDROME IN THE DEMYELINATING DISORDERS SPECTRUM

After the publication of a case relating subclinical MS,[13] few case reports have been published on first-degree relatives of patients with MS who were at a particular risk, demonstrating 10% of subclinical demyelination in asymptomatic siblings.[14–17] Two exploratory cohorts were published in less than 1 year: the French CFSEP and the UCSF cohorts of 30 patients each. A third of the patients developed a clinical event during the first 5 years of follow-up.[18,19] A Turkish-US American collaborative study followed by the French multi-center cohort study reported, respectively, 22 and 70 RIS patients.[20,21] From these studies, it has been learned that those individuals may have inflammatory cerebrospinal fluid (CSF), abnormal visual evoked potentials (VEP), and dissemination in time of follow-up scans such as Gd-enhancing or new T2 lesions. In European or North American observational studies, the authors found that up to 30% to 45% of patients presenting with RIS will have clinical symptoms within a range from 2.5 to 5 years.[18,19] Most patients who developed clinical symptoms had prior radiological progression. The presence of asymptomatic lesions in the cervical cord provided an increased risk of progression, either to relapsing or progressive MS (PP). It has been shown that after clinical conversion, RIS patients had the same clinical profile as classical MS patients, either relapsing or progressive.[20,22]

A formal description of RIS was first introduced in 2009 by Okuda and colleagues,[5] and defined a cohort of individuals who were at risk of future demyelinating events (**Box 1**). The Barkhof criteria for dissemination in space were considered (at least 3 out of 4 is defined as positive for DIS). The risk for clinical conversion from RIS to a clinical event and new MRI disease activity seems to be increased in the postpartum period, as it has been described in MS. In a prospective observational French study, a significantly shorter time of conversion to the first neurologic event was observed in the pregnant RIS group (15.3 months) compared with the nonpregnant controls (35.7 months), yielding an absolute difference of 20.4 months.[23] The first pediatric series have been reported for 52 children

---

Box 1
Radiologically isolated syndrome diagnostic criteria

1. Initial MRI demonstrating anomalies suggestive of demyelinating disease

2. Incidental anomalies identified on MRI of the brain or spinal cord with the primary reason for the acquired MRI resulting from an evaluation of a process other than a symptom suggesting a first clinical event of MS

3. CNS white matter anomalies meeting MRI criteria
   a. Ovoid, well-circumscribed, and homogeneous foci with or without involvement of the corpus callosum
   b. T2-hyperintensities measuring >3 mm^2 and fulfilling 3 of 4 Barkhof criteria for dissemination in space
   c. CNS anomalies not consistent with a vascular pattern
   d. Qualitative determination that CNS anomalies have a characteristic appearance of demyelinating lesions

4. MRI anomalies do not account for clinically apparent impairments

Data from Okuda DT, Mowry EM, Beheshtian A, et al. Incidental MRI anomalies suggestive of multiple sclerosis: the radiologically isolated syndrome. Neurology 2009;72(9):801; with permission.

---

from 2 to 13 years with the same prognostic factors for clinical conversion, adding the vitamin D low level.[24]

INSIGHTS FROM THE NEUROLOGIC COMMUNITY

Before considering the RIS diagnosis, a truly extensive review of the presenting MRI has to confirm the suggestive demyelinating nature of the T2-weighted hyperintensities because of the possible overdiagnosis issue.[25] The other thing is to confirm the normality of the neurologic examination, as it has been demonstrated that at their first clinical demyelinating event, about one-third of clinically isolated syndrome (CIS) patients had documented history of symptoms suggestive of MS.[26] In 2007, a task force worked on differential diagnosis in MS to develop a perspective that clinicians may use to address the concept of no better explanation for a suspected MS clinical presentation.[27] In their recommendations and consensus perspectives, they recognized an exceptional scenario in which a patient has no clinical presentation suggestive of a demyelinating disease, but an MRI suggestive of subclinical MS. The recognition of RIS was based on the fact that most patients presenting with a CIS have older lesions on MRI that did not account for the presenting syndrome. In 2011, the consortium studying the epidemiology of RIS worldwide (RISC) published its first retrospective cohort gathering 451 RIS subjects. The mean age at RIS diagnosis was 37.2 years with a mean clinical follow-up time of 4.4 years. The observed 5-year conversion rate to the first clinical event was 34%. In the multivariate model, age, sex (male), and lesions within the cervical or thoracic spinal cord were identified as significant predictors for the development of a first clinical event.[28] Evidence suggests that within 2 to 5 years after initial RIS detection, two-thirds of individuals show radiologic progression characterized by new lesions and/or gadolinium enhancement on MRI, and one-third exhibit neurologic symptoms consistent with conversion to MS. Nearly 12% of cases will evolve in PPMS, more commonly in men and at an older age, with more spinal cord lesions on MRI than in CIS/MS patients.[22] Despite these studies, in the 2013 revision of defining MS subtypes, it was declared that until more information is available from prospective RIS cohorts, RIS should not be considered as a distinct MS phenotype.[29]

EVIDENCE OF A PRECLINICAL DISEASE

The main condition for the diagnosis of RIS is the lack of neurologic history or complaint. A Norwegian study demonstrated on a historic cohort that preclinical MS can be documented decades before the first clinical symptom.[30] A systematic screening of individuals at the age of 18 to 19 years showed that those who will develop MS 20 years later, either RR or PP, scored lower on cognitive tests than those who will not. Other series showed that RIS patients could have abnormalities on VEP, OCT, or an inflammatory CSF.[21,31,32] It has been shown that they can also have either mild cognitive deficit or objective fatigue detected on extensive explorations without any complaint. In a first Italian report, 4 RIS patients suffered from a moderate deficit in attention/concentration and executive functions.[33] In the French cohort, it was shown that there was no correlation between clinical, biologic, and MRI results and cognitive dysfunctions.[34] When cognitive impairment is monitored, it demonstrates a significant proportion of patients with progressive cognitive decline compared with healthy controls.[35] A twin study has demonstrated that the asymptomatic twin differs less from his MS cotwin than from healthy controls on neurocognitive performances, independent from brain MRI, suggesting the role of genetic and environmental factors.[36] The question is if these patients could have an isolated cognitive form of MS or not.[37,38] The presence of psychiatric disturbances has also been detected in a Spanish cohort, with a high rate of anxiety or depression and somatization compared with CIS or controls.[39]

Fatigue and quality of life have been evaluated in RIS patients using the MSQOL-54, the EuroQOL 5D and modified fatigue impact scale (MFIS).[39,40] After 1 and 2 years follow-up, nonconverted RIS patients scored lower with the HRQOL compared with controls and without statistically differences to CIS patients. The association of fatigue with either or both physical and mental health composite summaries of HRQOL remained statistically significant between controls, RIS, and CIS.

EXPLORATORY MRI STUDIES

Apart from the analysis of usual surrogate markers such as T1 and T2 lesion load and brain atrophy, many nonconventional MRI techniques have explored the field of RIS. Cortical lesions are present in up to 40% of RIS patients, and their presence is more frequent in patients with oligoclonal band, cervical cord lesions, and dissemination in time on a follow-up brain MRI.[41] Interestingly, brain areas such as precentral gyrus or sensorimotor cortex are spared form cortical thickness, which may partially explain why neurologic examination of RIS patients remains normal.[42] Brain atrophy has also been documented in RIS, with normalized total brain volume and normalized cortical volume lower than in control subjects, but no difference in normalized white matter volume.[43,44] RIS patients with a high T1 lesion volume and low cortical volume were associated with worse cognitive performance.[45] More recently, the first evidence of thalamic atrophy in RIS that was consistent with previous reports in early MS stages was published.[42,46] It fits perfectly with a Canadian study conducted on young 18- to 25-year-old patients who will develop MS, in whose presymptomatic MRI indicated a failure in thalamic growth.[47] Evidence of diffuse metabolic damage was found among asymptomatic individuals, which was similar to the pathology observed in the early stages of MS. In contrast, healthy controls exhibited no such damage.[48] Despite what has been published about the early stages of MS, the decrease of Naa/Cr ratio was not correlated with other usual metrics, such as lesion load or atrophy, enhancing the fact that it is difficult to draw conclusions with a limited number of patients in this rare disease. All these reports documenting brain alterations could mean that the absence of symptoms in RIS patients could be due to the full capacity of plasticity and reorganization at the very early stage of inflammatory disease. This hypothesis is at least partially confirmed by the demonstration that RIS patients are similar to controls for normal-appearing white matter (NAWM) and cortical magnetization transfer compared with MS patients.[44] Long-term prospective studies are likewise needed to explain the clinical relevance of the nonconventional MRI findings with regard to the risk of MS conversion in individuals with RIS, as previous studies have shown the integrity of NAWM in RIS patients in contrast with CIS.

BIOLOGICAL SURROGATE MARKERS FOR CLINICAL EVENTS

Although some MRI abnormalities, such as cervical spinal cord lesions, hint that some individuals may be at a higher risk of conversion to MS than others, biological tools would be useful to more accurately discern the individuals with preclinical MS from those with just incidental radiologic findings. Oligoclonal bands and increased immunoglobulin G (IgG) index alone are useful to ensure organicity of the T2 lesions, but have not been demonstrated to be predictive of a seminal event when detected in CSF or in tears.[21,32,49] Interleukin (IL)-17 CSF levels are as increased as in CIS but not discriminant in serum, and cannot be used as a tool for limiting RIS overdiagnosis or to predict the risk in RIS for a clinical event.[50] In this spirit, CSF levels of IL-8 can add value to detect inflammation in the CNS, but as a nonspecific proinflammatory marker, will not increase specificity or accuracy for differentiating with other inflammatory conditions.[51] High CSF CHI3L1 levels associated with spinal cord lesions might help predict the risk of conversion from RIS to RRMS.[52] Changes in the serum proteome have been found in presymptomatic MS, especially in the glycoprotein spectrum.[53] The use of an antibody directed against sorcin, a membrane protein that regulates intracellular calcium homeostasis by modulating ryanodine receptor functions, is currently being investigated.[54]

FOLLOW-UP AND TREATMENT: A CONSENSUS TO CONSIDER

The diagnosis of RIS is rare, even in tertiary MS centers. Misdiagnosis has major consequences in RIS patients, as it has been demonstrated in MS.[55] The impact of medical error for these asymptomatic individuals has major psychological and economic consequences. After considering there is no suspicion of suggestive MS symptoms and a strictly normal neurologic examination, the neurologist has to look carefully at the MRI scans. The addition of a spinal MRI helps to consider if the Barkhof/Tintore criteria are truly reached.[19] If the RIS criteria are not met, it seems reasonable to consider either nonspecific white matter incidentaloma or to rule out other possible diseases involving the CNS.[25] It has to be emphasized here that RIS has been defined from 2005 MS criteria.[5] The 2010 revision could not be used while, with increasing the sensibility, there is a risk of decreasing specificity, as it was proposed to identify patients at high risk of MS after clinical presentations typical for demyelination. These 2010 criteria have been proposed to define DIS for MS with only 2 lesions in specific areas, but with the insistence that a lesion not be counted toward fulfillment of the DIS requirement if it was in the region responsible for the clinical symptomatology. Logically, until other studies demonstrate their accuracy, as the clinical symptom is by definition missing in RIS, using 2010 criteria is nonsense.[56] A 2016 revision goes forward in MS, suggesting that this requirement could be deleted, including the symptomatic lesion in DIS criteria could allow one to reduce the time for MS diagnosis.[57] In case of RIS diagnosis, it is important to clarify the use of other than recommended

DIS criteria on a large study, to exclude conditions that mimic T2 hyperintensities suggestive of MS.

Even if there has been some attempt in defining algorithms for management of RIS patients, treatment with disease-modifying therapies (DMTs) is not recommended for individuals given their asymptomatic state and the possibility that they may not progress to develop clinical symptoms, exposing them to unnecessary risk.[58] Individual initiatives are not recommended despite the extensive literature supporting the association of early MS treatment and reduction in the frequency of clinical attacks.[59,60] A US survey conducted twice in 2011 and in early 2014 among MS specialists demonstrated that on a daily practice basis, initiation of DMT for RIS patients would not be appropriate, but an annual follow-up including spinal cord MRI was highly recommended (94%).[61] There is also an increase of neurologists who would order a lumbar puncture. It is noticed that there is a significant increase of off-label prescriptions from 10% to 26% between the 2 surveys. A Medscape and a French MS Society initiative conducted in 2010 bring evidence that about 18% of RIS patients were on off-label DMT, and many have vitamin D supplementation.[62] On the other side, many MS specialists express that demonstration of more than 2 gadolinium-enhanced lesions on the follow-up MRI would be a strong argument for proposing DMT, despite phase III study showing benefit for these patients. Randomized controlled trials must be performed to address the possible efficacy of DMT in RIS in extending the time to a clinical event. Two clinical placebo-controlled trials are ongoing. The first began in 2015, with dimethyl fumarate as oral DMT (the ARISE Study); the second one is planned in 2017 in Europe, with teriflunomide (the TERIS Study).[63,64]

REFERENCES

1. Vernooij MW, Ikram MA, Tanghe HL, et al. Incidental findings on brain MRI in the general population. N Engl J Med 2007;357(18):1821–8.

2. Barkhof F, Filippi M, Miller DH, et al. Comparison of MRI criteria at first presentation to predict conversion to clinically definite multiple sclerosis. Brain 1997;120: 2059–69.

3. McDonald WI, Compston A, Edan G, et al. Recommended diagnostic criteria for multiple sclerosis: guidelines from the international panel on the diagnosis of multiple sclerosis. Ann Neurol 2001;50(1):121–7.

4. Polman CH, Reingold SC, Edan G, et al. Diagnostic criteria for multiple sclerosis: 2005 revisions to the "McDonald Criteria". Ann Neurol 2005;58(6):840–6.

5. Okuda DT, Mowry EM, Beheshtian A, et al. Incidental MRI anomalies suggestive of multiple sclerosis: the radiologically isolated syndrome. Neurology 2009;72(9): 800–5.

6. Castaigne P, Lhermitte F, Escourolle R, et al. Asymptomatic multiple sclerosis. Rev Neurol (Paris) 1981;137:729–37.

7. Engell T. A clinical patho-anatomical study of clinically silent multiple sclerosis. Acta Neurol Scand 1989;79:428.

8. Gilbert JJ, Sadler M. Unsuspected multiple sclerosis. Arch Neurol 1983;40:533.

9. Derwenskus J, Cohen BA. Clinically silent multiple sclerosis: description of a patient cohort without symptoms typical of MS but abnormal brain magnetic resonance imaging. Mult Scler 2007;13:1226–7.

10. Morris Z, Whiteley WN, Longstreth WT Jr, et al. Incidental findings on brain magnetic resonance imaging: systematic review and meta-analysis. BMJ 2009; 339:b3016.

11. Granberg T, Martola J, Kristoffersen-Wiberg M, et al. Radiologically isolated syndrome - incidental magnetic resonance imaging findings suggestive of multiple sclerosis, a systematic review. Mult Scler 2013;19(3):271–80.

12. Forslin Y, Granberg T, Jumah AA, et al. Incidence of radiologically isolated syndrome: a population-based study. AJNR Am J Neuroradiol 2016;37(6):1017–22.

13. DeSeze J, Vermersch P. Sequential magnetic resonance imaging follow-up of multiple sclerosis before clinical phase. Mult Scler 2005;11:395.

14. Tienari PJ, Salonen O, Wikstrom J, et al. Familial multiple sclerosis: MRI findings in clinically affected and unaffected siblings. J Neurol Neurosurg Psychiatry 1992;55:883.

15. Lynch SG, Rose JW, Smoker W, et al. MRI in familial multiple sclerosis. Neurology 1990;40:900.

16. Thorpe JW, Mumford CJ, Compston DA, et al. British Isles survey of multiple sclerosis in twins: MRI. J Neurol Neurosurg Psychiatry 1994;57:491.

17. De Stefano N, Cocco E, Lai M, et al. Imaging brain damage in first-degree relatives of sporadic and familial multiple sclerosis. Ann Neurol 2006;59(4):634–9.

18. Lebrun C, Bensa C, Debouverie M, et al, on behalf CFSEP. Unexpected multiple sclerosis: follow-up of 30 patients with magnetic resonance imaging and clinical conversion profile. J Neurol Neurosurg Psychiatry 2008;79(2):195–8.

19. Okuda DT, Mowry EM, Cree BA, et al. Asymptomatic spinal cord lesions predict disease progression in radiologically isolated syndrome. Neurology 2011;76(8):686–92.

20. Siva A, Saip S, Altintas A, et al. Multiple sclerosis risk in radiologically uncovered asymptomatic possible inflammatory-demyelinating disease. Mult Scler 2009;15(8):918–27.

21. Lebrun C, Bensa C, Debouverie M, et al, on behalf CFSEP. Association between clinical conversion to multiple sclerosis in radiologically isolated syndrome and magnetic resonance imaging, cerebrospinal fluid, and visual evoked potential: follow-up of 70 patients. Arch Neurol 2009;66(7):841–6.

22. Kantarci OH, Lebrun C, Siva A, et al, on behalf RISC and CFSEP. Primary progressive multiple sclerosis evolving from radiologically isolated syndrome. Ann Neurol 2016;79(2):288–94.

23. Lebrun C, Le Page E, Kantarci O, et al, on behalf CFSEP. Impact of pregnancy on conversion to clinically isolated syndrome in a radiologically isolated syndrome cohort. Mult Scler 2012;18(9):1297–302.

24. Makani N, Lebrun C, Siva A, et al. Comparison of MRI dissemination in space criteria for predicting a first clinical event in children with the radiologically isolated syndrome. AAN meeting, Boston, MA, 2017.

25. Lebrun C, Cohen M, Chaussenot A, et al. A prospective study of patients with brain MRI showing incidental T2 hyperintensities addressed as multiple sclerosis: a lot of work to do before treating. Neurol Ther 2014;3(2):123–32.

26. Gout O, Lebrun-Frénay C, Labauge P, et al, PEDIAS Group. Prior suggestive symptoms in one-third of patients consulting for a first event. J Neurol Neurosurg Psychiatry 2011;82(3):323–5.

27. Miller DH, Weinshenker BG, Filippi M, et al. Differential diagnosis of suspected multiple sclerosis: a consensus approach. Mult Scler 2008;14:1157–74.

28. Okuda DT, Siva A, Kantarci O, et al. Radiologically isolated syndrome: 5-year risk for an initial clinical event. PLoS One 2014;9(3):e90509.

29. Lublin FD, Reingold SC, Cohen JA, et al. Defining the clinical course of multiple sclerosis: the 2013 revisions. Neurology 2014;83:1–9.

30. Cortese M, Riise T, Bjørnevik K, et al. Pre-clinical disease activity in multiple sclerosis- a prospective study on cognitive performance prior to first symptom. Ann Neurol 2016;80(4):616–24.
31. Knier B, Berthele A, Buck D, et al. Optical coherence tomography indicates disease activity prior to clinical onset of central nervous system demyelination. Mult Scler 2016;22(7):893–900.
32. Gabelic T, Radmilovic M, Posavec V, et al. Differences in oligoclonal bands and visual evoked potentials in patients with radiologically and clinically isolated syndrome. Acta Neurol Belg 2013;113(1):13–7.
33. Hakiki B, Goretti B, Portaccio E, et al. Subclinical MS: follow-up of four cases. Eur J Neurol 2008;15:858.
34. Lebrun C, Blanc F, Brassat D, et al, on behalf CFSEP. Cognitive functions in radiologically isolated syndrome. Mult Scler 2010;16(8):919–25.
35. D'Anna L, Lorenzut S, Perelli A, et al. The contribution of assessing cognitive impairment in radiologically-isolated syndrome (RIS): a single case report follow-up study. Mult Scler 2014;20(14):1912–5.
36. Kuusisto S, Vahvelainen T, Hamalalnen P, et al. Asymptomatic subjects differ less from their twin sibling with MS than from healthy controls in cognition. Am Acad of Neurology Vancouver 2016. P500.
37. Pardini M, Uccelli A, Grafman J, et al. Isolated cognitive relapses in multiple sclerosis. J Neurol Neurosurg Psychiatry 2014;85(9):1035–7.
38. Assouad R, Louapre C, Tourbah A, et al. Clinical and MRI characterization of MS patients with a pure and severe cognitive onset. Clin Neurol Neurosurg 2014;126:55–63.
39. Labiano-Fontcuberta A, Aladro Y, Martínez-Ginés ML, et al. Psychiatric disturbances in radiologically isolated syndrome. J Psychiatr Res 2015;68:309–15.
40. Lebrun C, Cohen M, Clavelou P, on behalf CFSEP and RISC. Evaluation of quality of life and fatigue in radiologically Isolated syndrome. Rev Neuro 2016;172(6–7):392–5.
41. Giorgio A, Stromillo ML, Rossi F, et al. Cortical lesions in radiologically isolated syndrome. Neurology 2011;77:1886–99.
42. Labiano-Fontcuberta A, Mato-Abad V, Alvarez- Linera J, et al. Gray matter involvement in radiologically isolated syndrome. Medicine (Baltimore) 2016;95:e3208.
43. Amato MP, Hakiki B, Goretti B, et al. Association of MRI metrics and cognitive impairment in radiologically isolated syndromes. Neurology 2012;78:309–14.
44. De Stefano N, Stromillo ML, Rossi F, et al. Improving the characterization of radiologically isolated syndrome suggestive of multiple sclerosis. PLoS One 2011;6(4):e19452.
45. Rojas JI, Patrucco L, Míguez J, et al. Brain atrophy in radiologically isolated syndromes. J Neuroimaging 2015;25(1):68–71.
46. Aubert-Broche B, Fonov V, Narayanan S, et al, Canadian Pediatric Demyelinating Disease Network. Onset of multiple sclerosis before adulthood leads to failure of age-expected brain growth. Neurology 2014;83:2140–6.
47. Azevedo C, Overton E, Khadka S, et al. Early CNS Neurodegeneration in radiologically isolated syndrome. Neuroimmunol Neuroinflamm 2015;2:e102.
48. Stromillo ML, Giorgio A, Rossi F, et al. Brain metabolic changes suggestive of axonal damage in radiologically isolated syndrome. Neurology 2013;80(23):2090–4.

49. Lebrun C, Forzy G, Collongues N, et al, on behalf CFSEP and RISC. Tear analysis as a tool to detect oligoclonal bands in radiologically isolated syndrome. Rev Neurol (Paris) 2015;171(4):390–3.

50. Lebrun C, Cohen M, Pignolet B, et al, on behalf SFSEP, BIONAT Network, RISC. Interleukin 17 alone is not a discriminant biomarker in early demyelinating spectrum disorders. J Neurol Sci 2016;368:334–6.

51. Rossi S, Motta C, Studer V, et al. Subclinical central inflammation is risk for RIS and CIS conversion to MS. Mult Scler 2015;21(11):1443–52.

52. Thouvenot E, Hinsinger G, Demattei C, et al, on behalf of SFSEP and RISC. High CSF CH3L1 levels increase the risk of conversion from RIS to CDMS. ECTRIMS 2016, London.

53. Wallin MT, Oh U, Nyalwidhe J, et al. Serum proteomic analysis of a pre-symptomatic multiple sclerosis cohort. Eur J Neurol 2015;22(3):591–9.

54. Sehitoglu E, Çavus F, Ulusoy C, et al. Sorcin antibody as a possible predictive factor in conversion from radiologically isolated syndrome to multiple sclerosis: a preliminary study. Inflamm Res 2014;63(10):799–801.

55. Solomon AJ, Bourdette DN, Cross AH, et al. The contemporary spectrum of multiple sclerosis misdiagnosis: a multicenter study. Neurology 2016;87(13):1393–9.

56. Polman CH, Reingold SC, Banwell B, et al. Diagnostic criteria for multiple sclerosis: 2010 revisions to the McDonald criteria. Ann Neurol 2011;69:292–302.

57. Brownlee WJ, Swanton JK, Miszkiel KA, et al. Should the symptomatic region be included in dissemination in space in MRI criteria for MS? Neurology 2016;87:680–3.

58. Sellner J, Schirmer L, Hemmer B, et al. The radiologically isolated syndrome: take action when the unexpected is uncovered? J Neurol 2010;257(10):1602–11.

59. Bourdette D, Yadav V. Treat patients with radiologically isolated syndrome when the MRI brain scan shows dissemination in time: no. Mult Scler 2012;18(11):1529–30.

60. Brassat D, Lebrun C, On behalf of the CFSEP. Treat patients with radiologically isolated syndrome when the MRI brain scan shows dissemination in time: yes. Mult Scler 2012;18(11):1531–3.

61. Tornatore C, Phillips JT, Khan O, et al. Practice patterns of US neurologists in patients with CIS, RRMS, or RIS: a consensus study. Neurol Clin Pract 2014;2:48–57.

62. Medscape Great Debate: radiologically isolated syndrome. 2010. Available at: http://www.medscape.com/viewarticle/720673. Accessed March 4, 2012.

63. Okuda D, Lebrun Frenay C, Siva A, et al. [P7.207] Multi-center, randomized, double-blinded assessment of dimethyl fumarate in extending the time to a first attack in radiologically isolated syndrome (RIS) (ARISE Trial). 67th AAN Meeting 2015, Washington, DC.

64. Lebrun C, Siva A, Kantarci O, et al, RISC. Multi-center, randomized, double-blinded assessment of teriflunomide in extending the time to a first clinical event in radiologically isolated syndrome (RIS) (TERIS study). ECTRIMS Online Library. London. Sep 14, 2016; 145587.

Common Clinical and Imaging Conditions Misdiagnosed as Multiple Sclerosis

A Current Approach to the Differential Diagnosis of Multiple Sclerosis

Aksel Siva, MD, FEAN

KEYWORDS

- Multiple sclerosis • Differential diagnosis • Multiple sclerosis mimics
- Nonspecific white matter abnormalities • MRI

KEY POINTS

- The incidence and prevalence rates of multiple sclerosis (MS) are increasing; so are the number of misdiagnosed cases as MS. One major source of misdiagnosis is misinterpretation of nonspecific clinical and imaging findings and misapplication of MS diagnostic criteria resulting in an overdiagnosis of MS!
- The diagnostic spectrum of MS and related disorders includes the MS subclinical and clinical phenotypes, MS variants and inflammatory astrocytopathies, and other antibody-associated atypical inflammatory-demyelinating syndromes. The differential diagnosis of MS includes these disorders as well as some other diseases mimicking MS.
- There are several systemic diseases in which either the clinical or MRI or both findings may mimic MS; however, in most, a well-taken history and a through physical examination will reveal the symptoms and signs of the systemic disease and appropriate laboratory workup will confirm the non-MS diagnosis.
- Because nonspecific white matter abnormalities on brain MRI and other imaging findings that may mimic MS, as well as MS-nonspecific lesions, may be seen in people with MS, neurologists should be aware of all possibilities and they should be able to interpret the MRI findings independent of the radiology reports! Currently, the old school of taking a detailed history, a thorough neurologic examination, and a cerebrospinal fluid study are essential for the MS diagnosis. MRI is one other tool that is most often confirmatory, but may cause confusion at times too, necessitating a "think twice" approach before reaching a final diagnosis.

Department of Neurology, Istanbul University, Cerrahpaşa School of Medicine, Cerrahpaşa, Istanbul 34098, Turkey
E-mail address: akselsiva@gmail.com

Neurol Clin 36 (2018) 69–117
https://doi.org/10.1016/j.ncl.2017.08.014
0733-8619/18/© 2017 Elsevier Inc. All rights reserved.

neurologic.theclinics.com

INTRODUCTION

The prevalence of multiple sclerosis (MS) is on the increase,[1,2] which in large is likely to be due to an increased awareness both by the medical and nonmedical communities. Patients are self-admitted or referred for a neurology consultation either because of clinical symptoms and signs or cranial and spinal MRI findings that are suggestive of "MS" or because of both. The raised admittance rates with a presumed diagnosis of MS, in turn, also results in increased misdiagnosed cases. The problem of misdiagnosis and difficulties in diagnosing MS have been reported before the introduction or widespread use of diagnostic tools, such as imaging, evoked potentials, and cerebrospinal fluid studies in neurology,[3] which is certainly understandable. However, it seems that the most advanced tools that we have today have not changed this problem much. Indeed, in recent years, several studies confirmed this issue of incorrect MS diagnosis and further had emphasized that a significant number of these individuals who in fact did not have MS were even put on long-term MS treatments.[4–8]

Currently, the most common cause of MS misdiagnosis seems to be nonspecific white matter abnormalities on brain MRI and misinterpretation and misapplication of radiographic diagnostic criteria, as well as the presence of vague or nonspecific neurologic symptoms considered to be related to MS.[8,9] In fact, it has been shown that in up to one-third of "normal" people aged 20 to 45, transient neurologic symptoms, such as visual changes (including blurring, diplopia), weakness, poor balance and coordination, and speech difficulties of no clinical significance are reported without any underlying abnormality.[9,10] It is also not uncommon to see people with dizziness, numbness, and similar sensory symptoms, without any underlying disease in medical practice too. When people with such symptoms present and by coincidence turn out to have a number of nonspecific white spots on their brain MRI, they easily may be misdiagnosed as having MS by the unexperienced physician. Interestingly, most of these cases end up receiving a final diagnosis of a psychiatric disorder or migraine or fibromyalgia,[6,8] as most studies had shown psychiatric conditions are among the major causes of MS misdiagnosis.[3,4,6,9] It is not uncommon for someone to come to a clinician with the fear of having MS because of disease suggestive symptoms, which in fact are due to somatization or of no clinical significance. Many times, the final diagnosis will end up being hypochondriasis, a somatoform disorder with anxiety or depression or malingering. However, if the clinician does not concentrate well in such patients' history and examination in whom the MRI scan shows a few nonspecific white spots, then the psychiatric problem may be missed and the patient may be misdiagnosed as having MS. A well-taken history will reveal that psychiatric-based (somatic) symptoms cannot be easily localized and are not consistent with known neuroanatomical sites; they are multiple, show variations and fluctuations, but are always there! So, their symptoms will not be consistent with the classic definition of MS that is based on attacks being disseminated in time and space.[9]

Another major issue in the diagnosis and differential diagnosis of MS is a large number of other disorders that may mimic MS, such as the so-called atypical inflammatory-demyelinating diseases of the central nervous system (CNS) that include neuromyelitis optica spectrum disorders (NMOSD), acute disseminated encephalomyelitis (ADEM), and some other rare diseases within this group, several inherited disorders that have their onset at adolescent or adult age periods, as well as some infectious, neoplastic, or vascular disorders affecting mainly the young adult population.[9,11–15] These disorders and their differential diagnosis from MS have been reviewed in detail in several publications and although some also are reviewed here, further specific information can be found in those publications.[9,11–16]

The purpose of this review was not to cover all possible MS mimickers, but to present a clinician's point of view and approach in the diagnosis and differential diagnosis of MS on several conditions and diseases based on a combination of personal experience and published evidence. This review also does not include pediatric MS and its differential.

DIAGNOSIS OF MULTIPLE SCLEROSIS

MS is an immune-mediated neuroinflammatory and neurodegenerative disease of the CNS. By definition, dissemination of the disease process both in space and time should be shown within the CNS by clinical and neuroimaging findings. Dissemination in space (DIS) should be confirmed either by neuroimaging (MRI) or by clinical findings demonstrating multifocal involvement of the CNS at the designated sites. The criteria for dissemination in time (DIT) needs to be fulfilled clinically either by the presence of recurrent attacks or a steady progression and/or by neuroimaging showing asymptomatic enhancing lesions on the initial scan or the appearance of new lesions on follow-up scans. Finally, there should be no better explanation to account for symptoms and signs or MRI findings (no alternative neurologic disease).[17]

Steps to MS diagnosis starts with a detailed medical and neurologic history and examination in a patient who is admitted with a presumed diagnosis of MS or in whom the disease is suspected because of clinical or imaging findings that are suggestive of MS in the differential. In people who already have an MRI study, it is essential for the neurologists to study the images themselves and not solely depend on the radiology report, which sometimes may be misleading.

It is also essential to do a spinal tap and study the cerebrospinal fluid (CSF) in people who are suspected to have MS, even when the neurologist is comfortable with the diagnosis.[18] Unfortunately, a significant number of practising neurologists find a clinical history and MRI findings sufficient to make a diagnosis of MS. However, the CSF is not only important in supporting the diagnosis, but at times it may reveal unexpected findings, such as a high level of protein, a low glucose level, or elevated number of cells, when the diagnosis of MS then needs to be questioned! Besides, the CSF findings, including the presence of oligoclonal bands (OCBs), the immunoglobulin (Ig)G level, and IgG index may also guide physicians to decide the timing and type of treatment that they may plan. It is expected in the near future that several probable predictive biomarkers in the CSF will further help physicians in the care of their patients.[18,19]

THE DIAGNOSTIC SPECTRUM OF MULTIPLE SCLEROSIS

The diagnostic spectrum of MS and related disorders includes the MS subclinical and clinical phenotypes, MS variants and inflammatory astrocytopathies, and other antibody-associated atypical inflammatory-demyelinating syndromes[15,20] (Table 1). The differential diagnosis of MS includes these disorders as well as some other diseases mimicking MS.

The clinical phenotypes of MS include the clinical isolated syndromes (CISs), and the relapsing and the progressive forms of the disease. Although most CIS cases are considered as "early MS," not all are MS, and another 10% to 15% despite continuing MRI activity may not have further clinical episodes.[21] It is important to make a differential diagnosis of patients who present with "CIS," because most of the spectrum disorders, as well as some systemic disorders with CNS involvement may present as such and the correct diagnosis has important implications regarding what to do in these individuals.

Table 1		
The spectrum of MS and related disorders		
MS Subclinical and Clinical Phenotypes	**MS Variants**	**MS-Related Disorders (Once Upon a Time Ago Used to Be MS!)**
• RIS	• Tumefactive MS	• ADEM
• CIS	• Balo	• NMO/NMOSD
• SAMS	• Marburg	• aMOG-related syndromes
• SAPMS	• *Schilder?*	• Others (antibody unknown?
• RRMS		Atypical CNS inflammatory
• 2⁰ PMS		disorders?)
• PPMS		

Abbreviations: ADEM, acute disseminated encephalomyelitis; aMOG, anti myelin oligodendrocyte glycoprotein antibody; CIS, clinical isolated syndromes; CNS, central nervous system; MOG, myelin oligodendrocyte glycoprotein; MS, multiple sclerosis; NMOSD, neuromyelitis optica spectrum disorders; PPMS, primary progressive MS; RIS, radiologically isolated syndromes; RRMS, relapsing-remitting MS; SAMS, single attack MS; SAPMS, single attack progressive MS; 2⁰PMS, secondary progressive MS.

Modified from Siva A. The spectrum of multiple sclerosis and treatment decisions. Clin Neurol Neurosurg 2006;108(3):333-8.

The red flags in the differential diagnosis of MS are well known and have been listed in several publications by MS experts.[9,11,16] In this review, I favor to name some of them and some others as "think-twice flags," because many also can be seen in patients with MS. Indeed, when they are present, we need to "think twice" either before making or confirming a diagnosis of MS. These "think twice" warnings will be summarized as demographic, clinical, laboratory, and imaging possibilities and pitfalls!

DEMOGRAPHIC POSSIBILITIES AND PITFALLS IN THE DIFFERENTIAL DIAGNOSIS OF MULTIPLE SCLEROSIS
Age

Although up to 10% of patients with MS may have their disease onset before age 18,[22] the probability of other diseases such as genetic leukoencephalopathies, as well as non-MS acute demyelinating syndromes should be considered in the differential of a pediatric patient who presents with MS-suggestive clinical or imaging abnormalities (**Box 1**). The same "think twice" approach also should be considered in people who present with similar clinical/MRI findings after age 50.

Family History

It is well known that between 5% and 20% of patients with MS have another family member with MS.[23] However, it is less common to see more than 2 or 3 affected individuals with MS in the same family, and when this number is exceeded and these

Box 1
The "think twice" demographic and clinical possibilities and pitfalls in an individual who presents with MRI abnormalities suggestive of multiple sclerosis (MS)
All possible in MS, but other diseases should be ruled out first!
• *Childhood-onset (age <<16)* [consider the probability of dysmyelinating diseases]
• *Late-onset (age >>50)* [consider the probability of ischemic diseases and other vasculopathies with secondary demyelinating changes]
• *Strong family history ≥3 family members have identical MRI abnormalities* [consider genetic diseases]

family members have similar clinical symptoms and MRI appearances, the probability of genetic diseases should be considered first.

Race, Ethnicity, and Geography

MS is seen in almost all races and ethnic groups, but it is a disease affecting mostly White and people living in temperate and cold climates, although the latitude gradient is not as prominent as previously anticipated.[1] However, it is less likely to be seen in people in the tropical zones and it has a higher incidence in African American individuals compared with native Africans. So, when someone from equatorial Africa, the Seychelles, Central and South America, or from the west coast natives of the Pacific Northwest is admitted with a progressive spastic paraparesis and increased signal areas on T2-weighted cranial MRI, human T-lymphotropic virus (HTLV)-1 associated myelopathy/tropical spastic paraparesis should be the first differential over primary progressive MS (PPMS).[24] A similar race-geography–oriented differential diagnosis may be considered for neuro-Behçet disease (NBD) in a young adult of Middle East or eastern-Asian origin who presents with clinical symptoms and MRI changes suggestive of MS.[25]

CLINICAL POSSIBILITIES AND PITFALLS IN THE DIFFERENTIAL DIAGNOSIS OF MULTIPLE SCLEROSIS
Probability of the Presence of a Systemic Disease with Central Nervous System Involvement or as a Comorbid Disorder in the Differential Diagnosis of Multiple Sclerosis

Any patient who is admitted with a probable clinical and/or imaging diagnosis of MS should be interviewed in detail and investigated to rule out the presence of a systemic disease involving the CNS, which may be responsible for the neurologic manifestations or for comorbidity.

In patients who have any systemic symptoms suggestive of a connective-tissue disorder or a vasculitic syndrome, such as arthralgias, malaise, fever, oral ulcers, malar rash and skin lesions, photo-sensitivity, dry eyes or mouth, livedo reticularis, and other manifestations referable to any organ system, the differential should be extended to rule out a systemic autoimmune or autoinflammatory disease. There also are several hereditary or acquired vasculopathies of different etiologies, such as cerebral autosomal dominant arteriopathy with subcortical infarcts and leukoencephalopathy (CADASIL), Fabry, and Susac, which may also mimic MS.

Patients who have systemic symptoms suggestive of an infectious disease should be admitted for serologic studies to rule out infectious diseases, such as Lyme, tuberculosis, retroviral diseases, such as human immunodeficiency virus (HIV), HTLV-1 and HTLV-2, and others.

Some people may present with vague neurologic symptoms, who are found to have anxiety or appear to be depressed. Some believe that they might have MS and many of them reach their "diagnosis" through Internet-search and strange so-called medical Web sites! On the other hand, somatoform neurologic symptoms are not uncommon, and if some of these people get an MRI and have a number of white spots in their brains, they might be easily confused to have MS, as already noted. In these individuals, somatoform symptom and anxiety disorders or not well-defined rheumatologic disorders, such as fibromyalgia, may be the whole story! However, in my practice I have seen several patients who have both, a somatoform symptom disorder and MS too.

The "Think Twice" Neuro-Clinical Possibilities and Pitfalls in the Differential Diagnosis of Multiple Sclerosis When MRI Changes are in Part Suggestive of Multiple Sclerosis

The most common symptoms suggestive of MS are optic neuritis; diplopia of brainstem origin; facial numbness and other sensory symptoms consistent with intra-axial trigeminal involvement, sensory symptoms such as paresthesia, dysesthesia, allodynia in the extremities or part of body (within an anatomic distribution or not so clear cut!); the Lhermitte phenomenon; useless hand; weakness (in one or more extremities); gait problems and imbalance; and bladder and/or bowel dysfunction. When any of these symptoms develop subacutely in a young adult, MS becomes one of the major considerations in the differential diagnosis. Many times, the neurologic examination followed by an MRI study will help the physician to narrow the differential. Once it is confirmed that this is truly the first neurologic episode, a diagnosis of CIS is made. However, it should be kept in mind that not all CISs are MS related and may be due to some other disorders, and that not all CISs evolve in to clinically definite MS.[26–28] Therefore, it is of most importance to make a correct diagnosis in these patients. The problem increases when the clinical symptomatology and/or imaging findings are not typical or do not fulfill the MS diagnostic criteria. One diagnostic challenge is when a patient is admitted with some neurologic CNS symptoms and in whom the MRI changes are suggestive of MS, but that are not diagnostic. In these cases, the type and onset of the neurologic manifestations would be the best clues for our "think twice" neuro-clinical possibilities and pitfalls approach (**Box 2**).

An acute onset of a neurologic deficit that has its onset and full development within a few minutes or even hours in a young patient should alert the clinician for the probability of a vascular disorder before an inflammatory-demyelinating event. An acute hemiparesis is not expected in MS, and all other possibilities need to be excluded before narrowing the differential to it. The same should be considered for the differential of optic neuritis when such a patient presents with acute-onset visual loss. However, although quite uncommon, an acute-onset neurologic episode also may occur in patients with MS.

The nature and type of the neurologic symptoms also may guide us in our think twice approach in the differential diagnosis of MS. Symptoms of impaired consciousness or cognitive deficits, aphasia, apraxia, and seizures are unlikely to be seen at MS

Box 2
The "think twice" neuro-clinical possibilities and pitfalls

All possible in MS, but first other diseases should be ruled out!

- *Acute* (strokelike) onset (acute hemiparesis; acute optic neuropathy [ON])

- *Unexpected course!* [Fulminant/rapidly progressive course]

- *Onset with atypical symptoms for MS* [impaired consciousness, cognitive deficits, aphasia, apraxia, seizures, extrapyramidal symptoms and signs]

- *Clinical stereotype!* [Attacks originating always from the same central nervous system (CNS) region]

- *Progressive and lateralized/mono-symptomatic disease* [progressive mono/hemiparesis from onset; a cerebellar syndrome]

- *Lack of typical MS symptoms in a patient with a long-standing CNS disease* [eg, none of ON, bladder problems, sensory symptoms, Lhermitte]

- *No documented response to IVMP at any time* [likely to be noninflammatory disease, non-MS]

onset. The presence of such symptoms mainly in a young patient who turns out to have inflammatory-demyelinating–looking lesions, the more likely diagnosis would be either primary or secondary CNS vasculitis, CNS infections (ie, toxoplasmosis in a patient with HIV; progressive multifocal leukoencephalopathy and others), ADEM, or one of the autoimmune encephalopathies. A fulminant and rapidly progressive course is unexpected in MS and is more likely to be seen in other inflammatory or infectious disorders. Extrapyramidal symptoms and signs are also uncommon in MS, and their presence will indicate more the probability of some hereditary or metabolic neurodegenerative diseases.

On the other hand, there may be some patients who present with long-standing and/or progressive neurologic deficits and some limited MRI changes in whom (mostly progressive forms of) MS may be considered in the differential. The lack of typical MS symptoms, such as optic neuropathy (ON), bladder problems, sensory symptoms, Lhermitte phenomenon, and symmetricity of symptoms and signs rather than multifocality, together with some of the MRI diagnostic pitfalls that are discussed later in this article should raise the probability of other diagnoses before MS.

Attacks originating always from the same CNS region (clinical stereotype) are unlikely to be due to MS. In addition, there are a few patients who might have a very slowly progressive and lateralized mono-symptomatic disease in the form of a progressive monoparesis or hemiparesis from onset and some subtle MRI changes with a few small white matter lesions. Whether they do have true PPMS or another condition affecting the CNS is not easy to diagnose. The CSF may help only to a certain extent.

Finally, in patients in whom the clinician is already having difficulties confirming the diagnosis of MS, if there is no documented response to intra venous methylprednisolone (IVMP) at any time, this should also raise the probability that the underlying disease process might likely to be noninflammatory and non-MS.

LABORATORY POSSIBILITIES AND PITFALLS IN THE DIFFERENTIAL DIAGNOSIS OF MULTIPLE SCLEROSIS
Serum Studies

There are no blood or other tests that are diagnostic for MS. All the studies that we carry on in people with suspected MS are to exclude a number of systemic diseases with CNS involvement and a limited number of neurologic disorders that may mimic MS in addition to standard biochemistry.

Several systemic vasculitic and collagen vascular diseases, such as systemic lupus erythematosus (SLE), Sjögren, and Behçet disease (BD), are included in the differential of MS. Despite that in each of these diseases CNS involvement that mimics MS may occur, many times their systemic symptoms and signs are present by then, raising the probability of something other than MS. Besides, in most of such patients, the CSF and MRI findings are not consistent with MS and will provide clues to the clinician to think twice.

There may be some immune-system changes in patients with MS, including a high incidence of autoantibodies, but usually these are of no clinical significance.[9] Positive antinuclear antibody (ANA) testing was found in 22.5% to 30.4% of patients with MS, but the titers were mostly low ($\leq$1:320) and none of them had SLE or any of the other systemic autoimmune diseases.[29,30] In another study, 32.6% of patients with MS had either anti-cardiolipin antibodies and/or anti-beta2 glycoprotein-I antibodies, and, interestingly, in 59.0% of the same cohort the sera was positive for ANA.[31] Finally, in a more recent study, autoantibodies were detected in 38% of patients with MS and were not significantly associated with disease characteristics or severity and did not have any systemic autoimmune disease, including 4% with Sjögren syndrome A (SSA) antibodies, whom none met the diagnostic criteria for Sjögren syndrome.[32] It is a common practice to prioritize a diagnosis of a rheumatologic disease when any of these rheumatologic autoantibodies are found in patients who are worked up with a suspected diagnosis of MS. However, these autoantibodies are frequently found in patients with MS and have no diagnostic or specific meaning and should not exclude MS. We refer our patients for a rheumatologic consultation only when the ANA titer is higher than 1:320 and when 1 or more other rheumatologic autoantibodies is present for a probable comorbid rheumatologic disease. The probability of such a comorbid disease is more important in patients with a diagnosis or probable neuromyelitis optica (NMO)/NMOSD.

Some other laboratory tests that may cause confusion are low serum vitamin B12 levels, positive Lyme antibodies, and elevated angiotensin-converting enzyme (ACE) levels. Decreased levels of vitamin B12 have been reported in up to 19.4% of patients with MS, in the absence of B12 deficiency.[33] The finding of reactive Lyme serology in patients with MS has been shown to be up to 7% in one study with no suggestive features of the infection and is unlikely to indicate neurologic Lyme disease.[34] Elevated serum ACE levels were also reported in 23% of patients with MS and need not raise suspicions of alternative diagnoses such as "sarcoidosis" in a patient who is already highly suggestive of MS.[35]

In summary, the presence of abnormal laboratory tests in patients who are likely to have MS based on clinical judgment and imaging evidence should not change the clinical diagnosis of MS. In such instances, the abnormal laboratory result is either a false-positive finding or may indicate a comorbid condition.[9]

In patients who present with suspected atypical demyelinating syndromes, inflammatory astrocytopathies, or other inflammatory diseases mimicking MS, a set of selective antibodies may be studied only in the absence of clinical and imaging diagnostic evidence (**Box 3**).

Cerebrospinal Fluid Studies

A through workup of a patient suspected to have MS or related disorder should always include a spinal tap and a CSF study, as mentioned previously. Despite that in 90% to 95% of patients with MS either "oligoclonal IgG bands" (OCBs) or an elevated IgG level and/or increased IgG index are found in the CSF, neither is diagnostic. However,

---

Box 3
Selective autoantibodies (Abs) that may be studied in patients who present with suspected atypical demyelinating syndromes, inflammatory astrocytopathies, or other inflammatory diseases mimicking multiple sclerosis, depending on the clinical and imaging presentations

- AQP4-immunoglobulin (Ig)G

- aMOG-IgG

- aNMDAr-IgG and other Abs for autoimmune encephalopathies

- Antibody panel for vasculitic/collagen (rheumatologic) disorders (antinuclear antibodies, adsDNA; RF; Sjögren syndrome (SS)A and SSB; ACl)

- Antibody panel for paraneoplastic disorders

- Antibodies for infectious disorders

Abbreviations: aMOG, anti-myelin oligodendrocyte glycoprotein antibody; aNMDAr, anti N-methyl D-aspartate receptor; Abs, antibodies; RF, rheumatoid factor.

in a patient in whom the clinical and imaging findings are highly suggestive of CIS/MS, the presence and type of OCBs will assist the physician to confirm the diagnosis. However, in up to 10% of patients with MS, the CSF findings may remain normal.[19] It is essential to use the right methodology for detecting OCBs, which currently is isoelectric focusing with immunofixation.[18]

One should keep in mind that OCBs can be detected in approximately 4% to 5% of healthy individuals and in up to 20% of the healthy siblings of newly diagnosed patients with MS.[36] The rate of positive OCBs in some other inflammatory and noninflammatory neurologic disorders show a great variation.[37] In some systemic disorders that may mimic MS, such as NBD, they are positive in fewer than 15%, whereas in SLE or Sjögren with CNS involvement they may be seen in a slightly higher rate, and in neurosarcoidosis they may be positive in up to half of the cases.[19,38,39]

Not only the positivity of IgG-OCB, but also the type may provide further clues to the differential.[18,37,38] Type 1 is when there are no bands in the CSF and serum, which is the normal response, whereas in type 2, OCBs are present in the CSF with no corresponding abnormality in serum, indicating local intrathecal synthesis of IgG. Most patients with MS are type 2 positive. The remaining patients with MS are mostly type 3, in whom the IgG bands are found both in the CSF and serum, with additional bands in the CSF. In SLE with CNS involvement and in neurosarcoidosis, this pattern may be detected as well.[37] When OCBs are present in the CSF, which are identical to those in serum, it is type 4 positivity and it is more commonly seen in systemic inflammatory and infectious disorders affecting the CNS as well as in Guillain-Barré syndrome and ADEM. When this response is found, the clinicians should extend their differential to include systemic immune-mediated disorders or infections before MS. Type 5 is when there is a monoclonal IgG pattern in both CSF and serum, indicating the likelihood of myeloma or monoclonal gammopathy of undetermined significance.

A mild pleocytosis consisting mostly of lymphocytes and up to 50 cells/µL may be seen in MS; however, we start to "think twice" once a (nontraumatic) spinal tap reveals more than 20 to 30 cells and/or a protein level higher than 60 mg/dL (normal: <45 mg/dL), despite that up to 90 mg/dL has been reported in MS.[19,38] A CSF cell count greater than 50/µL should raise the suspicion of an infectious cause, or non-MS other inflammatory diseases such as ADEM, NMO, NBD, and neurosarcoidosis, in which a mild to moderately elevated protein is commonly seen and OCBs are less common. In NMO, the increased pleocytosis mostly consists of neutrophils and eosinophils, and in NBD, neutrophils dominate during the acute episode, later to be replaced by lymphocytes.[39] In diseases, such as SLE or Sjögren with CNS involvement, the CSF findings are similar to MS, with a variable rate of IgG-OCBs (**Box 4**).

The CSF albumin-serum ratio (Qalb) also can be used to evaluate blood-CSF barrier integrity, as the CSF protein is usually normal in MS, but may be slightly elevated in some.[19,37] However, the Qalb is influenced by age, body weight, sex, and some other variables. Measles–rubella–zoster (MRZ) reaction is considered the most specific test for MS diagnosis, which could be efficiently used to confirm MS in OCB-negative or in uncertain cases, but it is not used routinely due to its complexity and cost.[18]

In pediatric cases with MS, the pleocytosis may be slightly higher and rate of OCBs slightly lower than adult MS cases, but this issue is not discussed further here.

MRI DIAGNOSIS OF MULTIPLE SCLEROSIS

The current imaging diagnosis of MS according to McDonald 2010 diagnostic criteria[17] is based on the demonstration of MS-suggestive inflammatory-demyelinative lesions disseminated in time and space by MRI in an individual who reports

---

Box 4
The "think twice" cerebrospinal fluid (CSF) findings in MS differential diagnosis: possibilities and pitfalls

- Normal CSF (no oligoclonal bands [OCBs], normal IgG and IgG index): start thinking twice!
- *OCB* (−): less likely to be MS
- *Cells* up to 50/mL in MS, but already when more than 20 to 30 start thinking twice! 20 to 50 neuroinflammatory; >50: neuro-infectious!
- *Protein* up to 90 mg/dL in MS, but already when more than 60, start thinking twice! Neuroinflammatory diseases are more likely
- *Albumin CSF/serum ratio* (QAlb): normal or slightly increased, when elevated (together with increased cells) think more of infections or leptomeningeal metastases, as well as acute and chronic demyelinating polyneuropathies and spinal stenosis
- *Glucose:* normal in MS; if low, consider bacterial or viral meningo-encephalitis, also may be leptomeningeal metastatic infiltration

---

MS-suggestive symptoms and signs. The DIS requires ≥1 T2 lesions in ≥2 regions of the following CNS areas, which are juxtacortical (lesions should touch the cortex), periventricular (lesions should touch the ventricles), infratentorial, and the spinal cord.[17] Recently these criteria were slightly modified to add the optic nerve as a fifth site and including the cortex together with the juxtacortical site.[40] Although the requirements keep 2 or more of these 5 sites, the minimum number of lesions at the periventricular site has been increased to 3. These recommended criteria are expected to be incorporated into the upcoming new revision of the McDonald diagnostic criteria (**Box 5**). To fulfill DIT, the presence of 1 or more asymptomatic enhancing lesions in the initial MRI or the development of any new T2 lesions on follow-up MRI are required.

Box 5
Modified McDonald MRI (2010) criteria according to the recommended 2016 Magnetic Resonance Imaging in Multiple Sclerosis (MAGNIMS) criteria to establish disease dissemination in space in MS

Dissemination in space can be shown by involvement of at least 2 of 5 areas of the CNS as follows:

- Three or more periventricular lesions
- One or more infratentorial lesion
- One or more spinal cord lesion
- One or more optic nerve lesion
- One or more cortical or juxtacortical lesion

Dissemination in time: original 2010 criteria unchanged

- Simultaneous presence of asymptomatic gadolinium-enhancing and nonenhancing lesions at any time
- A new T2 and/or gadolinium-enhancing lesion(s) on follow-up MRI, with reference to a baseline scan irrespective of the timing of the baseline MRI

Adapted from Polman CH, Reingold SC, Banwell B, et al. Diagnostic criteria for multiple sclerosis: 2010 revisions to the McDonald criteria. Ann Neurol 2011;69:292–302; and Filippi M, Rocca MA, Ciccarelli O, et al. MRI criteria for the diagnosis of multiple sclerosis: MAGNIMS consensus guidelines. Lancet Neurol 2016;15:292–303; with permission.

In clinical practice, it is easier to make a diagnosis of CIS/early MS when the clinical presentation together with the MRI findings are highly consistent with a diagnosis of MS and confirmed by a CSF study. However, many times, neither one will be clear cut and either to make a diagnosis of MS or exclude it will become a challenge. The challenge is not limited only to the onset of the neurologic disease, but it may be considered for some patients who already have been diagnosed and even treated for MS for many years, despite that something is not right with that diagnosis! The number of misdiagnosed and treated cases are increasing and becoming a significant problem, with overreading and misinterpretation of the MRI findings being the major cause of misdiagnosis in most.[6,8] It should be kept in mind that MRI criteria for MS diagnosis are not developed to differentiate MS from other conditions, but to identify the patients with high-risk CIS who will convert to clinical MS in the setting of clinical findings suggestive of MS.[8]

In a patient who has been referred with a "clinical diagnosis" of probable MS, MRI may confirm the clinical diagnosis of MS, and may be suggestive of an alternative diagnosis, but at times it may cause further diagnostic confusion! The neurologist should not rely on a radiology report, especially when it is not from an expert neuroradiologist that the neurologist trusts. Neurologists should understand and interpret the MRI themselves. A proper reading of an MRI in an individual with questionable MS will be of great importance (**Box 6**). Another major problem in daily practice is the lack of standardization and proper MRI studies in individuals suspected to have MS or related disorders. Despite that a well-standardized protocol for brain MRI has been described,[41] its clinical implementation is not widespread globally! Neurologists should be aware of the protocol and may require the MRI centers to which they refer their patients to implement it.

Advanced Quantitative MRI Techniques and Multiple Sclerosis–Related Findings

In recent years, the development of high field-strength MRI machines and advanced quantitative MRI techniques has introduced several findings that enhance the imaging diagnosis of MS. The detection of increased iron deposition within MS-related lesions (most chronic and some acute focal MS lesions show increased iron deposition), the demonstration of cortical lesions (cortical lesions are abundant in patients with MS), and revealing the perivenular distribution pattern of MS lesions (most MS lesions show a central vein and a rim of hypointensity) are among such findings.[41] Of those, the "central vein sign" (CVS) is probably becoming a major marker for a reliable differential diagnosis between MS and MS-like syndromes or MS-like lesions.[42,43] In a recent consensus article, the limitations and recommendations have been outlined for the evaluation of the CVS in the diagnosis and differential diagnosis of MS.[44]

Box 6
The role of an MRI study in the differential diagnosis of MS

A proper (expert) MRI reading:

- *Confirmative:* may confirm the clinical diagnosis of MS

- *Suggestive:* may be suggestive but not confirmative, necessitating further workup and follow-up for MS

- *Explorative:* may not be conclusive and leads to further workup for non-MS other inflammatory or noninflammatory diseases

- *Eliminative:* may exclude the clinical diagnosis of MS and offer an alternative diagnosis

However, because currently these findings preferably require MRI systems that operate at higher magnetic-field strengths (≥3.0 T/with the exception of CVS that can now be shown with 1.5 T) and sophisticated software programs/sequences, and that their specificity needs to be validated and confirmed, they are yet not part of the routine practice.

Radiologically Isolated Syndrome

One exception to the role of MRI in the differential diagnosis of MS is when an MRI study is carried on for another clinical purpose and the MRI turns out to show MS-suggestive lesions. There are indeed some people who are referred for an MRI study due to non-MS symptoms or conditions (eg, migraine or other primary headaches, pituitary adenoma, syncope) and then are found to have incidental lesions that are consistent with MS, despite that they never had any symptom of the disease. These people are diagnosed as having the "radiologically isolated syndrome" (RIS). This topic is further discussed in the article by Christine Lebrun-Frenay and colleagues' article, "Anomalies Characteristic of Central Nervous System Demyelination: Radiologically Isolated Syndrome," in this issue.

IMAGING POSSIBILITIES AND PITFALLS IN THE DIFFERENTIAL DIAGNOSIS OF MULTIPLE SCLEROSIS

As already mentioned, a significant number of the misdiagnosed MS cases are due to misinterpretation of the MRI findings by the radiologist or by the neurologist or both! In an individual with MRI abnormalities suggestive of MS, there are some clues that will make the physician think twice before making a too-early diagnosis (**Box 7**)!

MRI Findings Atypical for Multiple Sclerosis or Less Likely to Be Multiple Sclerosis: Semisymmetric/Symmetric White Matter Involvement of the Cerebral Hemispheres, Lack of Ovoid Lesions, Very Small Lesions, Lack of Spinal Cord Involvement, and/or in Most Other Sites Consistent with Multiple Sclerosis

In individuals who are within their third and fourth decades, and are admitted with a suspected or definite diagnosis of MS mostly because of their MRI findings and vague/nonspecific neurologic symptoms, such as dizziness, numbness and tingling sensations, and headache, there are some "pink flags" that make us think twice. When the lesions are very small (<3 mm) and ovoid lesions are absent, these raise some suspicion on the possibility of MS. When white matter lesions are scattered mostly in a peripheric-subcortical distribution rather than periventricular localization, we start thinking twice too. Our suspicion raises further in these individuals when, despite the presence of a large number of subcortical lesions, there are no or only a few juxtacortical and/or periventricular lesions. Many times, the distribution of these lesions is almost in a symmetric/semisymmetrical pattern and more prominent within the frontal lobes. It is unlikely to observe posterior fossa, corpus callosum, and spinal cord lesions in these people. The physical and neurologic examinations are mostly found to be normal in these individuals; however, to rule out an underlying systemic disorder or a vasculopathy, we look for vascular and other risk factors and we carry on several laboratory tests, such as vitamin B12, homocysteine, ANA, anti double-stranded DNA (adsDNA), anticardiolipin antibodies (ACIs). In most of them, no abnormality is detected and our final diagnosis ends up being either a psychiatric (somatization) disorder with "nonspecific white matter abnormalities" (NSWMA), or an individual having NSWMA of no clinical significance (**Fig. 1**).

Box 7
MRI findings atypical for MS – less likely to be MS (in individuals ≤45 yrs old)[a]

- Very small lesions (<3 mm)
  [*NSWMA; Vasculopathies; Migraine*]

- Absence of ovoid lesions
  [*NSWMA; Vasculopathies; Migraine*]

- Peripheric – subcortical - localization of white matter lesions rather than periventricular
  [*NSWMA; Vasculopathies; Migraine*]

- Despite the presence of a large number of subcortical lesions either no or only a few juxta-cortical and/or periventricular lesions
  [*NSWMA; Vasculopathies; Migraine*]

- Absence of posterior fossa, corpus callosum and spinal cord lesions
  [*NSWMA*]

- Symmetrical/semi-symmetrical lesions
  [*NSWMA; inherited disorders including CADASIL*]

- Disproportionally large corpus callosum lesions
  [*Susac's; NMOSD; malignant primary bain tumors and lymphoma*]

- No change in successive MRIs – all MRIs are the same!
  [*NSWMA*]

- No gadolinium enhancement in any MRI
  [*NSWMA; Migraine, -most- genetic disorders*]

- Persistent gadolinium enhancement in all MRIs
  [*vascular lesions e.g., venous developmental anomalies*]

- Continuous gadolinium enhancement in successive MRIs over many months
  [*Neurosarcoidosis, some infectious diseases*]

- Family members with similar "identical" MRI!
  [*genetic disorders*]

- Lesions with prominent mass effect
  [*Tumors, AIIDLs; some infections; granulomatous disorders*]

- Up/downward (edematous) extension of large brainstem lesion/s
  [*NBD; tumors*]

- Longitudinally extensive spinal cord lesions
  [*NMOSD; MOG-myelopathies; Neuro-sarcoidosis;NBD; spinal cord vascular malformations/dural fistula; tumors*]

[a] Some of the other diagnostic probabilities with similar MRI findings are listed within brackets under each so MRI findings atypical for MS
Abbreviations: AIIDLs, atypical idiopathic inflammatory demyelinating diseases; CADASIL, Cerebral autosomal dominant arteriopathy with subcortical infarcts and leukoencephalopathy; CNS, central nervous system; MOG, myelin oligodendrocyte glycoprotein; NBD, Neuro-Behçet's Disease; NMOSD, Neuromyelitis optica spectrum disorder; NSWMA, Nonspesific white matter abnormalities.

Migraine and White Matter Lesions

It is well known that people with migraine headaches (mainly with aura) are more likely to have white matter abnormalities (WMA) that may be seen in the posterior fossa structures too[45] (**Fig. 2**). In a prospective study it was shown that these WMAs may increase in time but without having any clinical significance.[46] It is quite likely that it is this migraine subpopulation with such brain abnormalities that are commonly

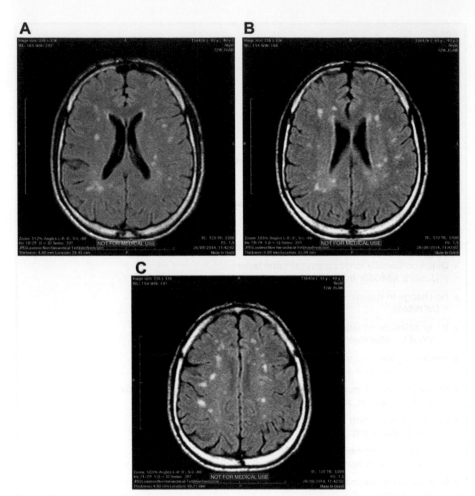

Fig. 1. (*A–C*) Nonspecific neurologic symptoms with NSWMAs on MRI. A young man with dizziness and numbness in hands and T2 lesions on MRI was admitted for a second opinion with a diagnosis of MS. His history revealed that he had received a diagnosis of MS based on his symptoms and an MRI study reported to be consistent with MS 4 years ago and was put on long-term treatment for MS. Over the next 4 years his "same" symptoms persisted and his follow-up MRI studies were also reported as being suggestive of MS. However, his evaluation in our center revealed a normal physical and neurologic examination. When his previous 3 MRI studies were compared, there were no changes in any, there was no gadolinium enhancement in any, and his T2-hyperintense lesions were almost semisymmetrical, mostly subcortical with only a very few being juxtacortical and periventricular. There were no posterior fossa, spinal cord, or corpus callosum lesions and no atrophy or T1 black holes could be detected. A repeat MRI was done in our center and was read as showing NSWMAs. His complete workup, including a CSF study, was normal. Psychiatric consultation was consistent with anxiety disorder and a tendency for somatization. Now after 10 years, he continues to be fine, with occasional complaints of dizziness and his last MRI done in 2015 remains the same.

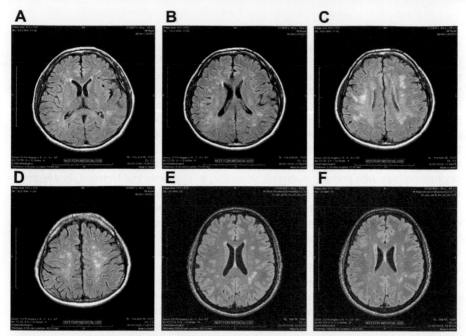

Fig. 2. (*A–F*) Two patients with migraine and NSWMAs on MRI. (*A–D*) A 40-year-old man with migraine with aura. An MRI study done for headaches and visual symptoms reveals bilateral mostly subcortical semisymmetrical NSWMAs in an umbrellalike distribution! An echocardiography discloses a large patent foramen ovale and an embolic shower test that was positive. (*E, F*) A 46-year-old woman with occasional migraine headaches. Her MRI shows similar NSWMA to the previous patient. She did not have any cardiac abnormality. The underlying pathology of these T2 hyperintensities are not clear but they are not suggestive of MS lesions, as discussed within the text.

mistaken for having MS! However, a well-taken medical history will reveal that the neurologic problem is migraine and that the nature of the MRI abnormalities when viewed in detail are not typical for MS. The supratentorial lesions in migraine are mostly subcortical, rather than periventricular and less likely to be juxtacortical, and it was recently shown that they lack the CVS expected to be seen in MS lesions.[47] In the migraineurs with WMAs, our diagnostic workup includes an echocardiography study and duplex ultrasonography for embolic shower in selected cases to rule out the probability of patent foramen ovale (PFO) or atrial septal defect (ASD) and related micro-emboli. One other but extremely low possibility is the coexistence of migraine with MS and the combination of lesions of both disorders.

Inherited Disorders and White Matter Lesions

Unless in the later stages of the disease, a symmetric/semisymmetrical distribution of white matter lesions is not expected in MS. When such a pattern is observed in a young adult with a recent-onset neurologic disease, there are several inherited disorders that should be included in the differential. Not uncommonly, the lesions of ADEM also may show a semisymmetrical distribution, but they tend to be larger and all or most will enhance, suggesting an acute inflammatory process of the same age. Besides, in ADEM the presence of an acute or subacute-onset encephalopathy is another and clinical clue to differentiate it from the inherited disorders. Finally, when such underlying diseases are ruled out, the previously discussed clinically innocent NSWMA will be at the top of remaining considerations.

The multisystem disorders caused by a variety of genetic defects will result in a number of inherited disorders, such as lysosomal storage disorders, several mitochondrial diseases, and several other neurometabolic disorders.[14] Multisystem involvement, a positive family history, involvement in some of both cortical and deep gray matter in a nonvascular pattern in addition to the semisymmetrical or symmetric white matter involvement, should raise the suspicion of such disorders. In some, calcified cerebral lesions or multiple cystic cavitations may be seen, which in that case will enhance the probability.[14] Of these genetic disorders affecting the white matter, the major groups to be included in the differential diagnosis of MS are the late-onset leukodystrophies, in which some also may involve the peripheral nervous system, and the genetic leukoencephalopathies with primary neuronal, vascular, or systemic involvement, in which the white matter changes are likely to be secondary[48] (**Box 8**).

Several leukodystrophies typically associated with onset in the pediatric age group can also present in older adolescents or throughout the adult decades and may have typical phenotypic presentations or may present with symptom complexes very different from their pediatric counterparts. In many of such cases, they present at disease onset with less confluent white matter changes on their MRIs than in pediatric cases and should be included within the differential diagnosis of MS and other disorders of abnormal white matter in adults.[49] In most of the leukoencephalopathies that have their onset in adolescence or at a later age, the CNS manifestations are gradually and very slowly progressive and therefore may be mistaken for PPMS. However, the MRI pattern that is mostly symmetric and has a semispecific pattern, no sign of inflammation in the CSF, a positive family history, and in some the genetic testing will help the physician to make the final diagnosis (**Fig. 3**).

Mostly the WMAs have a tendency to be symmetric with the presence of more or less bilateral confluent lesions and their predominant localization will lead to the diagnostic possibility in most.[48–51] The most common predominant patterns seen on MRI are frontal (eg, Alexander disease), parieto-occipital (eg, X-linked adrenoleukodystrophy),

---

Box 8
The MRI differential diagnosis of single gene disorders sharing clinical and radiologic characteristics with MS

Presence of the following findings: not suggestive of MS

- Symmetric-appearing white matter involvement of the cerebral hemispheres
- Cerebral involvement limited to long tracts (mostly within the post internal capsule and brain stem)
- Spinal cord involvement limited to long tracts: longitudinal lesions
- T1 hyperintensities of thalamic pulvinar
- T2 (symmetric) hyperintensities of dentate nucleus
- Multiple subcortical cystic cavitations

Absence of the following findings: not likely MS

- Lack of ovoid lesions
- Lack of spinal cord involvement
- Lack of gadolinium enhancement (exception: adrenoleukodystrophies)

Adapted from Weisfeld-Adams JD, Katz Sand IB, Honce JM, et al. Differential diagnosis of Mendelian and mitochondrial disorders in patients with suspected multiple sclerosis. Brain 2015;138:517–39; with permission.

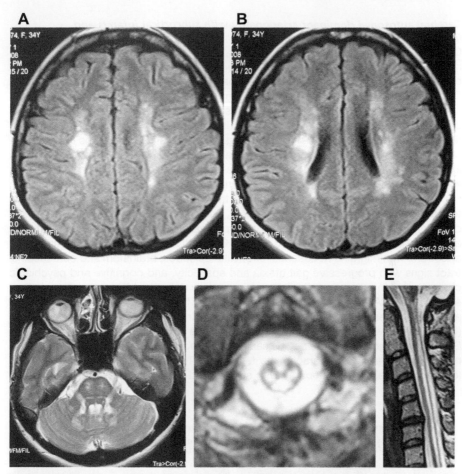

Fig. 3. (A–E) Leukoencephalopathy with brainstem and spinal cord involvement and high (or normal) lactate. A 32-year-old woman with subacute onset of paraparesis progressing to significant gait difficulty over a month; then having a fluctuating course with limited progression and major depression. Her MRI discloses inhomogeneous and spotty cerebral white matter abnormalities within the periventricular and deep cerebral white matter (A, B), sparing the temporal lobes and the U-fibers, posterior corpus callosum, and posterior internal capsule. Selective pyramidal tract involvement and cerebellar connections are involved as well as the intraparenchymal trajectories of the trigeminal nerve and long tract involvement of the spinal cord are almost diagnostic (C–E). The MR-spectroscopy may show high white matter lactate levels but not in all cases! This case was DARS2 gene positive (Van der Knaap, & G.C. Scheper Laboratory, Amsterdam). (*Courtesy of* Cengiz Yalcinkaya, Istanbul, Turkey and Aksel Siva, Istanbul, Turkey.)

periventricular (eg, metachromatic leukodystrophy), subcortical (eg, Canavan disease), diffuse cerebral (eg, vanishing white matter disease), or posterior fossa (eg, peroxisomal disorders), which will allow the experienced reader to make a proper diagnosis.[48,51] Enhancement is rare except in adrenomyeloneuropathy and Alexander disease. Additional imaging features, such as the presence of calcifications, macrocephaly, involvement of the cortex and deep basal ganglia, symmetric involvement within the cerebellum, and the descending white matter tracts are also important for further discrimination from MS and other inflammatory and infectious disorders that usually present with focal and not symmetric lesions.[48,50,51]

Cerebral autosomal dominant arteriopathy with subcortical infarcts and leukoencephalopathy

One of the other monogenic disorders caused by mutations in the NOTCH3 gene that may present in some young adults with episodic neurologic CNS symptoms and bilateral semisymmetrical white matter changes and therefore may mimic MS is CADASIL.[14,52,53] The primary disease process is a nonatheromatous, nonamyloid vasculopathy, and although the disease manifests itself as brain dysfunction due to cerebral small-vessel disease, the vasculopathy is systemic. The type of MRI involvement, the strong family history, and genetic testing are diagnostic. The lesions involve bilaterally the U-fibers, the basal ganglia, external capsule, insular regions, and commonly in the form of lacunarlike infarcts within the corona radiata and subcortical regions, with occasional microbleeds.[14,52] The anterior part of the temporal lobes, a location highly suggestive of CADASIL, as well as the frontal pole juxta-subcortical lesions together with external capsule involvement, should bring CADASIL to the top of the differential diagnosis list. Frequently the corpus callosum and cerebellum are spared, and spinal lesions are not expected (**Fig. 4**). CADASIL shows a heterogeneous clinical spectrum, with migraine headaches, strokelike episodes, brainstem and corticospinal tract signs with progressive gait ataxia and spasticity, and cognitive and psychiatric changes.[14,52] In some young individuals, especially when the MRI changes are in their early stages, CADASIL may be mistaken for MS. The recessively inherited "Cerebral autosomal recessive arteriopathy with subcortical infarcts and leukoencephalopathy" (CARASIL) shows a similar clinical picture and white matter changes as seen in CADASIL, but the cognitive decline begins earlier and, in addition, gait disturbance, low back pain, and alopecia are characteristic features.[54] The recently described CARASAL (cathepsin A–related arteriopathy with strokes and leukoencephalopathy) is another

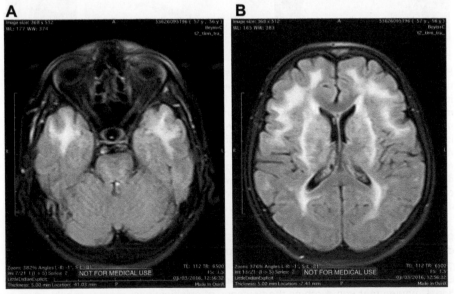

Fig. 4. (*A, B*) A 56-year-old woman with genetically proven CADASIL. Her MRI shows almost the typical imaging pattern of CADASIL, the lesions involve the anterior part of the temporal lobes, as well as the frontal pole juxta-subcortical lesions together with external capsule. The U-fibers and the basal ganglia, as well as the corona radiata and subcortical regions are also involved.

hereditary adult-onset cerebral small-vessel disease.[55] The MRI pattern was characterized by signal changes similar to CADASIL cases with bilateral patchy lesions in the frontoparietal periventricular and deep white matter, internal and external capsules, basal nuclei, thalami, and brainstem that that became diffuse, with acute infarcts and microbleeds in some.[55] However, the temporal white matter was relatively spared and the temporal poles were not affected. The disease seems to be extremely rare and further the MRI pattern should not be confused with MS by the expert.

Mitochondrial optic neuropathies

Recently, the term "mitochondrial ON" (MON) has increasingly been used to describe a group of optic neuropathies that exhibit mitochondrial dysfunction in retinal ganglion cells.[56] Leber hereditary ON (LHON), which is a maternally inherited bilateral ON, has its onset in teenage and is the most common of this group of disorders. Although the major neurologic manifestation in LHON is an acute or subacute onset of painless ON that affects both eyes successively, not uncommonly other neurologic features, such as myelopathy, ataxia, and other neurologic features, may be seen, sometimes accompanied by abnormal cranial MRI signal changes causing difficulty to distinguish both clinically and radiologically from MS. Besides, the probability of LHON and an MS-like illness (L-MS) to coexist is relatively high,[57] an association often referred as "Harding disease," causing further diagnostic confusion. In a recent study, it was shown that all patients with L-MS and approximately one-fourth of patients with LHON were found to have an MRI appearance typical of MS.[57] Female patients with LHON are likely to have a greater risk of having white matter lesions consistent with MS compared with male patients.[57,58] Because a number of toxins, antibiotics, and drugs may trigger the onset of LHON and that the presence of bilaterally symmetric optic neuropathies are most likely to be due to mitochondrial disease,[59] identifying these features helps with the diagnosis. A positive familial history, some features observed in the optic fundi examination, a normal CSF study, absence of gadolinium enhancement of brain lesions, and mitochondrial genetic testing are some features that will discriminate "isolated-LHON" from MS.

Fabry disease

Fabry disease (FD), which is due to mutations in the GLA gene, is another inherited multisystem X-linked disorder that is caused by deficiency of alpha-galactosidase.[60] It is characterized clinically by angiokeratoma, corneal and lenticular abnormalities, acroparesthesia, and renal and cardiac dysfunction, small fiber peripheral neuropathy, and stroke. It is listed among small-vessel diseases that may be confused both clinically and by MRI with MS due to the relapsing-remitting symptoms sharing characteristics with MS in some patients with FD, but the presence of large infarcts together with T1-hyperintense signal abnormalities in the pulvinar nuclei are characteristic.[61] Due to the systemic and other neurologic clinical manifestations, which also may include a painful neuropathy, it is unlikely to be mistaken with MS.

When family members of an individual in whom MS is considered within the differential diagnosis turn out to have similar "identical" MRI changes, an inherited disorder becomes more likely. In addition to hereditary disorders, metabolic and toxic disorders also have a tendency to be symmetric as well, with the presence of confluent lesions, whereas MS and other inflammatory and infectious disorders usually present with focal and not completely symmetric lesions.

Nonhereditary vasculopathies, which include some of the primary or systemic vasculitides and connective disorders and some other immune-mediated diseases involving the CNS, may present with MS-suggestive clinical manifestations and MRI abnormalities. Involvement of the U-fibers with the presence of juxtacortical lesions is a hallmark in MS, whereas this is absent in most acquired vasculopathies as well as in previously mentioned inherited leukoencephalopathies.

Disproportionally Large Corpus Callosum Lesions: Susac Syndrome and Other Conditions

Susac syndrome
Despite that they are not one of the regions included in the DIS criteria, corpus callosum lesions are common in MS and they are more frequently seen at the genu and body of the callosum with their origin at calloso-septal interface, and initially as small separate lesions that may enhance in the acute phase[62] (**Fig. 5**A). In an individual who presents with some CNS symptoms and some inflammatory-demyelinative–suggestive brain lesions on their MRI, MS is included as one of the major diagnoses. However, when such an individual turns out to have disproportionally large/cluster of corpus callosum lesions and limited hemispheric lesions, Susac syndrome should be a major consideration (**Fig. 5**B). Susac is an autoimmune endotheliopathy affecting the precapillary arterioles of the brain, retina, and inner ear presenting typically with a triad of encephalopathy, retinopathy, and hearing loss, but may have an atypical presentation as well.[63,64] Because the disease most often has its onset between the third and fourth decades of life and is more common in women, it can easily mimic MS. Besides, the probability that neurologic manifestations of Susac syndrome may appear before the ophthalmologic or inner ear manifestations, the steroid responsiveness, and that the spinal cord involvement also can be seen both clinically and by MRI, increase the difficulty to differentiate it from MS.[65] In addition to the clusters of snowball-like callosal lesions, the "string of pearls" appearance on MRI that is especially striking on diffusion-weighted imaging has been reported to be highly suggestive of Susac.[64] The lesions of Susac are likely to be the result of autoimmune-mediated occlusion of microvessels, and they lack the CVS contrary to the MS lesions, a finding that was confirmed in a high-field MRI study.[66] A perivascular setting is not typical for the lesions of Susac syndrome, and when they occur, coincidentally blood vessels are

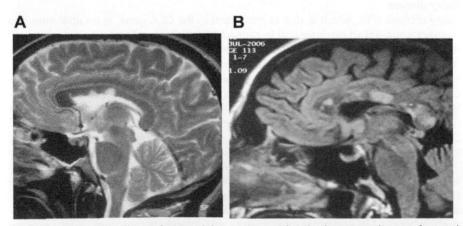

Fig. 5. (*A, B*) Corpus callosum lesions. (*A*) A patient with MS whose MRI shows a few and relatively small well-demarcated corpus callosum lesions (this patient had many hemispheric lesions and at other sites consistent for MS). (*B*) A patient with Susac disease, whose MRI shows disproportionally large and a cluster of corpus callosum lesions (he had a limited number of hemispheric lesions).

most likely located in the lesion's periphery.[66] It is well known that leptomeningeal enhancement can be observed in patients with MS,[67,68] a finding that also has been reported in Susac syndrome.[63] Recently, it was reported that the pattern of leptomeningeal enhancement may differ between the 2 diseases and that the varying enhancement pattern of vascular leakage in Susac may be helpful in differentiating it from the mostly stable enhancement pattern expected to be seen in MS.[69] In patients suspected to have Susac syndrome a standardized fundoscopy in conjunction with retinal fluorescein angiography, audiometry, neuropsychological examination, and MRI of the brain are required for the diagnostic workup.[63]

Other conditions

There are several other conditions whereby either predominant or isolated corpus callosum lesions may appear. Such lesions have been observed in some metabolic disorders or epileptic seizures, but generally they are transient and the etiology will be clear, not causing much confusion with MS. One such condition is the Marchiafava-Bignami disease, which is rare and mainly associated with alcoholism and thiamin deficiency and involves the middle layers of genu and splenium and in later stages resulting in the atrophy of the corpus callosum.[70] High-grade gliomas and brain lymphoma also may involve the corpus callosum and more frequently at the genu and splenium, they are large lesions extending across the corpus callosum and cross the midline from one hemisphere to the other, with the main lesion seen on one side and not likely to be confused with MS.[62,71] Gliomatosis cerebri also may involve the corpus callosum together by bilateral patchy or large brain lesions, but due to its infiltrative nature, it will not be confused with the inflammatory lesions of MS.

Brain NMO may also involve the entire corpus callosum (longitudinally extensive corpus callosum lesion!) but more frequently will affect the splenium and is not likely to mimic MS. ADEM is another atypical inflammatory disease that can involve the corpus callosum largely as well, but bi-hemispheric large demyelinative-inflammatory lesions, with most enhancing simultaneously, are expected to be seen. Occasionally, tumefactive demyelinating lesions may spread across the corpus callosum in a "butterfly" configuration, simulating an infiltrative astrocytoma or lymphoma.[72] In most of these previously mentioned disorders with large corpus callosum lesions, the clinical presentation will have at least some features of an encephalopathic syndrome, which are not expected to be seen in early MS.

Ischemic lesions mostly secondary to atherosclerotic disease may also involve the corpus callosum and may be difficult to differentiate from MS by imaging. They are small, usually central in the corpus callosum and the upper and lower margins are not involved. Because of the bilateral arterial supply of the corpus callosum, infarcts are usually confined to one side of the corpus callosum, with the exception in the acute stages when they may cross the midline.[71]

Small Vascular Disease: Could It Mimic Multiple Sclerosis on MRI?

One common condition that is mistaken for MS on MRI is "small vascular disease" (SVD) due to its multiplicity and dissemination in different sites.[51] SVD is the result of hypoxic-ischemic neurologic injury mainly due to arteriosclerosis and a number of other diseases affecting small blood vessels. It is most commonly seen in people older than 50 and is associated with the presence of vascular risk factors, such as hypertension, diabetes, smoking, and rarely the clinical presentation will be suggestive of MS. Lacunar infarcts are expected and the lesions of SVD are mostly subcortical and are not expected to involve the "U-fibers" (which is highly suggestive of MS), the corpus callosum, and the spinal cord. T2-hyperintense rims around the ventricles, known as "caps and bands" should not be confused with periventricular lesions of MS. SVD may involve the brainstem too, but the lesions are located centrally contrary to MS, where the lesions have a predilection to be more in the peripheral distribution. The white matter lesions seen in SVD do not have an ovoid shape and do not enhance unless in the acute/subacute phase. Microbleeds also can occur in SVD and these are best seen on either gradient echo or preferably susceptibility-weighted imaging (SWI).[51]

Nonatherosclerotic SVD may be seen in several other vasculopathies, as already discussed, such as CADASIL, Susac syndrome, and also in cerebral amyloid angiopathy.

The underlying pathology in NSWMA is not clear, and although SVD is suggested as one possibility, it is difficult to explain the whole pattern of involvement and shape of the lesions as a result of ischemic and hypoxic injury of small vessels. SVD should not be confused with RIS in asymptomatic individuals. But, as most people older than 50 already have several vascular risk factors, and do not present with MS-suggestive symptoms, SVD is not going to be a major problem for the differential diagnosis of MS. The only exception may be the individual who has late onset of MS with SVD comorbidity!

Perivascular Spaces

Perivascular spaces (PVSs) are anatomic structures that serve as drainage pathways surrounding small cerebral vessels as they penetrate the brain parenchyma. When they enlarge, they become visible, which is either due to aging and vasculo-degenerative changes or as an anatomic variation without any specific meaning. It was shown that patients with MS displayed more PVSs compared with healthy controls and likely to serve as a sign of neurodegeneration.[73] However, they should not be confused with MS lesions. PVSs that occur in almost all locations and most commonly in the deep gray matter, midbrain, fontal subcortical regions, but also in the corpus callosum, may cause some confusion at times and may be mistaken for MS lesions to the "unexperienced eye"! PVSs are hyperintense on T2-weighted imaging (T2WI), hypointense (isointense with CSF) on T1-weighted imaging (T1WI), and likely to be suppressed on fluid attenuation inversion recovery (FLAIR) images. They never enhance, are well demarcated, and some may have a mild mass effect.

A Few Imaging Clues to Avoid a Misdiagnosis of Multiple Sclerosis: No Change in Follow-up MRIs, No Gadolinium Enhancement in Any MRI, Continuous Enhancement of the Same Lesion

When the clinician is not comfortable with the clinical and MRI diagnosis of MS, there are a number of imaging clues that may help to exclude the probability of MS to a certain extent. In a patient with a certain duration of clinical symptoms and several MRI studies with white matter MS-suggestive lesions, but in whom the DIT and DIS criteria are not clear and the clinical manifestations are rather nonspecific, "the stability" of the MRI abnormalities should double the suspicion of an MS diagnosis. When there is no change in successive MRI studies of the same individual, all MRIs being the same, no spinal cord involvement and in addition if there has been no gadolinium enhancement in any of the MRI studies, MS is less likely to be the diagnosis. No evidence of atrophy and black holes further lessens the probability of MS. One exception is PPMS, the MS clinical phenotype in which some may have very low MRI activity or mainly spinal involvement.

MS lesions are not expected to enhance for more than a few weeks, and when there is a persistent enhancement beyond 3 months, other explanations should be considered. One common pitfall is the "persistent" gadolinium-enhancing lesion that may be mistaken for an MS-like lesion in an individual who is worked up for MS, or mainly in someone who already had received this diagnosis and has other MS-consistent lesions. When the same lesion continues to enhance in successive MR studies, the probability of a small vascular malformation, such a capillary telangiectasia, should be considered and not confused with an "active MS lesion." These lesions are mostly located in the brainstem and an SWI study may show the vascular pathology. Persistent gadolinium enhancement also may be seen in some of the inflammatory disorders such as granulomatous diseases as with the lesions of neurosarcoidosis or in infectious diseases such as (mostly HIV-related) cerebral toxoplasmosis! As such diseases may mimic MS, they need to be considered in its differential diagnosis in an individual whose MRI studies continue to show gadolinium enhancement in the same lesion/s on follow-up images.

Tumefactive Lesions, Imaging Conditions Misdiagnosed as "Not Multiple Sclerosis": The Tumefactive Demyelinative Lesions

Demyelinating-inflammatory lesions larger than 20 mm are referred to as tumefactive demyelinating lesions (TDLs).[72] TDLs may appear in patients with MS either at onset or during the course of the disease, which may be confused with gliomas or other brain tumors, abscesses, or other inflammatory disorders. When they occur at onset and in the absence of other demyelinative-inflammatory lesions, these other probabilities are considered first, which may lead to a diagnostic biopsy. Because the clinical presentations are largely dependent on lesion location and may include a variety of CNS symptoms, they are not helpful in the diagnosis. It has been shown that oligoclonal band positivity is less frequent in patients with tumefactive onset,[72,74] which lowers the supportive role of CSF in the differential. However, sometimes the imaging may provide some clues. TDLs are mostly focal, well-demarcated, hyperintense on T2WI, hypointense on T1WI, and in some T2WI, show a hypointense rim on MRI.[72,74] Most, if not all TDLs show gadolinium enhancement, with most having either an open-ring (with the open portion abutting the cortex or basal ganglia) or closed-ring pattern, and a few showing heterogeneous enhancement patterns, such as punctate and nodular or diffuse.[72,75] Although most TDLs are likely to have a mild to moderate mass effect and/or edema, when the mass effect is disproportionally less than expected from the lesion size, the probability of TDL should be borne to mind (**Fig. 6**) in a patient with a biopsy-proven tumefactive lesion! Decreased perfusion within the lesions, central diffusion restriction, and diffusion restriction in the periphery of the lesion and visualization of veins coursing through the lesion are not typical for tumors or abscesses and are more suggestive of TDLs, as observing rapid resolution of the lesion after high-dose intravenous steroids therapy.[75,76] Magnetic resonance spectroscopy is not expected to differentiate TDLs effectively from neoplasms.

In a patient with a new-onset neurologic episode and solitary tumefactive lesion in whom the probability of CNS lymphoma, brain tumor, or a specific infection cannot be ruled out, a diagnostic biopsy will be needed anyway. However, a biopsy may not be the final solution and also may be misleading, as the probability of a histologic misdiagnosis may be seen in up to one-third of patients with TDLs, with a significant number of these initial misreadings being low-grade or high-grade astrocytoma, and a few being lymphoma.[72] Therefore, the neurologist should remain alert and consider all probabilities at all times for such a subgroup of patients.

TDLs also may appear along the disease course in a patient with a well-established diagnosis of MS, and in such instances the diagnostic probabilities are less a

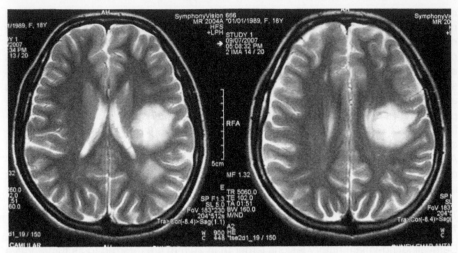

Fig. 6. MRI of a patient with biopsy-proven tumefactive lesion. An 18-year-old woman develops subacute right-sided hemiparesis, an MRI study shows a large tumefactive lesion, with very little perifocal edema and almost no mass effect. A biopsy confirms inflammatory-demyelinating pathology.

challenge. Yet, it should be kept in mind that MS and brain tumors, although highly unlikely, may be seen together in an unfortunate individual![77]

It has to be kept in mind that a heterogeneous group of atypical idiopathic inflammatory-demyelinating diseases of the CNS, including rare variants of MS such as Balo, ADEM, acute hemorrhagic leukoencephalitis, and NMO, can cause TDLs as well.[76]

Multiple Brain Lesions That May Mimic "Multiple Sclerosis" on MRI

Some patients may have multiple TDLs or large (close but <20 mm) demyelinative-inflammatory–looking lesions, and in such individuals the differential diagnosis will include pathologies with multiple CNS lesions such as metastatic tumors, CNS lymphoma, infectious and systemic inflammatory diseases involving the CNS, and atypical idiopathic inflammatory-demyelinating diseases, including ADEM. These diseases are listed in **Box 9** and only a few of the ones that cause the most confusion with MS diagnosis are discussed here.

Cerebral Vasculitic Disorders and Multiple Sclerosis

Vasculitis is inflammation of the blood vessels that may involve the CNS or the peripheral nervous system, or both.[78] Cerebral vasculitic disorders are either primary or secondary. Primary CNS vasculitis (PCNSV) (also called primary angiitis of the CNS) is an idiopathic vasculitis confined to the CNS. CNS vasculitis is considered secondary when it occurs in the setting of a multisystem inflammatory disease, such as a systemic vasculitis or connective-tissue disorder, including BD or lymphoproliferative diseases and other malignancies, some infections and related conditions, and drugs and substance abuse.[78]

CNS vasculitis is commonly included in the radiology reports among the differential imaging possibilities of the individuals with a number of white spots in their brains together with MS! These are generally reports written by radiologists who have an overload of work, who have too many MRI reports to write in a limited time, and feel

---

Box 9
Diseases with multiple CNS lesions that at times may mimic MS: what they might be?

Neoplastic and lymphoproliferative diseases
- Metastatic tumors
- Multifocal gliomas
- CNS lymphoma

Primary or secondary inflammatory diseases/autoinflammatory syndromes of the CNS
- Primary CNS vasculitis
- Systemic vasculitides involving the CNS
- Systemic autoinflammatory disorders with CNS involvement (ie, familial mediterranean fever and others)

Infectious diseases
- CNS toxoplasmosis (mostly human immunodeficiency virus [HIV]-related)
- Neuroborreliosis
- CNS tuberculosis
- CNS cysticercosis
- CNS hydatid cysts
- Progressive multifocal leukoencephalopathy
- Other CNS infections

Idiopathic granulomatous disorders
- Neurosarcoidosis

Idiopathic not well-defined (inflammatory) disorders
- CLIPPERS!!! (chronic lymphocytic inflammation with pontine perivascular enhancement responsive to steroids)

Atypical idiopathic inflammatory-demyelinating diseases of the CNS
  MS variants
- Balo concentric sclerosis
- Marburg MS
- Tumefactive MS
  Once upon a time ago MS-related: not anymore
- Acute disseminated encephalomyelitis (ADEM)
- Acute hemorrhagic leukoencephalitis
- Neuromyelitis optica/Neuromyelitis optica spectrum disorders (NMOSD)
- MOG-antibody related inflammatory-demyelinating syndromes
- Other autoantibody-mediated CNS conditions

---

obliged to write "*I may report everything I see, or I think I see, and will leave it to the clinician to decide what they are!*" without consideration of relevant clinical and laboratory data. Many times, these white spots are neither due to CNS vasculitis or MS, and are simply innocent NSWMAs.

Primary central nervous system vasculitis

PCNSV may involve both small and medium-sized leptomeningeal, cortical, and subcortical arteries, and to a lesser degree veins and venules. Its hallmark is a striking inflammatory alteration of the affected vessel wall resulting in infarcts and hemorrhages, as well as loss of myelin and axonal degeneration.[78] PCNSV can be seen at any age, but it occurs predominantly in the fourth to sixth decades and shows an equal sex ratio, and if angiographically documented so-called "benign" cases are included, then the gender dominance reverses in favor of women. The most common presentation is headache with encephalopathy accompanied by multifocal signs. Hemiparesis, strokelike episodes, visual symptoms, seizures, movement disorders, and progressive cognitive decline have all been reported.[78,79] The diagnosis is made with cerebral angiography and/or by CNS biopsy, the gold standard being histopathological confirmation.[78–80]

Although not common, the clinical presentation and MRI may be confused at times with MS; however, much less than discussed and seen in clinical practice. The most frequent type of lesions seen on MRI in PCNSV are bilateral cortical and subcortical multiple infarctions, within large-artery and branch-artery territories and others limited to small arteries, resulting in multiple subcortical infarctions.[79,80] Multiple microhemorrhages, multiple small/punctate enhancing lesions, large single-enhancing and multiple-enhancing mass/tumefactive lesions, and leptomeningeal enhancement all may be seen.[51,80] Spinal cord involvement, although not common, has been reported in patients with PCNSV.[81] PCNSV is a rare heterogeneous condition, and in most the clinical and many of the previously mentioned imaging findings are not to be confused with MS.

Secondary vasculitides of the nervous system
CNS inflammatory vasculitis, secondary to a known cause or underlying disease, are more commonly seen than the PCNSV. CNS vasculitis may develop in people with systemic immune-mediated disorders and autoinflammatory syndromes, granulomatous disorders, infectious diseases, lymphoproliferative diseases and other malignancies, and finally related to some drug and toxic substances.

Systemic immune-mediated disorders associated with nervous system vasculopathies
SLE, Sjögren syndrome, rheumatoid vasculitis, scleroderma, and dermatomyositis are among some of the systemic immune-mediated disorders associated with nervous system vasculopathies resulting in CNS and peripheral nervous system manifestations. When the CNS is involved in these disorders, both the clinical and the MRI abnormalities may mimic MS in some. However, a well-taken history will reveal the presence of non-neurologic symptoms and signs suggestive of a systemic disorder. On the other hand, when the MRI is highly suggestive of MS in a patient with such systemic symptoms, then the major question to be asked would be whether the CNS involvement is due to the systemic disease or whether we are dealing of a comorbidity of MS with a systemic vasculitic disorder. Clearly, in such cases, a correct diagnosis carries many important diagnostic and therapeutic consequences and we need to be aware of this possibility as well, which may not be so uncommon. As already discussed previously, the high rate of positive ANA serology in patients with MS, and a relatively high rate of OCBs in patients with SLE with neurologic involvement may further complicate the diagnostic process! One other challenge is the occurrence of the longitudinally extensive spinal lesion or longitudinally extensive optic nerve inflammatory lesion, mainly in patients with SLE and Sjögren syndrome, in whom the diagnosis then should include NMOSD, in which there will be a comorbidity of 2 diseases.[82]

Despite that the CNS lesions of SLE and other systemic immune-mediated vasculitic disorders may show DIT and DIS, in most these will be infarcts of any size, may be seen as multifocal gray matter and white matter hyperintensities, or may remain as focal inflammatorylike lesions or form confluent hyperintensities in the white matter.[83,84] Unlike MS, white matter lesions have a tendency to be within a vascular distribution and mainly in SLE the basal ganglia are frequently involved, with swelling and punctate enhancement.[51,84] Despite these well-described differences, there may remain some cases in whom the initial MRI findings may mimic more MS and may complicate the diagnosis, unless other clues to the systemic disease are identified.

In a subgroup of patients with immune-mediated inflammatory bowel diseases, CNS symptoms and white matter lesions on MRI may appear. Whether the CNS disease is a part of the systemic disease or a comorbid immune-mediated CNS disease within the MS spectrum is not clear.[85]

Neuro-Behçet disease

BD is an idiopathic chronic relapsing multisystem vascular-inflammatory disease of unknown origin affecting the CNS in approximately 5% to 10% of patients.[25] Currently the most widely used diagnostic criteria is the International Study Group's classification, according to which a definitive diagnosis requires recurrent oral ulcerations plus 2 of the following: recurrent genital ulcerations, skin lesions, eye lesions, and a positive pathergy test.[86] The primary neurologic involvement is NBD, and clinical and imaging evidence suggests that NBD may be subclassified into 2 major forms. The first, which is seen in most patients, may be characterized by a vascular-inflammatory CNS disease with focal or multifocal parenchymal involvement and therefore may be mistaken for MS.[25] The other form is caused by isolated cerebral venous sinus thrombosis and intracranial hypertension.

Despite that it is uncommon in the Western world, CNS-NBD is often included in the differential diagnosis of MS and in stroke in the young adult, especially when its known systemic symptoms and signs are mild and overlooked. Although the onset age of both disorders is approximately the same, NBD is more frequent in male individuals. The diagnostic criteria for NBD, although not validated, is "the occurrence of neurologic symptoms and signs in a patient that fulfills the International Diagnostic Criteria for BD that is not otherwise explained by any other known systemic or neurologic disease or treatment, and in whom objective abnormalities consistent with NBD are detected either on neurologic examination, MRI, and/or abnormal CSF examination."[87,88] Optic neuritis, sensory symptoms, and spinal cord involvement, which are common in MS, are rarely seen in NBD. The MRI is the gold-standard neuro-imaging tool for the diagnosis of NBD. Lesions are generally located within the brainstem, are large with no distinct borders and have a tendency to extend to the diencephalic structures and basal ganglia, and also, in some, downward, subcortical white matter lesions are not common[89] (**Fig. 7**). In the acute phase, they may show heterogeneous enhancement and, after the acute episode they show partial resolution, tumefactive lesions can also be seen. The MRI findings are clearly different in MS than CNS-NBD. The posterior fossa–brainstem lesions are more discrete and smaller in MS, whereas the MS diagnostic sites of the juxtacortical and periventricular regions and the ovoid shape of the lesions are less likely in CNS-NBD. Spinal cord involvement is rare in NBD, but when it occurs it is likely to show an extensively longitudinal myelitis pattern (but no AQP4-antibodies).[90] Recently, we have described the "bagel sign" pattern in patients with NBD, a central lesion with hypointense core and hyperintense rim with or without contrast enhancement to be observed in axial T2WIs of the spinal cord involvement, which is highly suggestive of NBD.[91] The CSF also reveals different patterns, with a more prominent pleocytosis, high protein levels, and a low rate of positivity (≤15%) for OCBs in CNS-NBD as compared with MS.

Autoinflammatory disease is a broad term used to describe disorders of uncontrolled and unprovoked inflammation driven by the innate immune system, including more commonly, the monogenetic periodic fever syndromes characterized by periodic fever and attacks of inflammation in the absence of an infectious trigger.[39] The prototypical disorder in the family is familial Mediterranean fever, one other being tumor necrosis factor–associated periodic syndrome, which may present with CNS involvement and multiple brain lesions, but the systemic symptoms will be overt and should alert the physician that a systemic disease is the cause.

Neurosarcoidosis

Sarcoidosis is a multisystem granulomatous disease of unknown etiology with approximately 10% of patients showing neurologic involvement.[92] The occurrence of the neurologic manifestations is called "neurosarcoidosis" (NS), a condition that

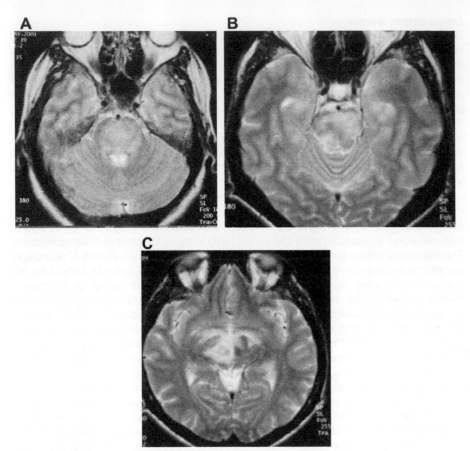

Fig. 7. (*A–C*) A case with CNS-NBD. MRI shows a large lesion with ill-defined borders involving the entire brainstem (*A*, *B*) and extending to the right diencephalic structures and basal ganglia (*C*).

develops mostly in patients who already have the systemic involvement of the disease. Clinically isolated neurosarcoidosis without signs or symptoms of systemic disease is possible but rare.[93]

The most commonly involved cranial nerve in patients with sarcoidosis is the facial nerve, but up to one-third of patients with NS may present with ON, with most being bilateral.[93,94] Because the intraorbital optic nerve and/or optic chiasm may be involved on MRI in these patients with NS, the differential diagnosis will include MS, NMOSD, lymphoma, and optic nerve tumors, if a diagnosis of sarcoidosis is not already made and in the absence of systemic symptoms of the disease.[94]

Meningeal involvement is a well-known form of NS with both leptomeningeal and pachymeningeal involvement with basal predilection, with multiple cranial involvement and other related clinical findings as well as diffuse and nodular enhancement of the leptomeninges on MRI, features not to be confused with MS. Parenchymal involvement may be seen in some patients with NS, not uncommonly involving the pituitary gland and the hypothalamus with its corresponding symptomatology, none suggestive of MS either; however, in a limited number of patients with NS, parenchymal lesions seen on MRI, which may be due to granulomas and ischemia or inflammation due to granulomatous vasculitis, may mimic MS plaques.[94] Although that the CSF in NS may show elevated CSF IgG index and OCBs similar to MS, a high level of protein, a low level of glucose, and a significant pleocytosis are clues that an alternative diagnosis other than MS is likely. CSF ACE may be elevated in NS but its sensitivity is not very high.

Spinal cord involvement is seen in approximately 10% of patients with NS, resulting in both parenchymal and meningoradicular forms.[93,94] The spinal involvement in NS is discussed later in this article.

The presence of peripheral lymphadenopathy and bilateral hilar lymph nodes on chest radiograph/chest computed tomography (CT), presence of panuveitis, other systemic manifestations of sarcoidosis, cranial neuropathies, (diffuse) meningeal enhancement, persistence of enhancement in parenchymal lesions, and, finally, pathologic examination of the noncaseating granulomatous lesions of sarcoidosis, will help in the differential diagnosis.[92,94]

Infectious diseases that may mimic multiple sclerosis

There are several infectious diseases in which either at onset or during the course of the disease there may be CNS involvement and multiple MRI white and gray matter lesions. But in most, the systemic symptoms and signs of the infection are expected to be present and the characteristics of CNS lesions are less likely to mimic MS. However, in a few such cases the clinician may remain puzzled! Lyme disease is commonly included in the differential of MS, but its probability to mimic MS is extremely low.[9] Both tuberculosis and varicella-zoster virus (VZV) can cause a granulomatous angiitis and therefore when involving the CNS may resemble MS. However, the major diagnostic confusion for tuberculosis involving CNS will be neurosarcoidosis rather than MS. The main neurologic syndromes related to primary acute varicella infections are encephalitis (VZV vasculopathy), acute cerebellar ataxia, myelitis, and meningitis, but none is likely to mimic MS and besides the VZV rash is expected to precede the neurologic complication of the infection in most. However, in some, the VZV vasculopathy, affecting the small (and large) vessels and mostly, but not exclusively in immunocompromised individuals may occur weeks to months after the zoster rash or even in the absence of it and therefore initially may create diagnostic problems.[95] The MRI abnormalities are multiple and likely to occur in both the gray and white matter and mainly at gray–white matter junctions and they may enhance.[95] However, even in the presence of confusing MRI findings, the encephalopathy and strokelike manifestations, as well as other neurologic features are not going to be suggestive of MS.

In rare instances, cerebral toxoplasmosis (neurotoxoplasmosis) mostly in relation to AIDS in the immunocompromised host may present with clinical and imaging findings mimicking MS or ADEM. Patients will often present with focal or multifocal CNS symptoms with severe headache and/or encephalopathy that may be confused with ADEM, but in a few with onset symptoms mimicking MS (**Fig. 8**). In MRI, the lesions of cerebral toxoplasmosis are hyperintense on T2/FLAIR images and hypointense on T1 images, often show ring-enhancement with perilesional edema.[96] They are likely to be in the juxta-cortical region and also frequently in the basal ganglia, but once the "eccentric target sign" is observed, it is highly suggestive of cerebral toxoplasmosis.[97] This lesion pattern is characterized by a ring-shaped zone of peripheral enhancement with a small eccentric nodule along the wall. Once it is seen, the diagnosis can be made easily.

In any patient who presents with multiple and small lesions with or without perilesional edema, scattered in the white matter and mainly at the white-gray matter junction and who also have leptomeningeal nodular enhancement, the probability of an infectious disorder (ie, CNS cryptococcosis) along with metastatic malignancies should be considered.

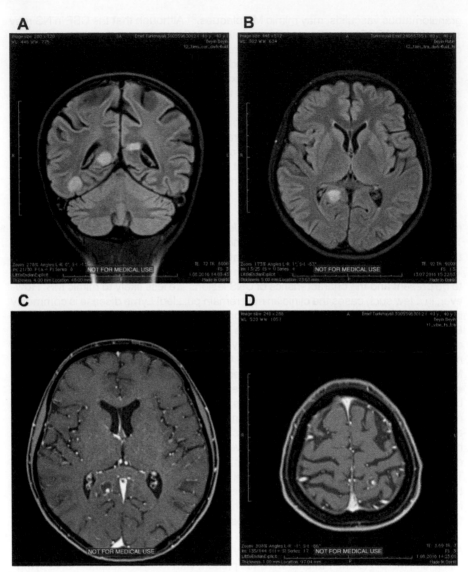

Fig. 8. (*A–D*) A young woman presenting with optic neuritis, multiple lesions, and disclosing multiple lesions with target sign. A 42-year-old woman develops visual loss on the right. Her MRI shows a longitudinally extensive optic nerve enhancement extending to the chiasma and multiple subcortical, periventricular, and juxtacortical lesions, as well as a central midbrain lesion. All lesions enhance simultaneously and most show the eccentric target sign (*C, D*) suggestive of cerebral toxoplasmosis. Her HIV test was positive.

Solitary or multifocal ring-enhancing lesions also may be seen in patients with CNS lymphoma, whether the abnormality is due to the infiltration of the lymphoma or an opportunistic infection in the setting of immunodeficiency is within the diagnostic spectrum to be considered in these patients. However, although not common such a patient, in the absence of other symptoms may present with some CNS symptoms and MRI that may include MS in the differential. Several clinical or imaging pitfalls will be expected in most of these individuals suggesting that not MS, but another diagnosis is more likely (**Fig. 9**).

Erdheim-Chester disease is a rare, non-Langerhans form of histiocytosis of unknown etiology that affects multiple organs. Approximately one-third have neurologic

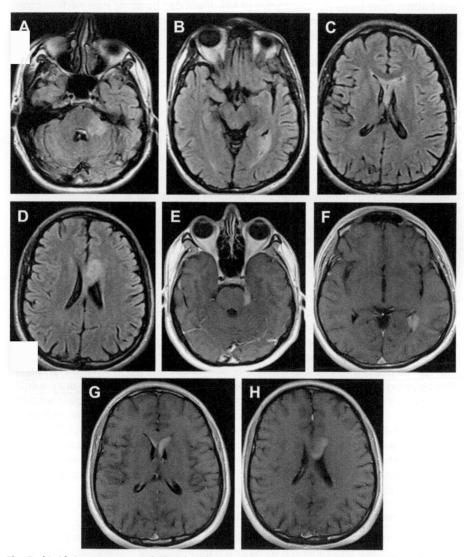

Fig. 9. (*A–H*) A young man admitted with neurologic symptoms and multiple brain lesions–biopsy-proven lymphoma. A 33-year-old man with a history of psoriasis after gradual onset of right hearing loss over 2 weeks followed by left facial numbness. His CSF study show no cells but a slightly elevated protein and positive OCB bands at pattern IV (similar bands both in serum/CSF). His MRI study shows multiple brainstem and periventricular lesions that all enhance. Extra-axial cranial nerve enhancement and intra-axial periventricular ependymal enhancement are all suggestive of infiltration (*E–H*). A brain biopsy reveals diffuse large cell–B-cell lymphoma. (*Courtesy of* Sabahattin Saip, Istanbul, Turkey.)

involvement with a wide range of neurologic manifestations with cerebellar and pyramidal syndromes being the most common ones, to be followed by seizures, headaches, and cranial nerve, neuropsychiatric, and neurocognitive symptoms.[98] Bone pain with other skeletal symptoms and diabetes insipidus are common. Although the MRI findings are more likely to show an infiltrative pattern with widespread lesions, nodules, or masses within the brainstem, cerebellum, and cerebrum, and/or a meningeal pattern most times not suggestive of MS, there can be some intermediate cases in whom both the clinical and imaging findings may mimic MS and therefore should be included in its differential diagnosis.[98,99]

Multiple Small/Punctate Enhancing Brain Lesions

There are several disorders of which the patients present with MS-like symptoms and an MRI showing a variety of lesions including multiple punctate enhancing lesions resulting in a diagnostic challenge. Such multiple punctate enhancing lesions are not expected in MS, although exceptions can occur. This type of lesion is more likely to be seen in cases of CNS vasculitis, neurosarcoidosis, CNS lymphoma, and chronic lymphocytic inflammation with pontine perivascular enhancement responsive to steroids (CLIPPERS).

Chronic lymphocytic inflammation with pontine perivascular enhancement responsive to steroids

CLIPPERS syndrome has been described as an inflammatory disorder of uncertain etiology with the characteristic imaging pattern of punctate and curvilinear-nodular enhancement peppering the pons with variable involvement of other infratentorial structures, spinal cord, basal ganglia, and corpus callosum whereby a subtler radiating pattern of similar enhancing lesions may be seen as well.[100] Clinically, these patients present with gait ataxia, diplopia, dysarthria, and also may have nonspecific dizziness, nausea, dysgeusia, pseudobulbar affect, tremor, nystagmus, paraparesis, sensory loss, and spasticity.[100] There are no systemic symptoms and the CSF will show the presence of pleocytosis, elevated CSF IgG, and OCBs suggestive of an autoimmune-inflammatory process. The rapid improvement in a patient's clinical course and imaging findings within a few weeks with glucocorticoid therapy and the likelihood of a relapse after stopping steroids confirms the diagnosis. Whether CLIPPERS is an unique entity or an unique expression of several autoimmune disorders or CNS lymphoma is not clear, despite that a recent neuropathologic study did not find an association with either.[101] Because MS-like lesions may be seen along with the typical lesions of CLIPPERS and an overlap with the anti–myelin oligodendrocyte glycoprotein (MOG) phenotype of NMOSD in a patient and similar imaging findings in another patient with a definite diagnosis of relapsing-remitting MS have been described, this relatively newly defined disorder needs to be included in the differential diagnosis of MS.[102,103]

Single Lesions Suggestive of Demyelinating-Inflammatory Disease

When a patient presents with a self-limited CNS neurologic episode or a progressive neurologic disease and turns out to have a nontumefactive solitary CNS lesion, the differential diagnosis may not be so easy. Depending on the clinical symptomatology and the site and type of the lesion in patients presenting with self-limited neurologic episodes, in most the clinical diagnosis will be "CIS" and its differential workup will suffice. Some of them may remain with this single lesion and a single episode, but many will develop further MRI lesions with or without further clinical episodes fulfilling a diagnosis of MS, or will develop other diseases.[21,26] However, when the neurologic symptoms and signs are progressive in patients with solitary lesions, the first probability would be still to rule out a tumor, despite not having tumefactive features, which is a difficult task. The differential will include, mostly, primary and, less, secondary neoplasia. Other probabilities are many and include a wide variety of inflammatory, autoimmune, metabolic, and infectious disorders. Once a workup for a systemic disease is done and such a probability is ruled out to a certain extent, a trial of pulse steroids may be tried and the clinical and imaging response may be monitored to further narrow the diagnostic probabilities. However, depending on the individual features of the patient and the clinical and MRI findings, a biopsy may be necessary in some.

Solitary demyelinating lesions that may produce a progressive myelopathy similar to primary progressive MS have been described and called "solitary sclerosis," with the lesion being in the upper cervical cord, cervico-medullary junction brainstem, or cerebral white matter.[104–107] These patients do not go on to develop other CNS lesions but show a clinical course consistent with PPMS, despite that they do not fulfill the diagnostic criteria for MS, suggesting that "solitary sclerosis" may be a focal form or subtype of MS. So "solitary sclerosis" should be included in the differential diagnosis of progressive myelopathies and other CNS progressive motor impairment for more than 1 year in patients with a single radiologically identified CNS demyelinating lesion along corticospinal tracts despite absence of DIS.[107]

ATYPICAL INFLAMMATORY-DEMYELINATING–LIKE LESIONS AND ATYPICAL INFLAMMATORY-DEMYELINATING SYNDROMES

Not uncommonly, there are patients who present with subacute onset of CNS symptoms suggestive but not always typical of MS or related disorders, and have atypical brain lesion/s that give the impression of being of inflammatory-demyelinating in nature, creating diagnostic challenges. Besides, a subgroup may have infiltrative type lesions difficult to rule out inflammatory disorders. Some of such cases turn out to have in fact MS, but most are MS variants, such as Baló concentric sclerosis (BCS), tumefactive MS, or non-MS inflammatory-demyelinating disorders such as ADEM, some belonging to the autoimmune astrocytopathies such as NMOSD, or MOG-antibody (MOG-Ab)–related oligodendrocytopathies, or related to a number of other autoimmune CNS diseases.[15,108,109] Besides, there will be some non–inflammatory-demyelinating diseases that their imaging findings may mimic MS or related disorders.

Clinically, the previously mentioned "atypical inflammatory-demyelinating syndromes" are rare disorders that differ from MS, due to their unusual clinical or imaging findings or poor response to MS treatments[15] (Box 10). Radiologically, despite that the definition of "atypical inflammatory-demyelinating lesion" is not clear, the current description for such an appearance includes lesions that have an unusual size (large with mass effect), unusual morphology (irregular appearance, indistinct borders, marked heterogeneity within a lesion), an intriguing pattern of contrast uptake of lesions, or other unusual features.[108]

BCS is considered to be a primary inflammatory CNS demyelinating disease that is a variant of MS having distinct imaging and pathologic features. Its lesions are characterized by alternating rings of demyelinated and myelinated (or partially demyelinated or intact) axons, resulting in concentrically multilayered ringlike lesions usually in the cerebral white matter, giving the so-called onion-bulb appearance.[110,111] Gadolinium enhancement is more likely to occur at the periphery, but occasionally enhancement of multiple layers also may be observed. Lesions of BCS may be either isolated or multiple, and many times are seen with other MS-suggestive lesions. The lesions of BCS may look like tumefactive lesions, but their concentric pattern will be

> **Box 10**
> **When to suspect atypical demyelinating syndromes, inflammatory astrocytopathies, or other diseases mimicking MS?**
>
> *In patients who present with the following:*
>
> - An atypical syndrome
>
> - Atypical MRI findings (eg, one large presumed demyelinating MRI lesion; a longitudinally extensive optic nerve, corpus callosum, or spinal lesions; or multiple demyelinatinglike lesions showing simultaneous gadolinium enhancement)
>
> - A typical syndrome with atypical MRI findings or an atypical syndrome with typical MRI findings!
>
> - An atypical course (eg, rapid and severe clinical deterioration)
>
> - Patients not responding or deteriorating following effective MS treatment
>
> *Adapted from* Hardy TA, Reddel SW, Barnett MB, et al. Atypical inflammatory demyelinating syndromes of the CNS. Lancet Neurol 2016;15:967–81; with permission.

diagnostic. Tumefactive demyelinization and other tumefactive lesions have been discussed previously.

Patients with NMOSD who have the "typically" longitudinally extensive spinal or optic nerve lesions, or corpus callosum involvement are discussed elsewhere in the text. However, after the definition of the AQP4 antibodies, several new clinical forms of NMOSD have been described, with some showing cerebral or brainstem atypical inflammatory-demyelinating lesions consistent with the previous description of atypical lesions.[112] Therefore, the clinician who sees patients with atypical brain/brainstem lesions, some of which are now described as being typical for NMOSDs (such as the diencephalic lesions) with symptomatic narcolepsy or acute diencephalic clinical syndromes, several cerebral syndromes, or with a variety of brainstem syndromes, should suspect NMOSD and look for the antibody.[112–114] If the antibody testing is not available or comes as negative, the probability of NMOSD still should be kept in mind.

It is now well known that in some of the patients with NMOSD-suggestive clinical and imaging findings who are seronegative for AQP4-Ab turn out to have serum antibodies directed against MOG-Ab. Adults with MOG-Ab–positive disease frequently have fluffy brainstem lesions, often located in the pons and/or adjacent to the fourth ventricle, have 3 or fewer lesions, and they are not likely to show ovoid lesions adjacent to the body of lateral ventricles, Dawson fingers, and T1-hypointense lesions that are more suggestive of MS, all imaging features helping to discriminate MOG-Ab disorder from MS.[115] The MOG-Ab longitudinally extensive transvers myelitis (LETM) cases are discussed later in this article.

Then there will be a few patients with other autoimmune CNS diseases who are positive for N-methyl-D-aspartate (NMDA) receptor or other antibodies, but because their clinical features commonly include cognitive, behavioral, and other psychiatric as well as extrapyramidal symptoms, they are not likely to be confused with MS.

PATIENTS PRESENTING WITH SPINAL CORD LESION/S SUGGESTIVE OF INFLAMMATORY-DEMYELINATIVE NATURE: IS IT MULTIPLE SCLEROSIS OR SOMETHING ELSE?

In patients who initially present with recent-onset spinal cord symptoms and parenchymal (intra-axial) spinal MRI abnormalities suggestive of an inflammatory pathology, the clinical and imaging features may provide some clues as to whether it is MS, another inflammatory-demyelinative disease, or something else. There are several questions to be addressed at the beginning regarding the imaging findings, such as the following: is this a solitary lesion or are there other similar spinal cord and/or brain lesions; is the length of the lesion a "short-segment spinal cord lesion" (involving <3 vertebral segments) or a "longitudinally extensive spinal cord lesion" (involving more than 3 vertebral segments) (**Box 11**); which spinal region is involved and what is the anatomic distribution of the lesion; is there mass effect and edema; is the lesion enhancing and if yes, what is the pattern of enhancement; and are there abnormal vascular structures associated with the lesion? Answers to each of these questions should be combined with the demographic and clinical characteristics of the patient and be supported with the CSF findings unless there is a contraindication to perform a spinal tap or the diagnosis is obvious, not necessitating further information.

The Differential Diagnosis of Short Spinal Lesions Suggestive of Multiple Sclerosis

When the spinal cord lesion is solitary, not extending more than 1 or 2 vertebral segments (short-segment spinal lesion), is peripherally located within the cord in a young individual in whom there is a subacute onset of spinal cord sensory symptoms such as numbness and a tingling sensation in the lower extremities, preceded by an upper respiratory tract or other infection, the most likely diagnosis will be isolated myelitis/CIS. These lesions commonly will show enhancement in an open ringlike or nodular pattern during the acute episode. In most of such cases, the neurologic examination will not disclose severe neurologic deficits and the patient may later develop Lhermitte phenomenon. Whether this will remain as a single event or is it the first attack of MS is difficult to say, and after a systemic disease or infection is ruled out by laboratory studies and a CSF study, no further diagnostic studies may be required. Such patients are to be followed clinically and by MRI. In people who recall earlier CNS neurologic

---

Box 11

The diagnostic possibilities in an individual with asymptomatic or recent-onset spinal cord symptoms and parenchymal spinal MRI abnormalities suggestive of inflammatory pathology

When it is a "short-segment spinal cord lesion" [fewer than 3 vertebral segments]
- Radiologically isolated syndromes (as incidental findings/asymptomatic)
- MS-myelitis
- Transverse myelitis (idiopathic inflammatory-demyelinative)
- Short-segment or recovering NMO/NMOSD: myelitis
- Myelitis associated with systemic vasculitic or collagen tissue disorders
- Tumors (ie, astrocytoma; ependymoma)
- Infectious disorders

When it is a "longitudinally extensive spinal cord lesion" [more than 3 vertebral segments]
- NMO/NMOSD: myelitis
- Transverse myelitis
- MS: multiple short-segment lesions in contiguity suggestive of a single longitudinally extensive transvers myelitis lesion
- Myelitis associated with systemic vasculitides and collagen tissue disorders (AQP4-Ab negative)
- Metabolic-toxic myelopathies (B12, Copper; alpha-tocopherol deficiencies)
- Granulomatous disorders (ie, sarcoidosis)
- Myelopathy associated with spinal venous dural fistula or other vascular malformations
- Tumors (ie, astrocytoma; ependymoma)
- Infectious disorders (ie, viral, tuberculosis, Lyme)

episodes consistent with MS, or already have a confirmed diagnosis of it, then the diagnosis is easily made to be MS-associated myelitis.

Most MS lesions occur in the cervical spinal cord region, some in the dorsal region and fewer in the caudal cord, predominantly in the dorsal and lateral columns and are peripherally located[116] (**Fig. 10**). The lesions are usually longitudinally oriented and their length as already mentioned do not extend 1 or 2 spinal segments and their width not more than half the diameter of the cord. The MS lesions are asymmetrically distributed within the cord and along the gray and white matters. Acute lesions may cause focal swelling of the cord with gadolinium enhancement.

In a patient presenting with symptoms consistent with partial myelopathy and showing multiple small (short-segment) asymptomatic spinal cord lesions other than the symptomatic one, as well some brain lesions fulfilling the DIS criteria of MS and a CSF study showing increased IgG production and/or OCBs, the diagnosis of MS is not much a challenge. However, this is not always the case, and there will be

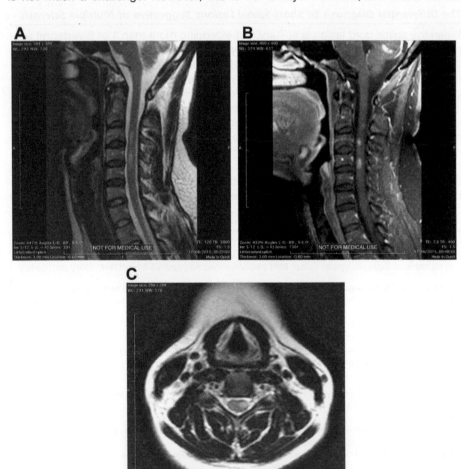

Fig. 10. (A–C) Spinal cord involvement in MS. One-segment to 2-segments-long short spinal cord–enhancing lesions, consistent with MS (A, B). Axial images show the peripherally located and small size lesion consistent with MS (C).

many patients in whom the findings will not be so clear cut and will present a diagnostic problem. In some patients, it may be difficult to differentiate from a short-length low-grade spinal cord tumor, such as an ependymoma or astrocytoma from a solitary spinal demyelinating-inflammatory lesion. Many times, neither the clinical symptomatology nor the CSF or any other laboratory study may add much to the differential diagnosis and initially a biopsy from a cord lesion unless critical is not a very desirable procedure. A therapeutic trial with high-dose intravenous methyl prednisolone and an MRI follow-up may be more informative in such cases. However, these tumors are likely to extend over many segments and are further discussed later.

One other probability to keep in mind is that in patients who present with short transverse myelitis, this can be the initial event of NMOSD. It was shown that in approximately 15% of the initial myelitis episodes of NMOSD, the length of the lesions was radiologically less than 3 vertebral segments.[117,118] This probability warrants the consideration of AQP4-IgG testing for cases with short transverse myelitis, mainly when they are centrally located and in whom there are no other clinical and imaging features consistent with MS.

Solitary and short-segment involvement of the spinal cord in infections, in vasculitic conditions, in hematologic and solid malignancies are rare, but despite their low probability should be kept in mind. There are also a large number of infectious agents that may cause both acute and chronic transverse myelitis with imaging appearance sometimes difficult to distinguish from MS (or NMOSD); however, they are not common and the clinical findings of fever, malaise, leukocytosis, and pain, as well as CSF findings and in some, the geographic background of the patient, are important in suspecting such a diagnosis.

The Differential Diagnosis of Long Spinal Lesions

The next diagnostic challenge is when a patient presents with a long spinal cord lesion extending over many vertebral segments (3 or more), which by definition is LETM. Currently, NMOSD is the first diagnostic probability to be considered when such lesions are detected on MRI. The clinical symptomatology may include sensory symptoms, such as numbness or a tingling sensation, which at times may be disturbing with allodynia: and/or motor symptoms that consist of a spastic paraparesis, tonic spasms, and bladder dysfunction. When these spinal cord symptoms develop acutely or subacutely, LETM due to neuromyelitis optica spectrum disorders (NMOD), other autoimmune, metabolic, vascular, and infectious myelopathies all are to be included in the differential.

LETM is the classic presentation of NMOSD and usually extends over 3 or more vertebral segments and affects the central cord. Spinal cord swelling is common, and the common form of gadolinium enhancement is longitudinally extensive or patchy and discontinuous, and may have a ringlike enhancement in some.[119] Lesions in the cervical cord may extend toward the area postrema but this is not specific for NMOSD.[119] Brighter T2-hyperintense spotty lesions (T1W-hypo) within the spinal cord lesion has been described for NMO and may help to differentiate it from MS[120] (Fig. 11). After the acute attack is treated, lesions tend to resolve with some residual T2-signal abnormalities and result in focal or longitudinally extensive atrophy. When such patients are AQP4-IgG seropositive, the diagnosis does not require much! However, despite being highly suggestive of NMOSD, there will be some patients who are AQP4-IgG seronegative, and if there is availability for testing serum antibodies directed against MOG in such cases, this may yield a small subgroup of patients with MOG related LETM. The MOG-positive cases have somewhat different imaging characteristics from NMO, as they show more deep gray matter and lower cord and conus involvement,[121] as well as presenting with short spinal lesions in approximately 40%.[122]

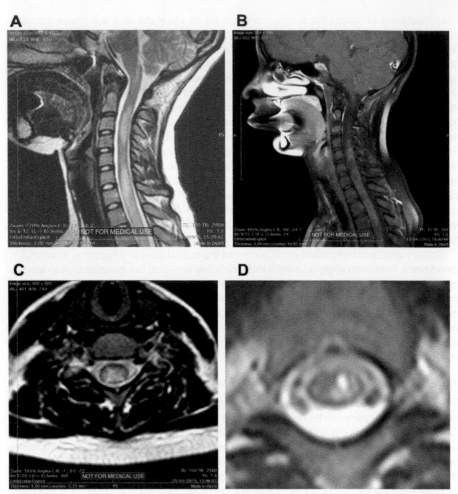

Fig. 11. (*A–D*) A patient with NMOSD presenting with LETM. An 18-year-old student develops intractable hiccups, nausea, and vomiting 6 weeks earlier that continues for approximately 3 weeks. No diagnosis is made and she is discharged from the hospital with partial improvement only to develop severe numbness and weakness below the neck. She is admitted to a neurology clinic where a diagnosis of NMOSD is made. Her MRI shows a heterogeneous long spinal cord lesion that enhances and a swollen cord (*A, B*). A (probably improved) lesion at the area postrema can be seen. Axial images show almost a holocord pattern of involvement (*C*) and a bright spotty lesion in the lower part of the lesion (*D*).

Sometimes confluent MS lesions in the spinal cord may give the appearance of a longitudinal cord lesion. However, axial scans will display the patchy distribution and peripheral localization of lesions, and although in a few patients such an image maybe seen at the time of the diagnosis, clinically most of them will have a relatively long history consistent with MS. Besides, long myelitis also has been reported in patients with conventional MS mimicking NMOSD, with most of such lesions being no longer than 3 to 4 segments and mostly localized within the lower cervical cord.[123,124]

Myelopathy associated with a longitudinally extensive spinal cord lesion has been reported to be the initial or sole clinical feature of sarcoidosis,[93,125] and in our practice, we also had a similar experience. The spinal cord involvement commonly is seen in both cervical and thoracic regions, followed by either of the thoracic or cervical regions according to the series reported.[93,94,125] The lesions are placed peripherally, been mostly in the dorsal part of the cord extending laterally at times as a crescent, but also can be in the anterior of the cord. Long linear subpial enhancement, and persistence of enhancement for many months or even up to a year despite pulse and/or oral corticosteroid treatment, is highly suggestive of spinal cord sarcoidosis (SCS), whereas a spinal cord ring-enhancement is seen in approximately one-third of NMOSD myelitis episodes and distinguishes it from SCS and other causes of longitudinally extensive myelopathies with the exception of MS.[125] Recently, central canal enhancement alone or in combination with dorsal-subpial enhancement resembling a trident head on axial sequences for SCS has been reported[126] (**Fig. 12**). An elevated ACE-level, hilar adenopathy shown by chest CT (or PET) followed by the pathologic verification of sarcoidosis through biopsy from an accessible lesion will confirm the diagnosis.[92]

Subacute combined degeneration of the spinal cord due to vitamin B12 (cobalamin) deficiency can result in symmetric high T2 signal in the posterior and lateral columns of the spinal cord, mainly of the cervical and upper thoracic segments and unlikely to enhance.[127] An inverted V-shape of affected areas of the dorsal spinal cord also has been reported in some cases[127] (**Fig. 13**). Rarely, early on in the disease process there may be cord swelling. A similar type of myelopathy with involvement of the dorsal column and corticospinal tracts also may be seen in copper deficiency myelopathy (CDM).[127–129] CDM most frequently presents in the fifth and sixth decades, is more common in women, with most cases developing as a neurologic complication of bariatric surgery, and MRI being abnormal in approximately half of the cases.[127,128] Finally, α-Tocopherol deficiency and some other metabolic-toxic myelopathies may disclose similar spinal MRI findings.[127]

Spinal cord dural arteriovenous fistulae are rare spinal arteriovenous malformations that can cause centromedullary high T2 signal, attributed to venous congestion, over multiple segments that can be accompanied by a hypointense rim. Because most of these patients will present with a progressive spastic paraparesis and gait disorder with other cord symptoms and a spinal cord image suggestive of an inflammatory-demyelinating lesion, they may mimic PPMS! But, a careful eye will recognize the draining dilated intramedullary and mostly the perimedullary veins as tortuous hypointense vascular structures surrounded by the high signal of the CSF on T2WIs[130] (**Fig. 14**).

Spinal cord primary tumors, mostly of higher grade, also can present with an image consistent with LETM, the cord may be swollen and the lesion might show a heterogeneous density with different patterns of enhancement, none of which are specific and therefore not helpful in differentiating a tumor from LETM or other cord pathologies. A trial of steroids and serial MRI follow-up is the common practice, with a spinal cord biopsy being the confirmatory diagnostic procedure when found necessary on individual basis. However, there are a few features that favor the probability of a tumor, such as the presence of intratumoral and/or juxtatumoral cysts, an associated syrinx, intralesional hemorrhages (more common with ependymomas than astrocytomas) and the so-called "cap sign" with a T2-hyopintense hemosiderin rim that is typical of an ependymoma.[131,132]

PROGRESSIVE CENTRAL NERVOUS SYSTEM SYMPTOMS MIMICKING MULTIPLE SCLEROSIS: THE VALUE OF NEGATIVE LABORATORY AND IMAGING FINDINGS

Several neurologic disorders that present with slowly progressive CNS symptoms, such as a progressive spastic paraparesis or spinocerebellar ataxia, may cause

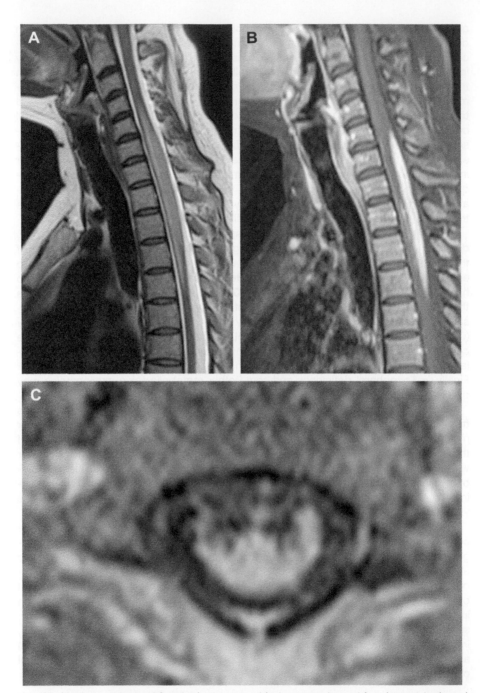

Fig. 12. (*A–C*) A patient with spinal neurosarcoidosis presenting with a long spinal cord lesion that continues to enhance over many months: a 52-year-old woman without any significant past medical history is admitted because of recent-onset disturbing paresthesias and mild weakness of lower extremities. Her spinal cord MRI shows a posteriorly located longitudinal lesion that enhances (*A, B*). Axial T1 gadolinium images disclose the so-called trident head sign (*C*).

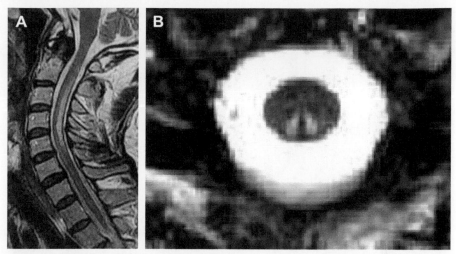

Fig. 13. (*A, B*) A patient with cobalamin deficiency presenting with a long spinal cord lesion and inverted V-shape pattern on axial images (*B*).

diagnostic uncertainties whether they are PPMS or something else. In such cases, the value of a negative workup that includes a normal CSF study and an MRI that does not show either cranial or spinal MS-consistent lesions will be supportive to rule out the possibility of MS. Hereditary spastic paraparesis and some types of spinocerebellar ataxias (SCAs) are such disorders that initially may result in some clinical difficulties, especially in the absence of a positive family history. However, the CSF will be normal and an MRI study of the brain and spine will be either normal or not reveal any lesion consistent with MS, with the exception of some localized atrophic changes in SCAs. Besides, in many, genetic testing will confirm the diagnosis. Primary lateral sclerosis is another disorder with progressive bilateral corticospinal tract involvement, but despite the progressive nature of the spastic paraparesis, there will be no bladder and sensory problems in addition to negative CSF, MRI, and visual evoked potentials (VEP) studies. However, in some patients later in the disease process, spinal cord imaging may show a nonspecific spinal cord atrophy and some signal hyperintensity on T2WIs, reflecting degeneration of pyramidal tracts with secondary demyelination.[127]

Compressive myelopathy due to cervical spondylotic myelopathy, mainly in the absence of disc herniation and cervical radiculopathy, also may cause a diagnostic problem, as the onset of symptoms, which includes corticospinal symptoms and signs with accompanying sensory and bladder dysfunction, are gradual and painless. The presence of myelopathic changes on MRI may further complicate the diagnosis, but the real challenge is when a patient has both MS and compressive myelopathy secondary to cervical spondylotic disease. In such patients, the patient needs to be studied in detail and decompressive surgery may be considered if found appropriate.

A FEW FINAL CLUES IN THE DIFFERENTIAL DIAGNOSIS OF MULTIPLE SCLEROSIS

As a clinician, in patients who we workup for the possibility of having MS or who were admitted with such a probable diagnosis, when the CSF is normal and does not show increased IgG and/or presence of OCBs, we need to think twice about the diagnosis; if the cranial and spinal MRIs are completely normal, then we need to think thrice; and when both the CSF and MRI are normal, the patent is likely not to have MS. On the

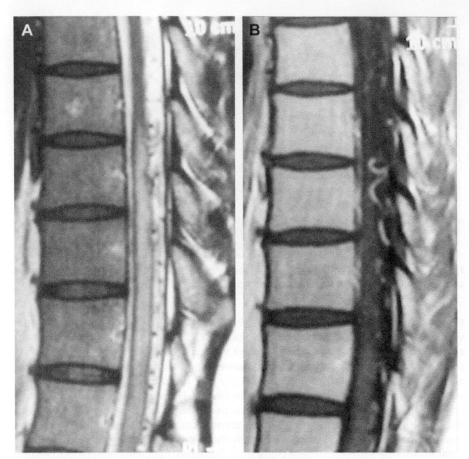

Fig. 14. (*A, B*) Spinal cord dural arteriovenous fistula. A 53-year-old man who presents with progressive spastic weakness of the legs and gait difficulty. He had received a diagnosis of MS 3 months previously and was put on long-term treatment with an MRI report of myelitis. However, the serpentlike draining dilated perimedullary veins, which also enhanced, were missed! His spinal angiography had confirmed spinal venous dural fistula and he was treated with embolization.

other hand, we should also keep in mind that an abnormal CSF or an abnormal MRI may not be always diagnostic.

SUMMARY: THE 2 SIDES OF THE COIN

Currently, as the incidence of MS increases, the number of misdiagnosed cases as MS (those who do not have the disease or have another disorder) and the patients who have the disease but are misdiagnosed for something else, is also arising. In a very recent national survey, conducted by The Health Union and named "MS in America 2017," including more than 5300 individuals diagnosed with MS, reveals that many people initially received an improper diagnosis.[133] Almost 50% of survey respondents reported having 5 or more office or hospital visits before obtaining their MS diagnosis, with most of them reported they were initially misdiagnosed with another condition, including depression (25%), migraine disease (15%), fibromyalgia (14%), psychiatric disorder (13%), B12 deficiency (11%), and chronic fatigue syndrome (10%). These diagnoses are quite interesting, because those are approximately the same diagnoses that were the "real" final diagnosis in patients initially misdiagnosed as having MS, of whom most had received unnecessary MS treatments! So, as physicians, we need to be highly alert and be aware of all clinical, laboratory, and imaging features and pitfalls that may assist us both in making a correct diagnosis or ruling out the possibility of an MS diagnosis. We also need to be extremely careful when we see a patient who already has received a diagnosis of MS, and first we should confirm that diagnosis ourselves, before proceeding further.

REFERENCES

1. Koch-Henriksen N, Sørensen PS. The changing demographic pattern of multiple sclerosis epidemiology. Lancet Neurol 2010;9(5):520–32.
2. Browne P, Chandraratna D, Angood C, et al. Atlas of multiple sclerosis 2013: a growing global problem with widespread inequity. Neurology 2014;83:1022–4.
3. Murray TJ, Murray SJ. Characteristics of patients found not to have multiple sclerosis. Can Med Assoc J 1984;131:336–7.
4. Carmosino MJ, Brousseau KM, Arciniegas DB, et al. Initial evaluations for multiple sclerosis in a university multiple sclerosis center. Arch Neurol 2005;62: 585–90.
5. Solomon AJ, Klein EP, Bourdette D. "Undiagnosing" multiple sclerosis: the challenge of misdiagnosis in MS. Neurology 2012;78:1986–91.
6. Solomon AJ, Bourdette DN, Cross AH, et al. The contemporary spectrum of multiple sclerosis misdiagnosis: a multicenter study. Neurology 2016;87:1393–9.
7. Solomon AJ, Weinshenker BG. Misdiagnosis of multiple sclerosis: frequency, causes, effects, and prevention. Curr Neurol Neurosci Rep 2013;13:403.
8. Toledano M, Weinshenker BG, Solomon AJ. A clinical approach to the differential diagnosis of multiple sclerosis. Curr Neurol Neurosci Rep 2015;15:57.
9. Rolak LA, Fleming JO. The differential diagnosis of multiple sclerosis. Neurologist 2007;13(2):57–72.
10. Levy DE. Transient CNS deficits: a common benign syndrome in young adults. Neurology 1988;28:831–6.
11. Miller DH, Weinshenker BG, Filippi M, et al. Differential diagnosis of suspected multiple sclerosis: a consensus approach. Mult Scler 2008;14:1157–74.
12. Rudick RA, Miller AE. Multiple sclerosis or multiple possibilities: the continuing problem of misdiagnosis [review]. Neurology 2012;78:1904–6.
13. Katz Sand IB, Lublin FD. Diagnosis and differential diagnosis of multiple sclerosis [review]. Continuum (Minneap Minn) 2013;19:922–43.
14. Weisfeld-Adams JD, Katz Sand IB, Honce JM, et al. Differential diagnosis of Mendelian and mitochondrial disorders in patients with suspected multiple sclerosis. Brain 2015;138:517–39.
15. Hardy TA, Reddel SW, Barnett MB, et al. Atypical inflammatory demyelinating syndromes of the CNS. Lancet Neurol 2016;15:967–81.
16. Rudick RA, Schiffer RB, Schwetz KM, et al. Multiple sclerosis: the problem of incorrect diagnosis [review]. Arch Neurol 1986;43:578–83.
17. Polman CH, Reingold SC, Banwell B, et al. Diagnostic criteria for multiple sclerosis: 2010 revisions to the McDonald criteria. Ann Neurol 2011;69:292–302.
18. Gastaldi M, Zardini E, Franciotta D. An update on the use of cerebrospinal fluid analysis as a diagnostic tool in multiple sclerosis. Expert Rev Mol Diagn 2016; 17(1):31–46.

19. Stangel M, Fredrikson S, Meinl E, et al. The utility of cerebrospinal fluid analysis in patients with multiple sclerosis. Nat Rev Neurol 2013;9(5):267–76.
20. Siva A. The spectrum of multiple sclerosis and treatment decisions. Clin Neurol Neurosurg 2006;108(3):333–8.
21. Chard DT, Dalton CM, Swanton J, et al. MRI only conversion to multiple sclerosis following a clinically isolated syndrome. J Neurol Neurosurg Psychiatry 2011;82: 176–9.
22. Waldman A, Ghezzi A, Bar-Or A, et al. Multiple sclerosis in children: an update on clinical diagnosis, therapeutic strategies, and research. Lancet Neurol 2014; 13(9):936–48.
23. Robertson NP, Fraser M, Deans J, et al. Age-adjusted recurrence risks for relatives of patients with multiple sclerosis. Brain 1996;119:449–555.
24. Bangham CR, Araujo A, Yamano Y, et al. HTLV-1-associated myelopathy/tropical spastic paraparesis. Nat Rev Dis Primers 2015;18(1):15012.
25. Siva A, Saip S. The spectrum of nervous system involvement in Behcet's syndrome and its differential diagnosis. J Neurol 2009;256(4):513–29.
26. Miller DH, Chard DT, Ciccarelli O. Clinically isolated syndromes. Lancet Neurol 2012;11(2):157–69.
27. Fisniku LK, Brex PA, Altmann DR, et al. Disability and T2 MRI lesions: a 20-year follow-up of patients with relapse onset of multiple sclerosis. Brain 2008;131: 808–17.
28. Tintore M, Rovira A, Rio J, et al. Defining high, medium and low impact prognostic factors for developing multiple sclerosis. Brain 2015;138:1863–74.
29. Barned S, Goodman AD, Mattson DH. Frequency of antinuclear antibodies in multiple sclerosis. Neurology 1995;45:384–9.
30. Cuadrad MJ, Khamasta MA, Ballesteros A, et al. Can neurologic manifestations of antiphospholipid syndrome be distinguished from multiple sclerosis? Medicine 2000;79:57–68.
31. Roussel V, Yi F, Jauberteau MO, et al. Prevalence and clinical significance of anti-phospholipid antibodies in multiple sclerosis: a study of 89 patients. J Autoimmun 2000;14:259–65.
32. Solomon AJ, Hills W, Chen Z, et al. Autoantibodies and Sjogren's Syndrome in multiple sclerosis, a reappraisal. PLoS One 2013;8(6):e65385.
33. Goodkin DE, Jacobsen DW, Galveze N, et al. Serum cobalamin deficiency is uncommon in multiple sclerosis. Arch Neurol 1994;41:1110–4.
34. Coyle PK, Krupp LB, Doscher C. Significance of a reactive Lyme serology in multiple sclerosis. Ann Neurol 1993;34:745–7.
35. Constantinescu CS, Goodman DBP, Grossman RI, et al. Serum angiotensin-converting enzyme in multiple sclerosis. Arch Neurol 1997;54(8):1012–5.
36. Haghighi S, Andersen O, Rosengren L, et al. Incidence of CSF abnormalities in siblings of multiple sclerosis patients and unrelated controls. J Neurol 2000;247: 616–22.
37. Deisenhammer F, Bartos A, Egg R, et al. Guidelines on routine cerebrospinal fluid analysis. Report from an EFNS task force. Eur J Neurol 2006;13:913–22.
38. Zettl UK, Tumani H. Multiple sclerosis & cerebrospinal fluid. Navarra (Spain): Blackwell Publishing Ltd; 2005. p. 1–116.
39. Miller JJ, Venna N, Siva A. Neuro-Behçet disease and autoinflammatory disorders. Semin Neurol 2014;34:437–43.
40. Filippi M, Rocca MA, Olga Ciccarelli O, et al. MRI criteria for the diagnosis of multiple sclerosis: MAGNIMS consensus guidelines. Lancet Neurol 2016;15: 292–303.

41. Rovira À, Wattjes MP, Tintore M, et al. Evidence-based guidelines: MAGNIMS consensus guidelines on the use of MRI in multiple sclerosis—clinical implementation in the diagnostic process. Nat Rev Neurol 2015;11:471–82.
42. Mistry N, Dixon J, Tallantyre E, et al. Central veins in brain lesions visualized with high-field magnetic resonance imaging: a pathologically specific diagnostic biomarker for inflammatory demyelination in the brain. JAMA Neurol 2013;70: 623–8.
43. Mistry N, Abdel-Fahim R, Samaraweera A, et al. Imaging central veins in brain lesions with 3-T T2*-weighted magnetic resonance imaging differentiates multiple sclerosis from microangiopathic brain lesions. Mult Scler 2016;22:1289–96.
44. Sati P, Oh J, Constable RT, et al. The central vein sign and its clinical evaluation for the diagnosis of multiple sclerosis: a consensus statement from the North American Imaging in Multiple Sclerosis Cooperative. Nat Rev Neurol 2016; 12(12):714–22.
45. Kruit MC, van Buchem MA, Launer LJ, et al. Migraine is associated with an increased risk of deep white matter lesions, subclinical posterior circulation infarcts and brain iron accumulation: the population-based MRI CAMERA study. Cephalalgia 2010;30(2):129–36.
46. Palm-Meinders IH, Koppen H, Terwindt GM, et al. Structural brain changes in migraine. JAMA 2012;308:1889–97.
47. Solomon AJ, Schindler KM, Howard DB, et al. "Central vessel sign" on 3T FLAIR* MRI for the differentiation of multiple sclerosis from migraine. Ann Clin Transl Neurol 2015;3(2):82–7.
48. Parikh S, Bernard G, Leventer RJ, et al. A clinical approach to the diagnosis of patients with leukodystrophies and genetic leukoencephelopathies. Mol Genet Metab 2015;114(4):501–15.
49. Vanderver A. Genetic leukoencephalopathies in adults. Continuum (Minneap Minn) 2016;22(3):916–42.
50. Schiffmann R, van der Knaap MS. Invited article: an MRI-based approach to the diagnosis of white matter disorders. Neurology 2009;72:750–9.
51. Aliaga ES, Barkhof F. MRI mimics of multiple sclerosis. In D.S. Goodin, Editor. Multiple Sclerosis and Related Disorders. Handb Clin Neurol 2014;122:291–316.
52. Chabriat H, Joutel A, Dichgans M, et al. CADASIL. Lancet Neurol 2009;8: 643–53.
53. Joshi S, Yau W, Kermode A. CADASIL mimicking multiple sclerosis: the importance of clinical and MRI red flags. J Clin Neurosci 2017;35:75–7.
54. Tikka S, Baumann M, Maija Siitonen M, et al. CADASIL and CARASIL. Brain Pathol 2014;24:525–44.
55. Bugiani M, Kevelam SH, Bakels HS, et al. Cathepsin A–related arteriopathy with strokes and leukoencephalopathy (CARASAL). Neurology 2016;87:1777–86.
56. Pilz YL, Bass SJ, Sherman J, et al. A review of mitochondrial optic neuropathies: from inherited to acquired forms. J Optom 2017;10(4):205–14.
57. Matthews L, Enzinger C, Fazekas F, et al. MRI in Leber's hereditary optic neuropathy: the relationship to multiple sclerosis. J Neurol Neurosurg Psychiatry 2015;86:537–42.
58. Harding AE, Sweeney MG, Miller DH, et al. Occurrence of a multiple sclerosis-like illness in women who have a Leber's hereditary optic neuropathy mitochondrial DNA mutation. Brain 1992;115(Pt 4):979–89.
59. Sadun AA, La Morgia C, Carelli V. Leber's hereditary optic neuropathy. Curr Treat Options Neurol 2017;13:109–17.

60. Schiffmann R. Fabry disease. In: Greenamyre JT, editor. MedLink neurology. San Diego (CA): MedLink Corporation; 2016. Available at: www.medlink.com.
61. Moore DF, Ye F, Schiffmann R, et al. Increased signal intensity in the pulvinar on T1-weighted images: a pathognomonic MR imaging sign of Fabry disease. AJNR Am J Neuroradiol 2003;24:1096–101.
62. Sarbu N, Shih RY, Jones RV, et al. White matter diseases with radiologic-pathologic correlation. Radiographics 2016;36(5):1426–47.
63. Rennebohm R, Susac JO, Egan RA, et al. Susac's syndrome–update. J Neurol Sci 2010;299(1–2):86–91.
64. Dörr J, Ringelstein M, Duning T, et al. Update on Susac syndrome: new insight in brain and retinal imaging and treatment options. J Alzheimers Dis 2014;42:S99–108.
65. Hua LH, Donlon S, Okuda DT. A case of Susac syndrome with cervical spinal cord involvement on MRI. J Neurol Sci 2014;337(1–2):228–31.
66. Wuerfel J, Sinnecker T, Ringelstein EB, et al. Lesion morphology at 7 Tesla MRI differentiates Susac syndrome from multiple sclerosis. Mult Scler 2012;18(11):1592–9.
67. Absinta M, Vuolo L, Rao A, et al. Gadolinium-based MRI characterization of leptomeningeal inflammation in multiple sclerosis. Neurology 2015;85(1):18–28.
68. Absinta M, Cortese ICM, Vuolo L, et al. Leptomeningeal gadolinium enhancement across the spectrum of chronic neuroinflammatory diseases. Neurology 2017;88:1439–44.
69. Engisch R, Titelbaum DS, Chilver-Stainer L, et al. Susac's syndrome: leptomeningeal enhancement on 3D FLAIR MRI. Mult Scler 2016;22(7):972–4.
70. Hillbom M, Saloheimo P, Fujioka S, et al. Diagnosis and management of Marchiafava-Bignami disease: a review Of CT/MRI confirmed cases. J Neurol Neurosurg Psychiatry 2014;85(2):168–73.
71. Friese SA, Bitzer M, Freudenstein D, et al. Classification of acquired lesions of the corpus callosum with MRI. Neuroradiology 2000;42(11):795–802.
72. Lucchinetti CF, Gavrilova RH, Metz I, et al. Clinical and radiographic spectrum of pathologically confirmed tumefactive multiple sclerosis. Brain 2008;131:1759–75.
73. Kilsdonk ID, Steenwijk MD, Pouwels PJ, et al. Perivascular spaces in MS patients at 7 Tesla MRI: a marker of neurodegeneration? Mult Scler 2015;21(2):155–62.
74. Altintas A, Petek B, Isik N, et al. Clinical and radiological characteristics of tumefactive demyelinating lesions: follow-up study. Mult Scler 2012;18(10):1448–53.
75. Kobayashi M, Shimizu Y, Shibata N, et al. Gadolinium enhancement patterns of tumefactive demyelinating lesions: correlations with brain biopsy findings and pathophysiology. J Neurol 2014;261:1902–10.
76. Frederick MC, Cameron MH. Tumefactive demyelinating lesions in multiple sclerosis and associated disorders. Curr Neurol Neurosci Rep 2016;16:26.
77. Abdoli M, Freedman MS. Neuro-oncology dilemma: tumour or tumefactive demyelinating lesion. Mult Scler Relat Disord 2015;4:555–66.
78. Siva A. Vasculitis of the nervous system. J Neurol 2001;248:451–68.
79. Salvarani C, Brown RD Jr, Calamia KT, et al. Primary central nervous system vasculitis: analysis of 101 patients. Ann Neurol 2007;62:442–51.
80. Powers WJ. Primary angiitis of the central nervous system: diagnostic criteria. Neurol Clin 2015;33(2):515–26.
81. Salvarani C, Brown RD Jr, Calamia KT, et al. Primary CNS vasculitis with spinal cord involvement. Neurology 2008;70:2394–400.

82. Wingerchuk DM, Lennon VA, Lucchinetti CF, et al. The spectrum of neuromyelitis optica. Lancet Neurol 2007;6:805–15.
83. Luyendijk J, Steens SC, Ouwendijk WJ, et al. Neuropsychiatric systemic lupus erythematosus: lessons learned from magnetic resonance imaging. Arthritis Rheum 2011;63(3):722–32.
84. Jeong HW, Her M, Bae JS, et al. Brain MRI in neuropsychiatric lupus: associations with the 1999 ACR case definitions. Rheumatol Int 2015;35(5):861–9.
85. Alkhawajah MM, Caminero AB, Freeman HJ, et al. Multiple sclerosis and inflammatory bowel diseases: what we know and what we would need to know! Mult Scler 2013;19(3):259–65.
86. Criteria for diagnosis of Behçet's disease. International Study Group for Behçet's disease. Lancet 1990;335:1078–80.
87. Siva A, Kantarci OH, Saip S, et al. Behçet's disease: diagnostic & prognostic aspects of neurological involvement. J Neurol 2001;248:95–103.
88. Kalra S, Silman A, Akman-Demir G, et al. Diagnosis and management of neuro-Behçet's disease: international consensus recommendations. J Neurol 2014; 261(9):1662–76.
89. Kocer N, Islak C, Siva A, et al. CNS involvement in neuro-Behcet's syndrome: an MR study. AJNR Am J Neuroradiol 1999;20:1015–24.
90. Uygunoglu U, Saip S, Siva A. Behcet's syndrome and nervous system involvement. In: Lisak RP, Truong DD, Carroll WM, et al, editors. International neurology. 2nd edition. Chichester, West Sussex, Hoboken, NJ: John Wiley & Sons, Ltd; 2016. p. 88–93. Chapter 28.
91. Uygunoglu U, Zeydan B, Ozguler Y, et al. Myelopathy in Behçet's disease: the bagel sign. Ann Neurol 2017. https://doi.org/10.1002/ana.25004.
92. Bagnato F, Stern BJ. Neurosarcoidosis: diagnosis, therapy and biomarkers. Expert Rev Neurother 2015;15(5):533–48.
93. Wegener S, Linnebank M, Martin R, et al. Clinically isolated neurosarcoidosis: a recommended diagnostic path. Eur Neurol 2015;73(1–2):71–7.
94. Agnihotri SP, Singhal T, Stern BJ, et al. Neurosarcoidosis. Semin Neurol 2014; 34(4):386–94.
95. Gilden D, Cohrs RJ, Mahalingam R, et al. Varicella zoster virus vasculopathies: diverse clinical manifestations, laboratory features, pathogenesis, and treatment. Lancet Neurol 2009;8:731–40.
96. Ramachandran TS. Cerebral toxoplasmosis. In: Greenamyre JT, editor. MedLink neurology. San Diego (CA): MedLink Corporation; 2015. Available at: www.medlink.com.
97. Kumar GG, Mahadevan A, Guruprasad AS, et al. Eccentric target sign in cerebral toxoplasmosis: neuropathological correlate to the imaging feature. J Magn Reson Imaging 2010;31(6):1469–72.
98. Lachenal F, Cotton F, Desmurs-Clavel H, et al. Neurological manifestations and neuroradiological presentation of Erdheim-Chester disease: report of 6 cases and systematic review of the literature. J Neurol 2006;253:1267–77.
99. Wright RA, Hermann RC, Parisi JE. Neurological manifestations of Erdheim-Chester disease. J Neurol Neurosurg Psychiatry 1999;66:72–5, 21.
100. Pittock SJ, Debruyne J, Krecke KN, et al. Chronic lymphocytic inflammation with pontine perivascular enhancement responsive to steroids (CLIPPERS). Brain 2010;133:2626–34.
101. Blaabjerg M, Ruprecht K, Sinnecker T, et al. Widespread inflammation in CLIPPERS syndrome indicated by autopsy and ultra-high-field 7T MRI. Neurol Neuroimmunol Neuroinflamm 2016;3(3):e226.

102. Ferreira RM, Machado G, Souza AS, et al. CLIPPERS-like MRI findings in a patient with multiple sclerosis. J Neurol Sci 2013;327(1–2):61–2.
103. Symmonds M, Waters PJ, Küker W, et al. Anti-MOG antibodies with longitudinally extensive transverse myelitis preceded by CLIPPERS. Neurology 2015; 84(11):1177–9.
104. Schmalstieg WF, Keegan BM, Weinshenker BG. Solitary sclerosis: progressive myelopathy from solitary demyelinating lesion. Neurology 2012;78:540–4.
105. Lattanzi S, Logullo F, Di Bella P, et al. Multiple sclerosis, solitary sclerosis or something else? Mult Scler 2014;20:1819–24.
106. Cohen M, Lebrun C, Ayrignac X, et al. Solitary sclerosis: experience from three French tertiary care centres. Mult Scler 2015;21:1216.
107. Keegan BM, Kaufmann TJ, Weinshenker BG, et al. Progressive solitary sclerosis: gradual motor impairment from a single CNS demyelinating lesion. Neurology 2016;87(16):1713–9.
108. Seewann A, Enzinger C, Filippi M, et al. MRI characteristics of atypical idiopathic inflammatory demyelinating lesions of the brain: a review of reported findings. J Neurol 2008;255(1):1–10.
109. Wallner-Blazek M, Alex Rovira A, Fillippi M, et al. Atypical idiopathic inflammatory demyelinating lesions: prognostic implications and relation to multiple sclerosis. J Neurol 2013;260:2016–22.
110. Karaarslan E, Altintas A, Senol U, et al. Baló's concentric sclerosis: clinical and radiologic features of five cases. AJNR Am J Neuroradiol 2001;22:1362–7.
111. Hardy TA, Miller DH. Baló's concentric sclerosis. Lancet Neurol 2014;13:740–6.
112. Pittock SJ, Lennon VA, Krecke K, et al. Brain abnormalities in neuromyelitis optica. Arch Neurol 2006;63:390–6.
113. Kremer L, Mealy M, Jacob A, et al. Brainstem manifestations in neuromyelitisoptica: a multicenter study of 258 patients. Mult Scler 2014;20:843–7.
114. Wingerchuk DM, Banwell B, Bennett JL, et al. International consensus diagnostic criteria for neuromyelitis optica spectrum disorders. Neurology 2015;85: 177–89.
115. Jurynczyk M, Geraldes R, Probert F, et al. Distinct brain imaging characteristics of autoantibody-mediated CNS conditions and multiple sclerosis. Brain 2017; 140(3):617–27.
116. Dekker I, Wattjes MP. Brain and spinal cord MR imaging features in multiple sclerosis and variants. Neuroimaging Clin N Am 2017;27(2):205–27.
117. Flanagan EP, Weinshenker BG, Krecke KN, et al. Short myelitis lesions in aquaporin-4-IgG-positive neuromyelitis optica spectrum disorders. JAMA Neurol 2015;72:81–7.
118. Huh SY, Kim SH, Hyun JW, et al. Short segment myelitis as a first manifestation of neuromyelitis optica spectrum disorders. Mult Scler 2017;23:413–9.
119. Flanagan EP, Weinshenker BG. Neuromyelitis optica spectrum disorders. Curr Neurol Neurosci Rep 2014;14(9):483.
120. Yonezu T, Ito S, Mori M, et al. 'Bright spotty lesions' on spinal magnetic resonance imaging differentiate neuromyelitis optica from multiple sclerosis. Mult Scler 2014;20:331–7.
121. Kitley J, Waters P, Woodhall M, et al. Neuromyelitis optica spectrum disorders with Aquaporin-4 and myelin-oligodendrocyte glycoprotein antibodies: a comparative study. JAMA Neurol 2014;71:276–83.
122. Jarius S, Ruprecht K, Kleiter I, et al. MOG-IgG in NMO and related disorders: a multicenter study of 50 patients. Part 2: epidemiology, clinical presentation,

radiological and laboratory features, treatment responses, and long-term outcome. J Neuroinflammation 2016;13:280.

123. Qiu W, Wu JS, Zhang MN, et al. Longitudinally extensive myelopathy in Caucasians: a West Australian study of 26 cases from the Perth Demyelinating Diseases Database. J Neurol Neurosurg Psychiatry 2010;81:209–12.

124. Whittam D, Bhojak M, Das K, et al. Longitudinally extensive myelitis in MS mimicking neuromyelitis optica. Neurol Neuroimmunol Neuroinflamm 2017;4: e333.

125. Flanagan EP, Kaufmann TJ, Krecke KN, et al. Discriminating long myelitis of neuromyelitis optica from sarcoidosis. Ann Neurol 2016;79(3):437–47, 18.

126. Zalewski NL, Krecke KN, Weinshenker BG, et al. Central canal enhancement and the trident sign in spinal cord sarcoidosis. Neurology 2016;87(7):743–4.

127. Hedera P. Hereditary and metabolic myelopathies. Handb Clin Neurol 2016;136: 769–85.

128. Kumar N, Ahlskog JE, Klein CJ, et al. Imaging features of copper deficiency myelopathy: a study of 25 cases. Neuroradiology 2006;48:78–83.

129. Jaiser SR, Winston GP. Copper deficiency myelopathy. J Neurol 2010;257(6): 869–81.

130. Saliou G, Krings T. Vascular diseases of the spine. Handb Clin Neurol 2016;136: 707–16.

131. Baruah D, Chandra T, Bajaj M, et al. A simplified algorithm for diagnosis of spinal cord lesions. Curr Probl Diagn Radiol 2015;44(3):256–66.

132. Pinter NK, Pfiffner TJ, Mechtler LL. Neuroimaging of spine tumors. Handb Clin Neurol 2016;136:689–706.

133. Available at: https://multiplesclerosisnewstoday.com/2017/05/01/survey-indicates-misdiagnosis-of-ms-and-ineffective-treatments-are common/. Accessed May 1, 2017.

New Concepts Related to Disease Appreciation in Multiple Sclerosis

Christina J. Azevedo, MD, MPH*, Amirhossein Jaberzadeh, PhD,
Daniel Pelletier, MD

KEYWORDS

- Multiple sclerosis • MRI • Neuroimaging • Central vein imaging • Cortical lesions
- Lesion probability mapping • Image subtraction • Brain volumetrics

KEY POINTS

- Central vein imaging, cortical lesion detection, and lesion probability mapping are emerging MRI techniques that have the potential to improve the accuracy of MRI in establishing a diagnosis of MS.
- Incorporating central vein imaging into clinical practice will require the adoption of a standardized and commercially available pulse sequence to detect central veins, a uniform definition of a central vein, and standard criteria to define the central vein sign as present or absent in an individual patient.
- Pulse sequences need to be optimized to ensure reliable detection of all cortical lesion types before incorporating cortical lesions into MS diagnostic criteria or clinical practice.
- The field needs to develop sophisticated image processing algorithms that are robust to large heterogeneity in MRI acquisition to derive useful information from the MRI scans that are collected in clinical practice.
- With some additional work, image subtraction and brain volumetrics are promising tools that could provide clinicians with quantitative metrics to monitor MS patients over time.

INTRODUCTION

In the past several decades, MRI has become an indispensable tool in the field of multiple sclerosis (MS) for clinicians and researchers alike. In addition to providing essential insights into MS pathophysiology, MRI plays an integral role in confirming

Disclosure Statement: Dr C.J. Azevedo has received consulting fees from Genzyme, Genentech, and Biogen. Dr D. Pelletier has received speaking and/or consulting fees from Novartis, Hoffman-La Roche, Sanofi Genzyme, and Vertex. Dr A. Jaberzadeh has nothing to disclose.
Department of Neurology, Keck School of Medicine, University of Southern California, 1540 Alcazar Street, Suite 206, Los Angeles, CA 90033, USA
* Corresponding author.
E-mail address: cazevedo@usc.edu

diagnosis of MS as well as monitoring disease activity and response to treatment once a diagnosis is established. The utility of MRI as a diagnostic and monitoring tool is due, in large part, to its high sensitivity to detect inflammatory demyelinating white matter lesions, which have long been considered the pathologic and imaging hallmark of MS.

The past several decades of progress notwithstanding, MS clinicians and researchers still face several challenges. Although MRI is highly sensitive to detect white matter lesions caused by MS, it is not wholly specific to MS; in other words, MRI is also highly sensitive to detect white matter lesions from other etiologies (eg, migraine or small vessel disease). Discriminating MS from other conditions is a challenge that is routinely faced by clinicians and is not addressed by current MRI criteria for MS. Moreover, once a diagnosis of MS has been established, clinicians lack standardized, quantitative methods to reliably measure changes in the disease over time, which may help guide treatment decisions.

This review highlights promising MRI and postprocessing techniques that have potential applications in these areas. With some further study, these tools could be usefully integrated into clinical care.

THE ROLE OF MRI IN ESTABLISHING A DIAGNOSIS OF MULTIPLE SCLEROSIS

MRI plays a fundamentally important role in establishing a diagnosis of MS. In the current version of the MS diagnostic criteria,[1] MRI can support, or even replace, clinical criteria for dissemination in space and time in patients with a clinical presentation suggestive of a demyelinating event. Dissemination in space can be demonstrated on MRI by the presence of greater than or equal to 1 T2 lesion in greater than or equal to 2 of 4 areas consistent with demyelination (periventricular, juxtacortical, infratentorial, and spinal cord). Dissemination in time can be satisfied by the simultaneous presence of asymptomatic gadolinium-enhancing and nonenhancing lesions at any time, or by a new T2 or gadolinium-enhancing lesion on any follow-up MRI. Compared with earlier versions of the MRI criteria,[2,3] the current version is simplified because it emphasizes lesion location rather than lesion counts, making it easier to apply in practice, and because it often allows a diagnosis of MS to be made with a single MRI scan rather than requiring a follow-up MRI after an arbitrary amount of time as in previous versions.[2,3]

When applied to patients who present with a clinical syndrome consistent with inflammatory demyelination of the central nervous system (CNS) (ie, optic neuritis, partial myelitis, or brainstem syndrome), the current version of the MRI criteria has been shown to have a sensitivity of 72% to 85% and a specificity of 67% to 92% to diagnose MS.[4–6] It has been emphasized that the MRI criteria are meant to be applied only in such patients with an appropriate clinical presentation,[1,7] and that they were not developed to differentiate MS from other conditions. The misinterpretation of MRI findings, including the inappropriate application of MRI criteria to patients with symptoms that are atypical or nonspecific for CNS demyelination, has been cited as a common cause of MS misdiagnosis,[8] an emerging area in the current MS literature. Cases in which white matter abnormalities are detected on an MRI that was obtained for atypical, nonspecific, or completely unrelated symptoms present a particular challenge for clinicians and highlight the need for advanced imaging techniques to be incorporated into clinical practice to aid the differentiation of inflammatory demyelination from other conditions. Central vein imaging, cortical demyelinating lesion detection, and lesion probability mapping are emerging MRI techniques that have the potential to improve the accuracy of MRI in establishing a diagnosis of MS.

Central Vein Imaging

In recent consensus statements, both the European Magnetic Resonance Imaging in MS research group and the North American Imaging in Multiple Sclerosis (NAIMS) Cooperative have suggested the central vein sign (CVS) as a potentially useful MRI marker that may improve the accuracy of MS diagnosis.[7,9] The observation that MS plaques tend to form around central blood vessels (small veins or venules) is a pathologic feature of the disease that was reported as early as the 1800s and can be observed in a majority of demyelinating white matter lesions yet remains poorly understood.[10]

It is possible to observe central veins in MS lesions in vivo using T2*-weighted MRI techniques.[11] T2*-weighted sequences take advantage of the magnetic field inhomogeneities from susceptibility differences among tissues, such as those caused by paramagnetic deoxyhemoglobin within veins. Deoxyhemoglobin disturbs the local magnetic field and causes faster T2* relaxation, resulting in a hypointense (dark) signal on T2*-weighted images.[11] The first in vivo observation of central veins within MS lesions was published in 2000 at 1.5T,[12] but they have also been demonstrated at 3T[13–15] and 7T[16–18] (Fig. 1). At 7T, several groups have shown that central veins are present in the majority (67%–80%) of white matter demyelinating lesions, in particular periventricular lesions,[12,17,19] but, strikingly, only in a minority (≤20%) of white matter lesions from other causes (migraine, small vessel disease, and so forth).[16–18] Although 7T is the most sensitive field strength to detect central veins,[20] detection rates of greater than 80% have been reported using optimized sequences at clinical field strengths (3T).[21] A standardized, commercially available imaging protocol or sequence to detect central veins is not yet adopted by the field, although recommendations toward this goal were recently proposed by the NAIMS Cooperative.[9]

A uniform radiological definition of a central vein has not been established but has been proposed.[9] An important task will be to establish criteria to classify the CVS as present or absent in an individual patient. The 40% rule has been proposed based on data suggesting that the presence of greater than 40% perivenous lesions is highly predictive of demyelinating disease,[22] with 100% positive and negative predictive value for a diagnosis of MS.[18] However, this approach requires counting all the lesions in the brain, which would be time consuming and impractical in patients with a high lesion burden, particularly in the clinical setting. Simpler criteria have, therefore, been proposed; in the same publication in which the 40% cutoff was originally tested, the investigators showed that if only 10 lesions per patient were sampled (in patients with ≥10 lesions), MS could be accurately discriminated from non-MS in 90% of

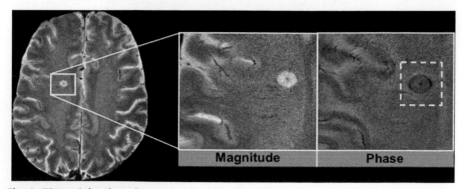

Fig. 1. T2*-weighted gradient-echo magnitude and phase images at 7T. A central vessel is visualized within the MS lesion (phase image [*dashed yellow box*]).

patients (44 of 45).[22] More recent data suggest that if 6 or more perivenous lesions are present or if fewer than 6 characteristic lesions are present but characteristic lesions outnumber nonperivenous lesions, the diagnosis is inflammatory demyelination; otherwise, inflammatory demyelination should not be diagnosed. This simple classification strategy was able to classify 20 MS/non-MS patients with 100% accuracy, in less than 2 minutes per case.[23]

The majority of studies evaluating the prevalence and diagnostic utility of the CVS are small, single-center, cross-sectional studies in subjects whose diagnoses are already known. Larger, prospective, multicenter studies in subjects presenting with their first clinical demyelinating event are necessary to evaluate the utility of the CVS in making a diagnosis of MS. Whether the CVS improves the accuracy of existing diagnostic criteria for MS[1] will be of interest. In addition, the ability of the CVS to discriminate between diseases will require further study.

Gray Matter (Cortical) Lesions

As with central vein imaging, the presence of gray demyelinating matter lesions, specifically cortical lesions, could help discriminate MS from other diseases and provide higher diagnostic accuracy for MS. The presence of cortical lesions in MS was described histopathologically several decades ago; in an early study of 60 MS brains, cortical lesions were present in 93%, and accounted for 59% of all brain lesions.[24] Cortical lesions have been classified into 3 types: leukocortical, or type I, lesions (34%), in which a single lesion involves both the juxtacortical white matter and cortex; intracortical, or type 2, lesions (16%), which are entirely within the cortex and often contain a central blood vessel (**Fig. 2**); and subpial, or type 3, lesions (50%), which extend from the pial surface into the cortex and commonly span multiple gyri.[25] Cortical lesions were initially reported to be less inflammatory than white matter lesions[25] and strongly associated with progressive phenotypes, occurring rarely or not at all in acute or relapsing disease[26]; however, subsequent work has demonstrated the presence of inflammatory cortical demyelination in en passant biopsy specimens at clinical presentation.[27] Given that biopsy was required to diagnose MS, the generalizability of these findings is a subject of debate, although a majority of subjects with available clinical follow-up had a typical MS course after a median of 3.5 years.[27]

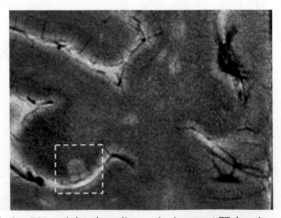

Fig. 2. High-resolution T2*-weighted gradient-echo image at 7T showing a type 2 (intracortical) lesion (*dashed yellow box*).

Histopathologically, cortical lesions are more challenging to visualize than white matter lesions likely because they are less inflammatory and not hypercellular and because cortical myelin does not stain as darkly as white matter myelin on routine staining.[28] Cortical lesions have also proved challenging to detect on conventional MRI, with intracortical lesion detection rates as low as 3% to 5% using conventional T2 and fluid-attenuated inversion recovery sequences at 1.5T.[29] Cortical lesion detection rates generally increase with field strength, particularly at 7T (see **Fig. 2**).[30–35] Technical challenges are that the cortex is thin (2–3 mm), cortical lesions are small, there is poor contrast between cortical lesions and surrounding gray matter, and there is often partial voluming from nearby cerebrospinal fluid. To overcome some of these challenges, newer pulse sequences have been tested, including double inversion recovery (DIR) and phase-sensitive inversion recovery (PSIR).

DIR is designed to suppress signals from both cerebrospinal fluid and white matter to facilitate visualization of gray matter. When applied to postmortem MS brains, DIR showed only 18% sensitivity to detect known cortical lesions, and subpial lesions, the most common subtype, were largely undetected.[36] Furthermore, DIR is typically plagued by artifacts in vivo and has a low signal-to-noise ratio, causing the interobserver agreement to be moderate at best.[37] PSIR has a higher signal-to-noise ratio and allows for clearer distinction between cortex and juxtacortical white matter and, therefore, more accurate classification of cortical lesion location compared with DIR.[38] However, subpial lesions remain largely undetected on PSIR as well.

Because of these limitations with current technology at 1.5T and 3T, it is premature to incorporate cortical lesions into clinical practice, including diagnosing MS and discriminating MS from other diseases. Further work needs to be done at 7T, which may become Food and Drug Administration–approved as a clinical field strength in the United States in the near future, to optimize pulse sequences to reliably visualize all cortical lesions, including subpial lesions. Once reliable detection is achieved, large, prospective, multicenter studies in subjects at first clinical presentation will be necessary to evaluate the utility of cortical lesions to aid in making a diagnosis of MS as well as studies focused on using cortical lesions to discriminate MS from other diseases.

Lesion Probability Mapping

MS clinicians and radiologists already assess lesion topography (ie, lesion location, shape, and distribution) qualitatively to interpret brain MRI scans for clinical purposes. However, a quantitative measure of white matter lesion distribution could provide additional evidence to confirm an MS diagnosis and/or discriminate MS from other diseases. Lesion probability mapping is a postprocessing technique that estimates the probability of a lesion occurring at each voxel in the brain (**Fig. 3**).[39–41] In theory, if the average distribution of white matter lesions in the common diseases (MS, migraine, small vessel disease, and so forth) was known, then a lesion probability map from an individual patient could be compared quantitatively to these reference distributions. The summary of this comparison could provide an additional piece of information to enhance the diagnostic accuracy of a clinical MRI interpretation.

In general, lesion probability mapping requires (1) segmenting white matter lesions and creating a binary lesion mask, such that each voxel in the brain is labeled as lesional or not; (2) registering, or aligning, each subject's MRI and lesion mask to a standard template; and (3) calculating the probability of a lesion being present at each voxel. Each voxel, therefore, contains its own probability distribution to contain a lesion, with possible values ranging between 0 and 1. A generalized linear model can then be performed at each voxel to measure the association between lesion probability and the outcome of interest. To minimize the number of statistical comparisons,

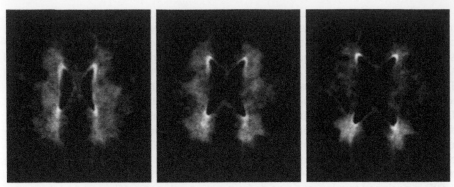

Fig. 3. Three representative high-resolution axial views of a white matter lesion probability map from 232 MS patients. The probability of a lesion at each voxel is represented visually by a gray-scale ranging from the lowest probability (*black*) to the highest probability (*white*).

voxels can be clustered together to make inference at the cluster level. Several investigators have taken this general approach to examine associations between lesion distribution and MS clinical outcomes (ie, Expanded Disability Status Scale or Multiple Sclerosis Functional Composite),[40,42,43] MS clinical subtype,[44–47] and genotype.[41,48]

Only 1 group has attempted to distinguish between demyelinating diseases using lesion probability mapping in a small, cross-sectional study of neuromyelitis optica and MS.[49] Further work is needed to expand this potentially useful and conceptually appealing technique, including the creation of reference lesion distributions for common MS mimickers, the refinement of postprocessing methods and statistical approaches to analyze such data, and more studies testing the discriminative value and operating characteristics (sensitivity, specificity, and so forth) of lesion probability mapping to diagnose MS.

THE ROLE OF MRI IN MONITORING MULTIPLE SCLEROSIS OVER TIME

In addition to its utility in diagnosing MS, MRI plays a fundamental role in monitoring the disease over time. The clinical significance of new white matter lesion accumulation over time is conclusive, with both short-term implications for risk of relapse[50,51] and long-term implications for disability accrual.[52–54] Despite this, no standardized method exists to detect new white matter lesions. Similarly, brain atrophy is a critically important element of the disease that is not routinely measured in clinical practice, despite its established clinical relevance[55] and face validity as an in vivo measure of neurodegeneration.[56] With some focused effort, many of the imaging and postprocessing tools that are commonly used in MS clinical research could be incorporated into routine clinical care to provide clinicians with standardized, quantitative metrics by which MS patients could be monitored over time.

A major hurdle to accomplishing this goal is the substantial heterogeneity in the MRIs that are collected clinically. In 2006, the Consortium of Multiple Sclerosis Centers MRI Task Force, an international group of neurologists and radiologists, recommended a standardized MRI protocol for the diagnosis and follow-up of MS,[57] which was recently revised in 2016.[58] Despite these guidelines, MRI scans in MS clinical practice are not standardized and are unlikely to become standardized in the near future. Perhaps a new concept in MS imaging is to accept this heterogeneity in MRI acquisition but create image-processing pipelines that are robust to the heterogeneity, to derive as much useful information as possible from the scans that are collected.

Heterogeneity in acquisition is less of an issue when MRIs are collected for diagnostic purposes but is a major concern for automated image-processing algorithms.

Developing image-processing algorithms that can accommodate heterogeneity in image acquisition is a fast-moving and complex field. There are several sources of heterogeneity in images collected on different magnetic resonance scanners, including differences in scanner hardware and pulse sequence parameters (eg, voxel size, echo time, and repetition time), which create variations in tissue contrasts between scans. The ideal postprocessing pipeline would normalize pixel intensity to mitigate these differences as well as correct magnetic field inhomogeneities, coregister scans, and harmonize across platforms. Such a pipeline would provide the backbone to perform automated image analysis, including lesion segmentation (and perhaps lesion probability mapping), automated detection of new lesions, and brain volumetrics. Because of their direct clinical utility, this review focuses on automated detection of new lesions and volumetrics.

Automated Detection of New Lesions

In current clinical practice, the identification of new MS lesions over time relies entirely on visual inspection by the treating neurologist and radiologist, a task that is time-consuming and can be particularly challenging when comparing heterogeneous scans with gaps between slices, different patient positioning in the scanner, motion or other artifacts, and lack of realignment of images. In addition to correcting for these differences, the ideal postprocessing pipeline could automatically identify new MS lesions and present the result to neurologists and radiologists along with the typical MRIs as an additional tool to assist the clinical interpretation of MS MRI scans (**Fig. 4**).

There are several approaches to detect changes in white matter lesions over time; interested readers are referred to reviews focused specifically on this topic.[59,60] This article's focus is on intensity-based image subtraction. Intensity-based image subtraction is a promising method to identify new, enlarging, shrinking, or resolved white matter lesions. As implied by its name, image subtraction essentially subtracts 2 images obtained from the same patient at different time points to identify areas where the lesions have changed. This generally requires (1) preprocessing of MRI, including removal of nonbrain tissue (ie, skull), intensity normalization, image coregistration, and white matter masking; (2) construction of a dissimilarity map between the 2 images analyzed; (3) segmentation of the dissimilarity map to create a change mask; and (4) postprocessing of the change mask to display the areas of interest.[60] In the postprocessing stage, true change can be attempted to be separated from systematic or analytical errors[61,62] by using automatic thresholding based on either intensity or size of the lesions. Intensity and size thresholds must be adjusted with respect to each other to achieve a good trade-off between sensitivity and specificity.[63]

Although subtraction methods can provide high sensitivity, they can also suffer from false-positive reults,[59] which can be mitigated by using more than one sequence to perform image subtraction.[63] Several image subtraction algorithms have been proposed in the MS literature.[61–67] Subtraction seems promising and potentially useful; in multicenter clinical trial datasets, subtraction was found to improve detection of lesion change compared with conventional methods[68] and to provide increased power to detect treatment efficacy compared with monthly serial gadolinium-enhanced T1-weighted imaging.[69]

Direct comparison between available subtraction methods is difficult due to variable preprocessing and postprocessing techniques and performance metrics used in the studies reported. In addition, existing studies have used different validation data

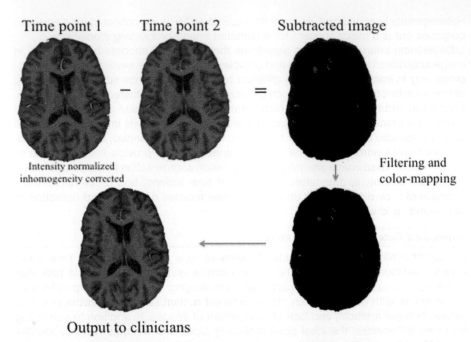

Time point 1   Time point 2   Subtracted image

Intensity normalized
inhomogeneity corrected

Filtering and
color-mapping

Output to clinicians

Fig. 4. Image subtraction demonstrating the automated detection of a new demyelinating lesion on a follow-up MRI scan, adjacent to the frontal horn of the R lateral ventricle. The new lesion is colored in red.

sets obtained from different ground truths, further complicating comparisons. One group has directly compared 3 methods in the literature against a single ground truth, with segmentations refined jointly until reaching a consensus.[60] In this study, subtraction-based dissimilarity maps with proposed automatic confidence level thresholdng[63] provided the best detection of lesion change in terms of Dice similarity and reliability. Further head-to-head studies of a similar nature are needed to help select the best image subtraction algorithm. In addition, the quality of the input images into image subtraction algorithms will likely influence their performance; one group has shown, for example, that image subtraction performed better with 3-D images than with 2-D images.[68] Given the aforementioned vast heterogeneity in image acquisition, this issue needs to be addressed prior to implementation of image subtraction into clinical practice. Finally, improvement in lesion size (ie, shrinkage or resolution) is an aspect of the MS disease process that is neither commonly studied nor routinely measured or reported in MS clinical trials and clinical research. Further work is necessary to understand the clinical relevance and effect of disease-modifying therapies on lesion improvement.

Brain Volumetrics

The net accumulation of tissue damage in MS, including gray matter, white matter, and nonlesional tissue, leads to permanent loss/degeneration of both gray matter and white matter. Neuroaxonal loss is a fundamentally important aspect of the disease and is thought to be the major pathologic substrate of irreversible physical and cognitive disability in MS.[70] Brain volume measurements on MRI can offer an in vivo measure of neurodegeneration and have been studied extensively in MS.

As opposed to regional measures, whole-brain volume is the most commonly used volumetric measure in MS clinical research and clinical trials. Whole-brain volume has face validity as a measure of neurodegeneration and is reproducible and its clinical relevance is established.[55] Many of the currently available disease-modifying therapies have been shown to slow the rate of whole-brain atrophy in MS.[55] As such, there is great interest in incorporating whole-brain volume measurements into routine clinical care. Several barriers exist, however, which are discussed in a recent review.[56] Such barriers include the lack of a standardized MRI protocol for MS, the lack of a gold-standard image processing software to measure whole-brain volume, and the lack of specific statistical methods to translate whole-brain volume measurements into clinically relevant metrics at the individual level. The heterogeneity in MRI acquisition, discussed previously, is a major issue in this context, due to the significant intrascanner and interscanner variability that can occur in brain volume measurements from different MRI scanners.[71] If and when brain volumetrics are ready to be incorporated into routine clinical care, the ideal image-processing pipeline, described previously, would need to be deployed as a preprocessing step to homogenize the images as much as possible, including across scanner platforms, prior to submitting them to a software to measure brain volume.

Currently, it remains unclear which brain region to measure to best estimate neurodegeneration. Whole-brain atrophy may not be abnormal in early phases of MS[72,73] and can fluctuate significantly due to edema associated with new white matter lesion formation or resolution thereof, corticosteroids or newly initiated disease-modifying therapies,[74] patient hydration status,[75] and time of day at which the MRI scan is performed.[76] Gray matter volume is less likely to be confounded by these factors and has been shown a better predictor of physical and cognitive disability and quality of life than white matter volume or whole-brain volume.[77–79] Among gray matter regions, the deep gray matter structures, in particular the thalamus, have been a topic of recent interest.[80] As a central relay nucleus with widespread incoming and outgoing projections, the thalamus may be particularly susceptible to MS pathology, especially downstream (wallerian) degeneration from axonal transection within white matter lesions in incoming tracts.[81] Thalamic atrophy has been observed in several early phases of CNS demyelinating disease, including clinically isolate syndrome at presentation,[72] pediatric MS,[82] and radiologically isolated syndrome.[73] Thalamic atrophy seems clinically relevant[83] and sensitive to change over time throughout the disease duration.[84] As such, the thalamus may be an appealing region to study throughout the disease, both as a potential primary MRI endpoint for clinical trial design and as a barometer of net tissue damage in MS.[80]

From a clinical standpoint, it would be ideal to define a region that can be used to estimate how much additional atrophy has occurred in an individual patient beyond what would have occurred with normal aging as a quantitative measure of disease severity. Once studied and validated appropriately, clinicians could apply this at the individual level to make treatment decisions. This would inherently require an understanding of normal aging, so that the atrophy observed in an individual patient could be separated into "normal aging atrophy" and "MS-specific atrophy" (**Fig. 5**). Ideally, this method would be based on a region with a large amount of MS-specific atrophy, because only the MS-specific portion of the atrophy is presumably modifiable with disease-modifying therapies and should be the target for therapeutic intervention. A better understanding of the relative contributions of normal aging and MS to regional and whole-brain atrophy is emerging and is highly relevant for this purpose.

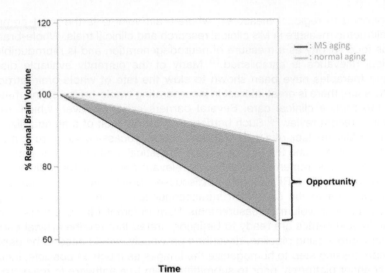

Fig. 5. The concept of MS-specific atrophy. Regional brain volume loss in healthy subjects (ie, normal aging) is depicted with the green line and in MS subjects with the red line. "MS-specific atrophy" (grey shaded area) refers to the additional brain volume loss that occurs beyond normal aging, which is presumably the opportunity for therapeutic intervention.

SUMMARY

As a marker, MRI has revolutionized the field of MS, both in clinical care and clinical research. There are still several challenges, however, and perhaps opportunities facing the field of MS imaging. Future work is likely to focus on incorporating quantitative imaging metrics and newer imaging acquisition methods into clinical care to increase the specificity of MRI in establishing a diagnosis of MS as well as using image processing methods to streamline the monitoring of MS patients over time in reproducible ways.

REFERENCES

1. Polman CH, Reingold SC, Banwell B, et al. Diagnostic criteria for multiple sclerosis: 2010 revisions to the McDonald criteria. Ann Neurol 2011;69:292–302.
2. Polman CH, Reingold SC, Edan G, et al. Diagnostic criteria for multiple sclerosis: 2005 revisions to the "McDonald criteria". Ann Neurol 2005;58:840–6.
3. McDonald IW, Compston A, Edan G, et al. Recommended diagnostic criteria for multiple sclerosis: guidelines from the international panel on the diagnosis of multiple sclerosis. Ann Neurol 2001;50:121–7.
4. Swanton JK, Fernando K, Dalton CM, et al. Modification of MRI criteria for multiple sclerosis in patients with clinically isolated syndromes. J Neurol Neurosurg Psychiatry 2006;77(7):830–3.
5. Swanton JK, Rovira A, Tintore M, et al. MRI criteria for multiple sclerosis in patients presenting with clinically isolated syndromes: a multicentre retrospective study. Lancet Neurol 2007;6(8):677–86.
6. Gomez-Moreno M, Diaz-Sanchez M, Ramos-Gonzalez A. Application of the 2010 McDonald criteria for the diagnosis of multiple sclerosis in a Spanish cohort of patients with clinically isolated syndromes. Mult Scler 2012;18(1):39–44.

7. Rovira A, Wattjes MP, Tintore M, et al, on behalf of the MAGNIMS study group. MAGNIMS consensus guidelines on the use of MRI in multiple sclerosis – clinical implementation in the diagnostic process. Nat Rev Neurol 2015;11:471–82.

8. Solomon AJ, Bourdette DN, Cross AH, et al. The contemporary spectrum of multiple sclerosis misdiagnosis: a multicenter study. Neurology 2016;87:1393–9.

9. Sati P, Oh J, Constable RT, et al, on behalf of the NAIMS Cooperative. The central vein sign and its clinical evaluation for the diagnosis of multiple sclerosis: a consensus statement from the North American Imaging in Multiple Sclerosis Cooperative. Nat Rev Neurol 2016;12(12):714–22.

10. Rae-Grant AD, Wong C, Bernatowicz R, et al. Observations on the brain vasculature in multiple sclerosis: a historical perspective. Mult Scler Relat Disord 2014;3(2):256–62.

11. Chavan GB, Babyn PS, Thomas B, et al. Principles, techniques, and applications of T2*-based MR imaging and its special applications. Radiographics 2009; 29(5):1433–49.

12. Tan IL, van Schijndel RA, Pouwels PJW, et al. MR venography of multiple sclerosis. AJNR Am J Neuroradiol 2000;21(6):1039–42.

13. Sati P, George IC, Shea CD, et al. FLAIR*: a combined MR contrast technique for visualizing white matter lesions and parenchymal veins. Radiology 2012;265(3): 926–32.

14. Sati P, Thomasson DM, Li N, et al. Rapid, high-resolution, whole-brain, susceptibility-based MRI of multiple sclerosis. Mult Scler 2014;20(11):1464–70.

15. Kau T, Taschwer M, Deutschmann H, et al. The "central vein sign": is there a place for susceptibility weighted imaging in possible multiple sclerosis? Eur Radiol 2013;23(7):1956–62.

16. Hammond KE, Metcalf M, Carvajal L, et al. Quantitative in vivo magnetic resonance imaging of multiple sclerosis at 7 Tesla with sensitivity to iron. Ann Neurol 2008;64:707–13.

17. Tallantyre EC, Brookes MJ, Dixon JE, et al. Demonstrating the perivascular distribution of MS lesions in vivo with 7-Tesla MRI. Neurology 2008;70(22):2076–8.

18. Mistry N, Dixon J, Tallantyre E, et al. Central veins in brain lesions visualized with high-field magnetic resonance imaging. JAMA Neurol 2013;70(5):623–8.

19. Kilsdonk ID, Lopez-Soriano A, Kuijer JP, et al. Morphological features of MS lesions on FLAIR* at 7T and their relation to patient characteristics. J Neurol 2014;261(7):1356–64.

20. Tallantyre EC, Morgan PS, Dixon JE, et al. A comparison of 3T and 7T in the detection of small parenchymal veins within MS lesions. Invest Radiol 2009; 44(9):491–4.

21. Dixon JE, Simpson A, Mistry N, et al. Optimisation of T2*-weighted MRI for the detection of small veins in multiple sclerosis at 3T and 7T. Eur J Radiol 2013; 82:719–27.

22. Tallantyre EC, Dixon JE, Donaldson I, et al. Ultra-high-field imaging distinguishes MS lesions from asymptomatic white matter lesions. Neurology 2011;76(6):534–9.

23. Mistry N, Abdel_Fahim R, Samaraweera A, et al. Imaging central veins in brain lesions with 3T T2*-weighted magnetic resonance imaging differentiates multiple sclerosis from microangiopathic brain lesions. Mult Scler 2016;22(10):1289–96.

24. Lumsden CE. The neuropathology of multiple sclerosis. In: Vinken PJ, Bruyn GW, editors. Handbook of clinical neurology. Amsterdam (Netherlands): Elsevier; 1970. p. 217–309.

25. Peterson JW, Bö L, Mörk S, et al. Transected neurites, apoptotic neurons, and reduced inflammation in cortical multiple sclerosis lesions. Ann Neurol 2001;50: 389–400.
26. Kutzelnigg A, Lucchinetti CF, Stadelmann C, et al. Cortical demyelination and diffuse white matter injury in multiple sclerosis. Brain 2005;128:2705–12.
27. Lucchinetti CF, Popescu BFG, Bunyan RF, et al. Inflammatory cortical demyelination in early multiple sclerosis. N Engl J Med 2011;365:2188–97.
28. Dutta R, Trapp BD. Pathogenesis of axonal and neuronal damage in multiple sclerosis. Neurology 2007;68(Suppl 3):S22–31.
29. Guerts JJ, Bö L, Pouwels PJ, et al. Cortical lesions in multiple sclerosis: combined postmortem MR imaging and histopathology. AJNR Am J Neuroradiol 2005;26(3): 572–7.
30. Metcalf M, Xu D, Okuda DT, et al. High-resolution phased-array MRI of the human brain at 7 tesla: initial experience in multiple sclerosis patients. J Neuroimaging 2010;20(2):141–7.
31. Tallantyre EC, Morgan PS, Dixon JE, et al. 3 Tesla and 7 Tesla MRI of multiple sclerosis cortical lesions. J Magn Reson Imaging 2010;32(4):971–9.
32. Nielsen AS, Kinkel RP, Tinelli E, et al. Focal cortical lesion detection in multiple sclerosis: 3 Tesla DIR versus 7 Tesla FLASH-T2. J Magn Reson Imaging 2012; 35(3):537–42.
33. Maniero C, Benner T, Radding A, et al. In vivo imaging of cortical pathology in multiple sclerosis using ultra-high field MRI. Neurology 2009;73:941–8.
34. Pitt D, Boster A, Pei W, et al. Imaging cortical lesions in multiple sclerosis with ultra-high-field magnetic resonance imaging. Arch Neurol 2010;67:812–8.
35. Graaf WL, Kilsdonk I, Lopez-Soriano A, et al. Clinical application of multi contrast 7T MR imaging in multiple sclerosis: increased lesion detection compared to 3T confined to gray matter. Eur Radiol 2013;23:528–40.
36. Seewan A, Kooi EJ, Roosendaal SD, et al. Postmortem verification of MS cortical lesion detection with 3D DIR. Neurology 2012;78(5):302–8.
37. Guerts JJ, Roosendaal SD, Calabrese M, et al, for the MAGNIMS Study Group. Consensus recommendations for MS cortical lesion scoring using double inversion recovery MRI. Neurology 2011;76(5):418–24.
38. Sethi V, Mulhert N, Ron M, et al. MS cortical lesions on DIR: not quite what they seem? PLoS One 2013;8(11):e78879.
39. Narayanan S, Fu L, Pioro E, et al. Imaging of axonal damage in multiple sclerosis: spatial distribution of magnetic resonance imaging lesions. Ann Neurol 1997;41: 385–91.
40. Charil A, Zijdenbos AP, Taylor J, et al. Statistical mapping analysis of lesion location and neurological disability in multiple sclerosis: application to 452 patient data sets. Neuroimage 2003;19:532–44.
41. Gourraud PA, Sdika M, Khankhanian P, et al. A genome-wide association study of brain lesion distribution in multiple sclerosis. Brain 2013;136(Pt 4):1012–24.
42. Vellinga MM, Geurts JJ, Rostrup E, et al. Clinical correlations of brain lesion distribution in multiple sclerosis. J Magn Reson Imaging 2009;29:768–73.
43. Kincses ZT, Ropele S, Jenkinson M, et al. Lesion probability mapping to explain clinical deficits and cognitive performance in multiple sclerosis. Mult Scler 2011; 17:681–9.
44. Di Perri C, Battaglini M, Stromillo ML, et al. Voxel-based assessment of differences in damage and distribution of white matter lesions between patients with primary progressive and relapsing-remitting multiple sclerosis. Arch Neurol 2008;65:236–43.

45. Ceccarelli A, Rocca MA, Pagani E, et al. The topographical distribution of tissue injury in benign MS: a 3T multiparametric MRI study. Neuroimage 2008;39: 1499–509.
46. Bodini B, Battablini M, De Stefano N, et al. T2 lesion location really matters: a 10 year follow-up study in primary progressive multiple sclerosis. J Neurol Neurosurg Psychiatry 2001;82:72–7.
47. Giorgio A, Gattaglini M, Rocca MA, et al. Location of brain lesions predicts conversion of clinically isolated syndromes to multiple sclerosis. Neurology 2013;80: 234–41.
48. Sombekke MH, Vellinga MM, Uitdehaag BM, et al. Genetic correlations of brain lesion distribution in multiple sclerosis: an exploratory study. AJNR Am J Neuroradiol 2011;32:695–703.
49. Matthews L, Marasco R, Jenkinson M, et al. Distinction of seropositive NMO spectrum disorder and MS brain lesion distribution. Neurology 2013;80:1330–7.
50. Sormani MP, Bonzano L, Roccatagliata L, et al. Magnetic resonance imaging as a potential surrogate for relapses in multiple sclerosis: a meta-analytic approach. Ann Neurol 2009;65:268–75.
51. Sormani MP, Stubinski B, Cornelisse P, et al. Magnetic resonance active lesions as individual-level surrogate for relapses in multiple sclerosis. Mult Scler 2011; 17(5):541–9.
52. Rio J, Rovira A, Tintore M, et al. Relationship between MRI lesion activity and response to IFN-beta in relapsing-remitting multiple sclerosis patients. Mult Scler 2008;14(4):479–84.
53. Propserini L, Gallo V, Petsas N, et al. One-year MRI scan predicts clinical response to interferon beta in multiple sclerosis. Eur J Neurol 2009;16(11): 1202–9.
54. Fisniku LK, Brex PA, Altmann DR, et al. Disability and T2 MRI lesions: a 20-year follow-up of patients with relapse onset of multiple sclerosis. Brain 2008;131: 808–17.
55. De Stefano N, Airas L, Grigoriadis N, et al. Clinical relevance of brain volume measures in multiple sclerosis. CNS Drugs 2014;28:147–56.
56. Azevedo CJ, Pelletier D. Whole-brain atrophy: ready for implementation into clinical decision-making in multiple sclerosis? Curr Opin Neurol 2016;29(3):237–42.
57. Simon JH, Li D, Traboulsee A, et al. Standardized MR imaging protocol for multiple sclerosis: consortium of MS Centers consensus guidelines. AJNR AM J Neuroradiol 2006;27:455–61.
58. Traboulsee A, Simon JH, Stone L, et al. Revised recommendations of the Consortium of MS Centers Task Force for a standardized MRI protocol and clinical guidelines for the diagnosis and follow-up of multiple sclerosis. AJNR AM J Neuroradiol 2016;37(3):394–401.
59. Lladó X, Oliver A, Cabezas M, et al. Segmentation of multiple sclerosis lesions in brain MRI: a review of automated approaches. Inf Sci 2012;186:164–85.
60. Lesjak Ž, Pernuš F, Likar B, et al. Validation of white matter lesion change detection methods on a novel publicly available MRI image database. Neuroinformatics 2016;14:403–20.
61. Tan IL, van Schijndel RA, Fazekas F, et al. Image registration and subtraction to detect active T2 lesions in MS: an interobserver study. J Neurol 2002;249:767–73.
62. Moraal B, Meier DS, Poppe PA, et al. Subtraction MR images in a multiple sclerosis multicenter clinical trial setting. Radiology 2009;250(2):506–14.

63. Ganiler O, Oliver A, Diez Y, et al. A subtraction pipeline for automatic detection of new appearing multiple sclerosis lesions in longitudinal studies. Neuroradiology 2014;56:363–74.
64. Sweeney EM, Shinohara RT, Shea CD, et al. Automatic lesion incidence estimation and detection in multiple sclerosis using multisequence longitudinal MRI. AJNR Am J Neuroradiol 2013;34(1):68–73.
65. Battaglini M, Rossi F, Grove RA, et al. Automated identification of brain new lesions in multiple sclerosis using subtraction images. J Magn Reson Imaging 2014;39(6):1543–9.
66. Horsfield MA, Rocca MA, Pagani E, et al. Estimating brain lesion volume change in multiple sclerosis by subtraction of magnetic resonance images. J Neuroimaging 2016;26(4):395–402.
67. Cabezas M, Corral JF, Oliver A, et al. Improved automatic detection of new T2 lesions in multiple sclerosis using deformation fields. AJNR Am J Neuroradiol 2016; 37(10):1816–23.
68. Moraal B, Wattjes MP, Guerts JJ, et al. Improved detection of active multiple sclerosis lesions: 3D subtraction imaging. Radiology 2010;255(1):154–63.
69. Moraal B, van den Elskamp IJ, Knol DL, et al. Long-interval T2-weighted subtraction magnetic resonance imaging: a powerful new outcome measure in multiple sclerosis trials. Ann Neurol 2010;67(5):667–75.
70. Bjartmar C, Wujek JR, Trapp BD. Axonal loss in the pathology of MS: consequences for understanding the progressive phase of the disease. J Neurol Sci 2003;206(2):165–71.
71. Biberacher V, Schmidt P, Keshavan A, et al. Intra- and interscanner variability of magnetic resonance imaging based volumetry in multiple sclerosis. Neuroimage 2016;142:188–97.
72. Henry RG, Shieh M, Okuda DT, et al. Regional grey matter atrophy in clinically isolated syndromes at presentation. J Neurol Neurosurg Psychiatry 2008;79: 1236–44.
73. Azevedo CJ, Overton E, Khadka S, et al. Early CNS neurodegeneration in radiologically isolated syndrome. Neuroimmunol Neuroinflamm 2015;2:e102.
74. Miller DH, Soon D, Fernando KT, et al, for the AFFIRM investigators. MRI outcomes in a placebo-controlled trial of natalizumab in relapsing MS. Neurology 2007;68:1390–401.
75. Nakamura K, Brown RA, Araujo D, et al. Correlation between brain volume change and T2 relaxation time induced by dehydration and rehydration: implications for monitoring atrophy in clinical studies. Neuroimage Clin 2014;6:166–70.
76. Nakamura K, Brown RA, Narayanan S, et al, Alzheimer's Disease Neuroimaging Initiative. Diurnal fluctuations in brain volume: statistical analyses of MRI from large populations. Neuroimage 2015;118:126–32.
77. Roosendaal SD, Bendfeldt K, Vrenken H, et al. Grey matter volume in a large cohort of MS patients: relation to MRI parameters and disability. Mult Scler 2011;17:1098–106.
78. Mowry EM, Beheshtian A, Waubant E, et al. Quality of life in multiple sclerosis is associated with lesion burden and brain volume measures. Neurology 2009;72: 1760–5.
79. Fisher E, Lee JC, Nakamura K, et al. Gray matter atrophy in multiple sclerosis: a longitudinal study. Ann Neurol 2008;64:255–65.
80. Minagar A, Barnett MH, Benedict R, et al. The thalamus and multiple sclerosis: modern views on pathologic, imaging and clinical aspects. Neurology 2013;80: 210–9.

81. Henry RG, Shieh M, Amirbekian B, et al. Connecting white matter injury and thalamic atrophy in clinically isolated syndromes. J Neurol Sci 2009;282:61–6.
82. Aubert-Broche B, Fonov V, Ghassemi R, et al. Regional brain atrophy in children with multiple sclerosis. Neuroimage 2011;58:409–15.
83. Houtchens MK, Benedict RH, Killiany R, et al. Thalamic atrophy and cognition in multiple sclerosis. Neurology 2007;69:1213–23.
84. Azevedo C, Khadka S, Liu S, et al. Thalamic atrophy over time in relapsing forms of MS: a large, 5-year, observational MRI study. Neurology 2015;84(14 Supplement) [abstract: S29.006;1526-632X].

Pediatric Multiple Sclerosis

From Recognition to Practical Clinical Management

Cynthia X. Wang, MD, Benjamin M. Greenberg, MD, MHS*

KEYWORDS

- Multiple sclerosis • Children • Demyelination • Diagnosis • Treatment

KEY POINTS

- Pediatric multiple sclerosis (MS) (before age 18) makes up approximately 5% to 10% of MS.
- Risks factors for pediatric MS are similar to those of adults, and include vitamin D deficiency, history of Epstein-Barr virus exposure, obesity, and exposure to cigarette smoke.
- Characteristics that argue against a diagnosis of MS include history of developmental delay, progressive course, encephalopathy, monofocal lesion, and prepubertal onset.
- Children with MS take longer to acquire significant disability but arrive at significant disability at a chronologically younger age compared with adults with MS.
- Selection of disease-modifying therapies should focus on compliance, safety, and impact of therapies on a developing central nervous system and immune system.

INTRODUCTION

There has been increasing recognition that multiple sclerosis (MS) can present in childhood, prompting growing efforts to characterize the spectrum of pediatric-onset disease. This chronic inflammatory, demyelinating disease of the central nervous system is thought to develop when genetically susceptible individuals are exposed to specific environmental factors at a critical time in development. Recent studies have explored the similarities and differences in pediatric versus adult-onset MS, and elucidated early risk factors in disease pathogenesis. Recognition and diagnosis of pediatric MS can be challenging given a broad differential of possible MS mimics. There has also been concern about the safety and generalizability of using immunomodulatory treatments, studied almost exclusively in adults, in children.

Disclosures: Dr B.M. Greenberg has received research funding from the NIH (5R01NS071463-02), PCORI, MedImmune, Chugai, Genentech and the Guthy Jackson Charitable Foundation. He has received consulting fees from Novartis, Alexion and EMD Serono. C.X. Wang: No disclosures.
Department of Neurology and Neurotherapeutics, UT Southwestern Medical Center, 5323 Harry Hines Boulevard, Dallas, TX 75390-8806, USA
* Corresponding author.
E-mail address: Benjamin.greenberg@utsouthwestern.edu

Neurol Clin 36 (2018) 135–149
https://doi.org/10.1016/j.ncl.2017.08.005   neurologic.theclinics.com

In this review, we discuss the epidemiology, clinical presentation, diagnostic evaluation, and treatment approach to pediatric MS. In particular, we highlight the areas in which pediatric disease may differ from adult-onset MS and review the differential diagnoses for MS in the pediatric population. We discuss the management of acute relapses and explore the potentially difficult long-term therapy decisions in patients with immature and developing nervous and immune systems. Last, we will discuss supportive care for patients with pediatric MS, with attention to how symptoms including fatigue, cognitive impairment, and mood dysfunction can manifest and impact younger patients.

EPIDEMIOLOGIC FACTORS

Although fewer than 10% of individuals with MS experience their first clinical demyelinating event before the age of 18, exposure to key environmental factors leading to an eventual adult diagnosis of MS likely occur during childhood.[1,2] Past studies have found that individuals carry the MS risk profile of their place of residence during childhood and that there is a latitude gradient to MS incidence, perhaps explained by direct sunlight exposure and vitamin D level.[3,4] Early viral exposures, specifically Epstein-Barr virus (EBV) infections, appear to confer increased MS risk in both children and adults.[4] In contrast, early exposure to cytomegalovirus may be protective against development of MS.[5] The genetic locus HLA DRB1*15 in children, like adults, appears to increase risk of developing MS, up to twofold to fourfold.[6] Disease pathogenesis likely involves interaction of multiple risk factors, as evidenced by observations that remote infection with HSV-1 can increase MS risk in HLA DRB1*15 negative individuals, but attenuate MS risk in DRB1*15 positive individuals.[7]

It is rare for demyelinating events to begin before puberty and only 20% of pediatric MS is diagnosed before age 10.[8] Before puberty, the ratio of females to males with MS is roughly even, but increases to 2 to 3:1 in adolescents.[9] This observation suggests that hormonal changes, menarche in particular, may play an important role in the pathogenesis of MS. Obesity has been associated with higher risk for MS,[10] although this may be somewhat confounded by its association with lower bioavailability of vitamin D and a younger age of menarche.[11] Vitamin D level appears not only to determine risk of developing MS but also influence relapse risk.[12,13] Children with MS are exposed to passive smoking twice as frequently as a control population.[14] Initial studies of gut microbiota in children with MS show a perturbation in flora indicative of a proinflammatory milieu.[15] Dietary intake of salt has yielded mixed results.[16]

CLINICAL PRESENTATION

The heralding event of pediatric multiple sclerosis can involve gait disturbance, vision loss, weakness, or sensory change, among other symptoms. Children may present with forms of clinically isolated syndrome, including optic neuritis, transverse myelitis, and cerebellar, brainstem, and cerebral hemispheric lesions. Approximately one-third of children who have an acute demyelinating event are later diagnosed with a relapsing disease such as MS or neuromyelitis optica spectrum disorder (NMOSD).[17] Encephalopathy, seizures, and polyfocal symptoms, which can be atypical for adult MS, can be seen in children. At onset, pediatric MS is nearly universally relapsing-remitting (85%–100% of cases)[18]; a progressive disease course should raise suspicion for an alternative diagnosis.

DIAGNOSIS

Similar to adult MS, making a diagnosis of pediatric MS is centered on identifying recurrent demyelinating events separated in space and time. The International

Pediatric Multiple Sclerosis Study Group originally proposed operational definitions for acquired demyelinating syndromes (ADS) in 2002 to facilitate diagnosis and improve communication between providers about these conditions.[19] It was later revised in to incorporate new developments including updated McDonald criteria.[20] Notably, the last revision of the McDonald criteria in 2010 made it possible to diagnosis MS at the first event if neuroimaging demonstrates silent lesions in 2 of the 4 regions (periventricular, juxtacortical, infratentorial, and spinal cord) characteristic for MS with at least 1 silent gadolinium-enhancing and nonenhancing lesion.[21] This can be applied to a pediatric population but should be implemented more cautiously as polyfocal syndromes such as acute disseminated encephalitis (ADEM) may satisfy some of these features (**Box 1**). When the initial event does not meet criteria for MS, subsequent clinical attacks or serial MRI showing new lesions assist in confirming the diagnosis.

NEUROIMAGING

MRI of brain and spinal cord has been very helpful to identify and monitor demyelinating activity as well as predict risk for an ultimate diagnosis of MS. The risk of MS is dramatically higher if a child has evidence of white matter brain lesions at time of first attack. Specifically, lesions oriented perpendicularly to the long axis of the corpus callosum and well-demarcated lesions argue for MS.[22] The central vein sign is an

---

Box 1
Diagnosis of pediatric multiple sclerosis

Summary of 2012 International Pediatric Multiple Sclerosis Study Group definitions for pediatric multiple sclerosis (MS) and immune-mediated central nervous system (CNS) demyelinating disorders

Pediatric clinically isolated syndrome (CIS) (all are required)
• A clinical CNS event with presumed inflammatory demyelinating cause.
• Absence of a clinical history of CNS demyelinating disease (if any, see pediatric MS).
• No encephalopathy except as readily explained by fever.
• Criteria for MS diagnosis on baseline MRI are not met.

Pediatric acute disseminated encephalomyelitis (ADEM) (all are required)
• A first polyfocal, clinical CNS event with presumed inflammatory demyelinating cause.
• An encephalopathy that cannot be explained by fever.
• No new clinical or MRI findings 3 months or more after onset.
• Brain MRI is abnormal during the acute (3 months) phase with typically diffuse, poorly demarcated large lesions involving predominantly the cerebral white matter.

Pediatric MS
• Two or more CIS separated by more than 30 days involving more than 1 area of the CNS.
• One CIS associated with MRI findings consistent with criteria of dissemination in space (DIS) and in which a follow-up MRI shows at least 1 new lesion consistent with dissemination in time (DIT) criteria.
• One ADEM attack followed by 1 CIS 3 or more months after symptom onset that is associated with new MRI findings consistent with criteria for DIS.
• A CIS with MRI findings that are consistent with criteria for DIS and DIT (at least 1 T2 lesion in at least 2 of 4 areas: spinal cord, infratentorial, juxtacortical, and periventricular [DIS] associated with a simultaneous presence of asymptomatic gadolinium-enhancing and nonenhancing lesions [DIT] if the patient is ≥12 years old) (revision proposed).

Data from Krupp LB, Tardieu M, Amato MP, et al, International Pediatric Multiple Sclerosis Study Group. International Pediatric Multiple Sclerosis Study Group criteria for pediatric multiple sclerosis and immune-mediated central nervous system demyelinating disorders: revisions to the 2007 definitions. Mult Scler 2013;19(10):1261–7.

imaging feature that is suggestive of MS.[23] MRI is also a sensitive modality for surveillance of new and potentially subclinical disease activity.

CEREBROSPINAL FLUID ANALYSIS

Cerebrospinal fluid analysis (CSF) can also be valuable in establishing a diagnosis of MS. In children, like adults, oligoclonal bands and immunoglobulin G index may be elevated in those with MS. Unmatched oligoclonal bands (OCB) in CSF compared with serum have been detected in 92% of children with MS[24]; in contrast, only 5% to 30% of children with monophasic ADEM were positive for OCBs.[25,26] The "MRZ reaction" (MRZR) a polyspecific, intrathecal humoral immune response against measles, rubella, and varicella zoster virus is present in most patients with MS (70%), although significantly less frequent in neurosarcoidosis (9%), autoimmune encephalitis (11%), and ADEM (0%). The specificity of MRZR for MS was 92% in the study cohort.[27] Pleocytosis and elevated protein can also be seen, but significant elevation of these parameters should be cues to consider alternate infectious and inflammatory conditions. In a study of 136 children with ADS, 66% had mild pleocytosis, defined as CSF nucleated cells exceeding 5 cells/m, although no child exceeded 60 cells/mm^3.[24] Cytology and flow cytometry should be completed if suspicion for malignancy is high.

ANCILLARY STUDIES

Other adjunctive studies include antibody testing, particularly assessment for anti-aquaporin 4 antibodies. The presence of antibodies to this water channel expressed on astrocytes is diagnostic of NMOSD, which requires a different therapeutic approach from MS. A growing literature suggests that children with antibodies to myelin oligodendrocyte glycoprotein (MOG) will have a clinical course more like NMOSD than relapsing-remitting MS, so testing should be considered.[28–31] Autoimmune encephalitis and paraneoplastic antibody panels also may be helpful, especially if a child presents with encephalopathy or has a known history of malignancy, respectively.

Visual-evoked potentials (VEP), brainstem auditory evoked potentials, and somatosensory potentials may be useful to look for evidence of past injury, and provide objective measures of injury in younger children who cannot verbalize their symptoms. In their cohort of 85 childhood patients with MS, Pohl and colleagues[32] detect dissemination in space with multimodal evoked potentials in 46% of the children before a second clinical attack. VEPs can be abnormal in up to 95% of children with a history of optic neuritis and even up to 60% of children with MS without known history of optic nerve dysfunction.[33] Optical coherence tomography (OCT) has been used in children with MS, and like adults, retinal nerve fiber layer atrophy occurs over time and is accelerated by optic neuritis.[34]

DIFFERENTIAL DIAGNOSIS

The differential diagnosis for MS in children is broad, especially in prepubertal children. Features that should prompt consideration of alternate causes include young age, fever, encephalopathy, progressive course, and systemic involvement of disease. Acute demyelinating syndromes other than MS are relatively more common in children compared with adults.

ACUTE DISSEMINATED ENCEPHALOMYELITIS

In young children, encephalopathy and polyfocal symptoms are most indicative of ADEM, especially if MRI demonstrates diffuse, asymmetric, and poorly demarcated

T2/fluid attenuated inversion recovery hyperintensities affecting deep white and gray nuclei. ADEM is classically described as having a monophasic course, although 6% to 18% of children presenting with ADEM will go on to have future relapses that confirm the diagnosis of MS.[13,35] Any recurrence or worsening of neurologic symptoms within 90 days of initial symptom onset is considered part of the first attack. However, continued episodes beyond this time course are rare and considered by some to be a subtype of ADEM called multiphasic ADEM. However, this is a controversial entity and children with relapsing course likely have an underlying systemic condition and should probably be considered for immunosuppression.

NEUROMYELITIS OPTICA SPECTRUM DISORDER

NMOSD has been reported in children as young as 23 months.[36] NMOSD may present similarly to MS, but can be distinguished with anti-AQP4 antibody testing. Although the historic description of NMO has been of predominantly spinal cord and optic nerve attacks, many patients can also have brain and brainstem involvement. The AQP4 protein, which is highly expressed within astrocyte foot processes, is critical for formation of the blood brain barrier. Autoantibodies that bind to this target can lead to astrocytic dysfunction and a cascade of inflammation that promotes demyelination and necrosis. If initial testing is negative, we typically repeat AQP4 testing once more after 6 months. Excluding this diagnosis is essential, as NMOSD has a distinct pathogenesis, and individuals with NMOSD may actually worsen on MS therapies, including interferon beta, natalizumab, and fingolimod.[37–39]

ANTI-MYELIN OLIGODENDROCYTE GLYCOPROTEIN–ASSOCIATED DISEASE

Recent reports also implicate MOG antibody in syndromes mimicking MS, including ADEM, NMOSD, optic neuritis (ON), and longitudinally extensive transverse myelitis (LETM). MOG is expressed on the outer myelin membrane and MOG antibodies are increasingly being identified in younger children with acute demyelinating syndrome, often associated with encephalopathy. Ketelslegers and colleagues[28] presented data that anti-MOG antibody positivity argues against MS. Although previously considered as having a relatively benign and nonrelapsing course, new studies of MOG-positive adults with NMOSD have shown contradictory findings of high disease burden and relapse rate.[40] Anti-MOG antibody testing can be completed on research basis and it should be commercially available in the near future.

OTHER

Neoplastic and infectious etiologies should always remain on the differential similar to adults. Large, tumefactive MS lesions may be challenging to distinguish from neoplasm, and sometimes tissue sampling is necessary to establish the correct diagnosis.

Additionally, genetic and metabolic diseases may manifest in or resemble an acute demyelinating event. Inherited white matter disorders, including the leukodystrophies, such as X-linked adrenoleukodystrophy and metachromatic leukodystrophy, are distinguished from MS by more diffuse and symmetric white matter involvement. Mitochondrial disorders, such as Leber hereditary optic neuropathy, can cause chronic progressive external ophthalmoplegia, and appear similar to some brainstem syndromes caused by MS.

Systemic inflammatory vasculopathies or vasculopathies isolated to the central nervous system (CNS) can present with headache and multifocal neurologic deficits. Primary angiitis of the CNS or CNS vasculitis may be occult on vascular imaging and conventional angiogram, and require brain biopsy for confirmation. Sarcoidosis, although rare in children, can have protean manifestations and is often mistaken for MS. It can present with cranial nerve (CN) deficits, especially CN VII palsy, leptomeningeal involvement, and basilar meningitis. Chest imaging to evaluate perihilar lymphadenopathy should be considered (**Table 1**).

TREATMENT
Acute Management of Relapses

The mainstay for treatment of acute MS relapses are high-dose corticosteroids, which have class I and II evidence in accelerating functional recovery after acute attacks in adult MS populations.[41] This often is administered as intravenous methylprednisolone (20–30 mg/d for 3–5 days), sometimes followed by a gradual taper of oral prednisone over 2 to 6 weeks. Corticosteroids also can be prescribed as oral prednisone, methylprednisolone, or dexamethasone, but must be in equivalent doses to 30 mg/kg of methylprednisolone. For relapses that do not respond sufficiently to steroids, especially relapses involving significant impairment in ambulation and/or vision, we consider concurrent or consecutive treatment with therapeutic plasma exchange

Table 1 Differential diagnoses of pediatric MS	
Autoimmune/ immune-mediated	ADEM, ON, TM, NMOSD, CRION, MOG SLE, sarcoid, Behcet, Sjogren, Susac NMDA, GAD, VGKC, OMAS
Vascular	Arterial ischemic stroke, DVST, PRES, RCVS, Primary angiitis of central nervous system, granulomatosis with polyangiitis, sickle cell disease, CADASIL, moyamoya disease or syndrome
Infectious/ postinfectious	Viral: HSV, EBV, HIV, JCV/PML, CMV, HTLV Bacterial: mycoplasma, TB, Lyme, Syphilis, Bartonella, Listeria Fungal: crypto, endemic mycoses (histo, blasto, coccidio) Postinfectious: AIDP, PANS/PANDAS
Metabolic/Genetic	Mitochondrial: MELAS, MERRF, LHON, Leigh, Alpers, NARP, Kearn-Sayre Leukodystrophies: X-linked ALD, metachromatic, Alexander, Canavan, Krabbe, Pelizaeus-Merzbacher Aicardi-Goutierres, X-linked CMT
Neoplastic	Glioma, central nervous system Lymphoma
Nutritional/Toxic/ Drug-induced	B12 deficiency, folate deficiency, CPM, amphetamines, anti-TNFa

Abbreviations: ADEM, acute disseminated encephalomyelitis; AIDP, acute inflammatory demyelinating polyneuropathy; ALD, adrenoleukodystrophy; CADASIL, cerebral autosomal dominant arteriopathy with subcortical infarcts and leukoencephalopathy; CMT, charcot marie tooth; CMV, cytomegalovirus; CPM, central pontine myelinolysis; CRION, chronic inflammatory relapsing optic neuropathy; DVST, deep vein sinus thrombosis; EBV, Epstein barr virus; GAD, glutamic acid decarboxylase; HIV, human immunodeficiency virus; HSV, herpes simplex virus; HTLV, human T cell lymphotrophic virus; JCV, JC virus; LHON, lebers hereditary optic neuropathy; MELAS, mitochondrial encephalomyopathy, lactic acidosis, and stroke-like episodes; MERRF, myoclonic epilepsy with ragged red fibers; NARP, neuropathy, ataxia and retinitis pigmentosa; NMDA, N-Methyl-D-aspartic acid; NMOSD, neuromyelitis optica spectrum disorder; OMAS, opsoclonus myoclonus ataxia syndrome; ON, optic neuritis; PANS/PANDAS, pediatric acute onset neuropsychiatric syndrome/pediatric autoimmune neuropsychiatric disorders associated with streptococcal infections; PML, progressive multifocal leukoencephalopathy; PRES, posterior reversible encephalopathy syndrome; RCVS, reversible cerebral vasoconstriction syndrome; SLE, systemic lupus erythematosus; TNFa, tumor necrosis factor alpha; TM, transverse myelitis; VGKC, voltage gated potassium channel.

(typically 5 single volume exchanges, every other day) or intravenous immune globulin (2 g/kg divided over 2–5 days). During treatment for the acute relapse, involvement of physical, occupational, and speech therapy may be helpful in supporting a child's initial recovery and for recommendations on the acuity, frequency, and potential duration of inpatient or outpatient therapy needs.

25-hydroxyvitamin D level should be assessed in all children presenting with acute demyelinating syndromes or newly diagnosed MS, as it is one of the only modifiable risk factors for MS development and relapse. Mowry and colleagues[12] reported in their cohort of 110 subjects with pediatric-onset MS, every 10 ng/mL increase in the adjusted 25-hydroxyvitamin D3 level was associated with a 34% decrease in the rate of subsequent relapses. Cholecalciferol (D3) should be used to correct vitamin D deficiency, preferably to a level of 60 to 100 ng/mL.

Chronic Immunomodulatory Treatments

There are now 15 different medications approved by the Food and Drug Administration (FDA) for treatment of adult MS, although none are approved for use in children (**Table 2**). Many of these disease-modifying treatments have unique mechanisms of action and vary in route of administration, efficacy, tolerability, and safety. Most of our knowledge about application of these treatments in children with MS comes from anecdotal experience, case reports and case series, and retrospectives analyses.

The approach to rational selection of an initial immunomodulatory treatment has been controversial. The traditional approach with so-called first-line therapies of interferon beta and glatiramer acetate is justified by their more extensive safety data and longer duration of experience with these medications.[42] This "step-up" approach involves escalating immunomodulatory treatment only after patients have clinical relapses or new demyelinating lesions despite sufficient duration of treatment and validation of compliance from the patient. This approach is potentially appealing in children, given our poor understanding of how newer immunomodulatory therapies impact an immature nervous and immune system.

Others argue for an induction or "step-down" approach, using the most potent treatments first, despite the potential for some to cause serious adverse events. This approach is relevant especially with fulminant demyelinating events causing significant residual deficits. The notion that quelling any inflammatory activity and exacting a state of no evidence of disease activity has emerged as a primary goal in treatment of MS. This state of freedom from disease activity is characterized by the absence of relapses, absence of Expanded Disability Status Scale progression, lack of new/enlarging T2 lesions on MRI, and lack of gadolinium-enhancing lesions on MRI.[43]

Currently, interferon beta-1a/1b agents have among the best safety and efficacy data in children.[44,45] Interferon agents can be delivered intramuscularly or subcutaneously, at frequencies ranging from daily to every 2 weeks. Side effects of interferons include flulike symptoms, headache, injection-site reactions, leukopenia, and transaminitis. Thus, before initiation of medication, a complete blood cell count and comprehensive metabolic panel should be assessed and then every 6 months. Interferon may lead to mood side effects and should be used with caution in children and adolescents with a known history of depression.

Glatiramer acetate is another MS therapy with an established safety profile.[46,47] It is a synthetic amino acid polymer resembling myelin basic protein and is thought to inhibit specific effector T-lymphocytes, antigen-presenting cells, and suppressor T-lymphocytes. It may be suitable in the pediatric population because there is no need for surveillance laboratory studies. It is offered in subcutaneous daily or 3 times

Table 2
Table of drugs, dosing regimen, mechanism, side effects, SAE, monitoring

Drug	Dosing Regimen	Side Effects	Adverse Events	Monitoring
Interferon beta-1a	30 μg IM once a week 22–44 μg SC 3 times a week	Flulike symptoms, headache, injection-site reactions	Abnormal LFTs, cytopenias	CBC, CMP every 6 mo
Interferon beta-1b	250 μg SC every other day			
Glatiramer acetate	20 mg SC once a day 40 mg SC 3 times a week	Dyspnea, flushing, injection-site reactions	Systemic reactions	None
Natalizumab	3–5 mg/kg (up to 300 mg) IV	Headache, fatigue, diarrhea, rash	PML, hepatotoxicity, development of neutralizing antibodies	CBC, CMP JCV IgG and index every 6 mo
Fingolimod	0.5 mg PO once a day	Headache, flu, diarrhea	Bradyarrhythmias, macular edema, skin cancer, increased infections/ sinusitis, PML, cryptococcal and VZV infections, abnormal LFTs	T/B cell subsets, CBC, CMP
Teriflunomide	7 and 14 mg PO once a day	Hair thinning, diarrhea, nausea,	Birth defects (Preg Category X), abnormal LFTs	T/B cell subsets, Quantiferon Gold, Hepatitis, CBC, CMP
Dimethyl fumarate	120–240 mg PO twice a day	Flushing, nausea, diarrhea, abdominal pain	PML, lymphopenia, severe allergic reactions	T/B cell subsets, CBCPD, Comp
Rituximab	375–500 mg/m² (500–1000 mg) once or given biweekly for 2 wk or weekly for 4 wk	Headache, nausea,	Severe allergic reaction, PML, increased infections	T/B cell subsets, CBC, CMP
Ocrelizumab	600 mg IV every six months with the first dose split in half (2 doses of 300 mg IV separated by 2 weeks)	Headache, infusion reactions	Severe allergic reactions, increased infections	Quantiferon Gold, Hepatitis B, CBC and CMP

Abbreviations: CBC, complete blood count; CMP, complete metabolic panel; IgG, immunoglobulin G; IM, intramuscular; IV, intravenous; kg, kilogram; mg, milligram; PO, per os; SC, subcutaneous.

a week injection. Possible side effects include injection-site reactions, including redness, pain, and swelling.

Many providers have used the newer oral and infusion medications, so-called second-line therapies, in pediatric patients with favorable results. There are currently randomized controlled phase III clinical trials for the oral agents, fingolimod, teriflunomide, and dimethyl fumarate[48] under way, but none have completed. Fingolimod may lead to serious adverse events, including bradycardia and macular edema. A first-dose observation with electrocardiogram before and 6 hours after administration, and hourly blood pressure and heart rate evaluation, is required. Dimethyl fumarate is a twice-a-day oral medication and can cause flushing and gastrointestinal issues. Teriflunomide requires monitoring of liver function, especially during the first 6 months of use and has an absolute contraindication in pregnancy.

Infusion medications have the advantage of infrequent dosing and allow accurate assessment of compliance. Natalizumab is among the most efficacious therapies available in reducing relapse rate. Several case and cohort studies have discussed its use as a second-line therapy in children.[49,50] However, it has been associated with potentially devastating development of progressive multifocal leukoencephalopathy in a small subset of patients. The risk of developing progressive multifocal leukoencephalopathy (PML) is influenced by john cunningham virus (JCV) seropositivity, duration of time on natalizumab, and history of prior immunosuppression. Alemtuzumab is a monoclonal antibody against CD52 and leads to depletion of mature lymphocytes. There are no published accounts of its use in pediatric MS and it has potential to give rise to secondary autoimmunity, such as autoimmune thyroid disease and idiopathic thrombocytopenic purpura. Rituximab is a chimeric CD20 monoclonal antibody that has been used off-label in both adult and pediatric patients with MS. Although safety and efficacy data in childhood-onset MS is still limited, several groups have reported positive experiences, including reductions in relapses and rare serious adverse events.[51,52] A related agent, ocrelizumab, is a humanized form of the monoclonal antibody that was recently approved by the FDA for relapsing-remitting MS, and is the first-ever therapy to be approved for use for progressive forms of MS.

Ultimately, the approach to drug selection should be discussed in depth with the patient and patient's family to gain understanding of what treatments may lead to highest rates of compliance and best preserve the child's quality of life. There has been a shift to personalized medicine and prioritizing patient-centered outcomes. It is important to engage patients and their families in shared decision making, as these early decisions may influence lifelong treatment.

Surveillance for Treatment Failure

Typically, we acquire a brain MRI 3 to 4 months after initiation of immunomodulatory treatments to use as a baseline to compare with future studies. We then usually continue MRI brain imaging at 6-month to 12-month frequencies. If clinical relapses or new enhancing or nonenhancing MRI brain lesions appear after this baseline, the possibility of treatment failure should be discussed with the patient and family. It is important to assess compliance, and create a comfortable environment for the patient and family to discuss this. If noncompliance exists, then it is critical to address barriers to compliance, and if it is not realistic to overcome these issues, then a transition to alternate agent should be carefully considered. If compliance was good, then it is vital to begin discussion of transitioning to a treatment with a different and potentially more efficacious mechanism.

Neuroimaging is not the only method for tracking MS-related impairment over time. Clinical tools include the Multiple Sclerosis Functional Composite, which consists of brief assessment gross motor function (25-foot timed walk), fine motor function (9-hole board), and attention/processing speed (Paced Auditory Serial Addition test). OCT can be used to track for evidence of changes in optic nerve health and examine for evidence of occult optic neuritis events. Binocular low-contrast visual acuity and symbol digit modalities have also been helpful in characterizing MS-related disability.[53]

Symptomatic Management

Receiving a diagnosis of a chronic disease can have a significant impact on a child's and the family's sense of well-being. Krupp and colleagues[54] interviewed children with MS and their families, many of whom expressed a sense of loss and worry about the future. The process to being diagnosed with MS may be frustrating and lengthy, given the likelihood of initial misdiagnosis of the condition in children. Thus, this provides an opportunity to provide support and reassurance to the family and address potential misconceptions about the condition. MS can influence a child's psychosocial, emotional, and cognitive development. As such, involving a multidisciplinary team of specialists, including physical medicine and rehabilitation, neuropsychology, physical therapy, social work, school liaison, and nutrition, may be extremely helpful in optimizing a child's care in all domains that may be affected by MS.

Discussion of the specific symptoms related to MS that diminish a child's quality of life is very important. This information can often be elicited from the child and family, although younger individuals may lack insight or not be able to articulate their concerns, and older individuals may be uncomfortable in talking about sensitive issues in front of their parents.

As children enter adolescence, we stress the importance of their communicating to their medical providers individually so they can speak more freely about issues concerning bowel, bladder, and sexual function. Establishing this level of comfort with their medical provider also helps to ease with their transition to adult care.

SPECIFIC AREAS OF CONCERN
Cognition

Children with MS have a wide range of cognitive deficits. These involve attention, working memory, processing speech, and executive functioning.[55–57] Neuropsychological testing is a very valuable tool to identify a child's relative strengths and weaknesses. Children and their families benefit from receiving a direct feedback session about the testing results, and should be provided specific recommendations for accommodations at school. A school liaison and social worker may help assist in the implementation of these recommendations through individualized education plans and 504 plans. Potential accommodations include preferential seating, additional time with assignments and tests, flexibility in bathroom breaks, and allowing school absences for medical issues. Children may also benefit from school-based physical therapy, occupational therapy, and speech language pathology.

Mood

Children and families should be made aware that MS is associated with mood disorders given the potential for physical disability, feelings of alienation, and poor academic performance. Independent of an individual's level of functioning, MS may increase risk of mood disorders on a biological level. Mood symptoms, such as anxiety and depression, may present differently in younger children. Irritability, oppositional behavior, and social withdrawal may be early signs of a mood disorder. Counseling, such as cognitive behavioral therapy and pharmacologic interventions, such as selective serotonin reuptake inhibitors, may be helpful in addressing mood symptoms.

Many children and families with MS derive great benefit from participation in support and educational groups about pediatric MS. These activities can decrease the feelings of isolation and help normalize the condition. Through attending local MS chapter meetings, camps, walks, and advocacy programs, a child may gain a sense of self-efficacy, self-esteem, and autonomy, which are valuable not only in management of their MS but also in their personal and psychosocial development.

Pain

Management of pain related to MS has not been well studied in the pediatric population. Fortunately, it does not seem to be as prominent of an issue as often is the case in adults. If pain is reported, detailed history taking on the quality and characteristics of pain can assist in identification and development of strategies to most effectively manage pain. Centralized, neuropathic pain may have a more burning, electrical, or tingling quality and be associated with objective sensory abnormalities on examination. Neuropathic pain may respond to medications, including gabapentin, pregabalin, tricyclic antidepressants, and serotonin-norepinephrine reuptake inhibitors.

In contrast, pain related to spasticity may lead to description of tonic or phasic spasms, and respond to antispasmodic agents, such as baclofen, tizanidine, or dantrolene. Localized areas of spasticity may respond well to onabotulinum toxin injections. Musculoskeletal pain can result from poor walking mechanics. Careful gait assessment by physical medicine and rehabilitation (PM&R) and physical therapy can identify orthotic needs.

Fatigue

Like in the adult population, fatigue is a major symptom in children with MS that may lead to poor quality of life. It is important to first assess for likely contributors to fatigue, including sleep and mood disorders. Once these are addressed, residual fatigue symptoms may respond to stimulant medications (especially if impacting cognition) and wakefulness-promoting agents (modafinil). There have been positive reports of use on L-carnitine and high-dose biotin (300-mg daily) in the adult population. Walking fatigue may respond to aminopyridine (4-AP).

Bladder and Bowel Management

Urinary dysfunction can be quite disabling to school-age children. Milder symptoms can be managed with regular intake of fluids and scheduled voids. More severe urinary retention and incontinence may result in urinary tract infections and require intermittent catheterization. If symptoms do not respond to conservative management, then evaluation by a urologist and urodynamic testing can be helpful in characterizing the type of urinary dysfunction, such as detrusor hyperactivity or detrusor sphincter dyssynergia.

Urinary dysfunction can in turn lead to constipation, as fear of accidents can lead to water restriction. Spinal cord lesions may affect the enteric nervous system and cause decreased gastric motility. Constipation can be managed with dietary fiber, bulking agents, stool softeners, promotility agents, osmotic agents, enemas, and suppositories. Finding a regimen may be challenging and require and trial-and-error approach.

Prognosis

Fortunately, the vast majority of children with MS do not accrue any significant disabilities in the first 5 years after their initial demyelinating event.[58]

Paradoxically, children often experience a more inflammatory disease at onset, characterized by a higher relapse rate and shorter duration between relapses compared with adults. The slower accrual of disability may relate to neurologic reserve, neuronal plasticity, or the severity and location of demyelination. A less favorable course may result from polyfocal involvement, progression of disability between relapses, and frequent relapses within the first 2 years of disease.[58,59]

Although children with MS may have a longer latency period between the initial demyelinating event and entry into the progressive disease, they are more likely to experience significant disability at a younger age compared with adults. A study of 116 children with MS found that 50% of the cohort entered the secondary progressive phase of MS after 23 years[59] versus adult studies suggesting that this transition may occur after 10 years.

It is worrisome that brain atrophy can be seen in children with MS even in the earliest stages of the disease and lead to failure of age-expected brain growth.[60] Multiple studies have described decreased thalamic and corpus callous volume in pediatric patient with MS, as well as smaller head size compared with healthy controls.[61]

FUTURE DIRECTIONS

Despite the acceleration of research into pediatric-onset MS, many questions remain. There is a need for continued international, multicenter, and collaborative studies given the rarity of this condition. Understanding pediatric MS will yield important insights into the natural history of MS and identify key genetic and environmental factors during the earliest stages of disease pathogenesis. In particular, studying the effect of MS and MS therapies on a developing immune and nervous system is crucial. Until we have more knowledge, caution should be taken with generalizing adult MS practices to children.

REFERENCES

1. Ferreira ML, Machado MI, Dantas MJ, et al. Pediatric multiple sclerosis: analysis of clinical and epidemiological aspects according to National MS Society Consensus 2007. Arq Neuropsiquiatr 2008;66(3B):665–70.
2. Belbasis L, Bellou V, Evangelou E, et al. Environmental risk factors and multiple sclerosis: an umbrella review of systematic reviews and meta-analyses. Lancet Neurol 2015;14(3):263–73.
3. Simpson S, Blizzard L, Otahal P, et al. Latitude is significantly associated with the prevalence of multiple sclerosis: a meta-analysis. J Neurol Neurosurg Psychiatr 2011;82(10):1132–41.
4. O'Gorman C, Lucas R, Taylor B. Environmental risk factors for multiple sclerosis: a review with a focus on molecular mechanisms. Int J Mol Sci 2012;13(9): 11718–52.
5. Waubant E, Mowry EM, Krupp L, et al. Common viruses associated with lower pediatric multiple sclerosis risk. Neurology 2011;76(23):1989–95.
6. Waubant E, Ponsonby AL, Pugliatti M, et al. Environmental and genetic factors in pediatric inflammatory demyelinating diseases. Neurology 2016;87(9 Suppl 2): S20–7.
7. Waubant E, Mowry EM, Krupp L, et al. Antibody response to common viruses and human leukocyte antigen-DRB1 in pediatric multiple sclerosis. Mult Scler 2013; 19(7):891–5.
8. Chitnis T. Pediatric multiple sclerosis. Neurologist 2006;12(6):299–310.

9. Pohl D, Hennemuth I, Von kries R, et al. Paediatric multiple sclerosis and acute disseminated encephalomyelitis in Germany: results of a nationwide survey. Eur J Pediatr 2007;166(5):405–12.

10. Langer-gould A, Brara SM, Beaber BE, et al. Childhood obesity and risk of pediatric multiple sclerosis and clinically isolated syndrome. Neurology 2013;80(6): 548–52.

11. Wortsman J, Matsuoka LY, Chen TC, et al. Decreased bioavailability of vitamin D in obesity. Am J Clin Nutr 2000;72(3):690–3.

12. Mowry EM, Krupp LB, Milazzo M, et al. Vitamin D status is associated with relapse rate in pediatric-onset multiple sclerosis. Ann Neurol 2010;67(5):618–24.

13. Banwell B, Bar-or A, Arnold DL, et al. Clinical, environmental, and genetic determinants of multiple sclerosis in children with acute demyelination: a prospective national cohort study. Lancet Neurol 2011;10(5):436–45.

14. Mikaeloff Y, Caridade G, Tardieu M, et al. Parental smoking at home and the risk of childhood-onset multiple sclerosis in children. Brain 2007;130(Pt 10):2589–95.

15. Tremlett H, Fadrosh DW, Faruqi AA, et al. Gut microbiota in early pediatric multiple sclerosis: a case-control study. Eur J Neurol 2016;23(8):1308–21.

16. Mcdonald J, Graves J, Waldman A, et al. A case-control study of dietary salt intake in pediatric-onset multiple sclerosis. Mult Scler Relat Disord 2016;6:87–92.

17. Yeshokumar AK, Narula S, Banwell B. Pediatric multiple sclerosis. Curr Opin Neurol 2017;30(3):216–21.

18. Renoux C, Vukusic S, Mikaeloff Y, et al. Natural history of multiple sclerosis with childhood onset. N Engl J Med 2007;356(25):2603–13.

19. Krupp LB, Banwell B, Tenembaum S. Consensus definitions proposed for pediatric multiple sclerosis and related disorders. Neurology 2007;68(16 Suppl 2): S7–12.

20. Krupp LB, Tardieu M, Amato MP, et al. International Pediatric Multiple Sclerosis Study Group criteria for pediatric multiple sclerosis and immune-mediated central nervous system demyelinating disorders: revisions to the 2007 definitions. Mult Scler 2013;19(10):1261–7.

21. Polman CH, Reingold SC, Banwell B, et al. Diagnostic criteria for multiple sclerosis: 2010 revisions to the McDonald criteria. Ann Neurol 2011;69(2):292–302.

22. Sati P, Oh J, Constable RT, et al. The central vein sign and its clinical evaluation for the diagnosis of multiple sclerosis: a consensus statement from the North American Imaging in Multiple Sclerosis Cooperative. Nat Rev Neurol 2016; 12(12):714–22.

23. Banwell B, Arnold DL, Tillema JM, et al. MRI in the evaluation of pediatric multiple sclerosis. Neurology 2016;87(9 Suppl 2):S88–96.

24. Pohl D, Rostasy K, Reiber H, et al. CSF characteristics in early-onset multiple sclerosis. Neurology 2004;63(10):1966–7.

25. Mikaeloff Y, Suissa S, Vallée L, et al. First episode of acute CNS inflammatory demyelination in childhood: prognostic factors for multiple sclerosis and disability. J Pediatr 2004;144(2):246–52.

26. Dale RC, De sousa C, Chong WK, et al. Acute disseminated encephalomyelitis, multiphasic disseminated encephalomyelitis and multiple sclerosis in children. Brain 2000;123 Pt 12:2407–22.

27. Hottenrott T, Dersch R, Berger B, et al. The intrathecal, polyspecific antiviral immune response in neurosarcoidosis, acute disseminated encephalomyelitis and autoimmune encephalitis compared to multiple sclerosis in a tertiary hospital cohort. Fluids Barriers CNS 2015;12:27.

28. Ketelslegers IA, Van pelt DE, Bryde S, et al. Anti-MOG antibodies plead against MS diagnosis in an Acquired Demyelinating Syndromes cohort. Mult Scler 2015; 21(12):1513–20.
29. Hacohen Y, Absoud M, Deiva K, et al. Myelin oligodendrocyte glycoprotein antibodies are associated with a non-MS course in children. Neurol Neuroimmunol Neuroinflamm 2015;2(2):e81.
30. Huppke P, Rostasy K, Karenfort M, et al. Acute disseminated encephalomyelitis followed by recurrent or monophasic optic neuritis in pediatric patients. Mult Scler 2013;19(7):941–6.
31. Reindl M, Jarius S, Rostasy K, et al. Myelin oligodendrocyte glycoprotein antibodies: how clinically useful are they? Curr Opin Neurol 2017;30(3):295–301.
32. Pohl D, Rostasy K, Treiber-held S, et al. Pediatric multiple sclerosis: detection of clinically silent lesions by multimodal evoked potentials. J Pediatr 2006;149(1): 125–7.
33. Ghezzi A, Pozzilli C, Liguori M, et al. Prospective study of multiple sclerosis with early onset. Mult Scler 2002;8(2):115–8.
34. Yilmaz Ü, Gücüyener K, Erin DM, et al. Reduced retinal nerve fiber layer thickness and macular volume in pediatric multiple sclerosis. J Child Neurol 2012; 27(12):1517–23.
35. Mikaeloff Y, Caridade G, Husson B, et al. Acute disseminated encephalomyelitis cohort study: prognostic factors for relapse. Eur J Paediatr Neurol 2007;11(2): 90–5.
36. Yuksel D, Senbil N, Yilmaz D, et al. Devic's neuromyelitis optica in an infant case. J Child Neurol 2007;22(9):1143–6.
37. Shimizu J, Hatanaka Y, Hasegawa M, et al. IFNβ-1b may severely exacerbate Japanese optic-spinal MS in neuromyelitis optica spectrum. Neurology 2010; 75(16):1423–7.
38. Barnett MH, Prineas JW, Buckland ME, et al. Massive astrocyte destruction in neuromyelitis optica despite natalizumab therapy. Mult Scler 2012;18(1):108–12.
39. Min JH, Kim BJ, Lee KH. Development of extensive brain lesions following fingolimod (FTY720) treatment in a patient with neuromyelitis optica spectrum disorder. Mult Scler 2012;18(1):113–5.
40. Jarius S, Ruprecht K, Kleiter I, et al. MOG-IgG in NMO and related disorders: a multicenter study of 50 patients. Part 2: epidemiology, clinical presentation, radiological and laboratory features, treatment responses, and long-term outcome. J Neuroinflammation 2016;13(1):280.
41. Goodin DS, Frohman EM, Garmany GP, et al. Disease modifying therapies in multiple sclerosis: subcommittee of the American Academy of Neurology and the MS Council for Clinical Practice Guidelines. Neurology 2002;58(2):169–78.
42. Chitnis T, Tenembaum S, Banwell B, et al. Consensus statement: evaluation of new and existing therapeutics for pediatric multiple sclerosis. Mult Scler 2012; 18(1):116–27.
43. Havrdova E, Galetta S, Stefoski D, et al. Freedom from disease activity in multiple sclerosis. Neurology 2010;74(Suppl 3):S3–7.
44. Banwell B, Reder AT, Krupp L, et al. Safety and tolerability of interferon beta-1b in pediatric multiple sclerosis. Neurology 2006;66(4):472–6.
45. Tenembaum SN, Segura MJ. Interferon beta-1a treatment in childhood and juvenile-onset multiple sclerosis. Neurology 2006;67(3):511–3.
46. Kornek B, Bernert G, Balassy C, et al. Glatiramer acetate treatment in patients with childhood and juvenile onset multiple sclerosis. Neuropediatrics 2003; 34(3):120–6.

47. Chitnis T. Disease-modifying therapy of pediatric multiple sclerosis. Neurotherapeutics 2013;10(1):89–96.
48. Chitnis T, Tardieu M, Amato MP, et al. International pediatric MS Study Group Clinical Trials Summit: meeting report. Neurology 2013;80(12):1161–8.
49. Ghezzi A, Moiola L, Pozzilli C, et al. Natalizumab in the pediatric MS population: results of the Italian registry. BMC Neurol 2015;15:174.
50. Huppke P, Stark W, Zürcher C, et al. Natalizumab use in pediatric multiple sclerosis. Arch Neurol 2008;65(12):1655–8.
51. Beres SJ, Graves J, Waubant E. Rituximab use in pediatric central demyelinating disease. Pediatr Neurol 2014;51(1):114–8.
52. Dale RC, Brilot F, Duffy LV, et al. Utility and safety of rituximab in pediatric autoimmune and inflammatory CNS disease. Neurology 2014;83(2):142–50.
53. Waldman AT, Chahin S, Lavery AM, et al. Binocular low-contrast letter acuity and the symbol digit modalities test improve the ability of the Multiple Sclerosis Functional Composite to predict disease in pediatric multiple sclerosis. Mult Scler Relat Disord 2016;10:73–8.
54. Krupp LB, Rintell D, Charvet LE, et al. Pediatric multiple sclerosis: perspectives from adolescents and their families. Neurology 2016;87(9 Suppl 2):S4–7.
55. Amato MP, Goretti B, Ghezzi A, et al. Cognitive and psychosocial features of childhood and juvenile MS. Neurology 2008;70(20):1891–7.
56. Banwell BL, Anderson PE. The cognitive burden of multiple sclerosis in children. Neurology 2005;64(5):891–4.
57. Macallister WS, Christodoulou C, Milazzo M, et al. Longitudinal neuropsychological assessment in pediatric multiple sclerosis. Dev Neuropsychol 2007;32(2):625–44.
58. Mikaeloff Y, Caridade G, Assi S, et al. Prognostic factors for early severity in a childhood multiple sclerosis cohort. Pediatrics 2006;118(3):1133–9.
59. Gusev E, Boiko A, Bikova O, et al. The natural history of early onset multiple sclerosis: comparison of data from Moscow and Vancouver. Clin Neurol Neurosurg 2002;104(3):203–7.
60. Aubert-broche B, Fonov V, Narayanan S, et al. Onset of multiple sclerosis before adulthood leads to failure of age-expected brain growth. Neurology 2014;83(23):2140–6.
61. Kerbrat A, Aubert-broche B, Fonov V, et al. Reduced head and brain size for age and disproportionately smaller thalami in child-onset MS. Neurology 2012;78(3):194–201.

Ethnic Considerations and Multiple Sclerosis Disease Variability in the United States

CrossMark

Erica Rivas-Rodríguez, MD, Lilyana Amezcua, MD, MS*

KEYWORDS

- Ethnicity • Race • Hispanic • African American • Health disparity
- Genetic admixture

KEY POINTS

- Hispanics and African Americans are at risk of greater MS disease burden early on the disease course.
- Hispanics, African Americans, and Asians are more likely to develop opticospinal MS than Caucasians, a phenotype that can lead to greater ambulatory disability.
- The HLA region is the most important MS susceptibility locus in Caucasians and other minority populations.
- Minority populations are overrepresented in socioeconomically disadvantaged groups and disproportionately face barriers to health care and access to MS specialists.

INTRODUCTION

There is a general sense that minority populations in the United States are less frequently affected with multiple sclerosis (MS). These minority populations include individuals of African American, Hispanic, and Asian backgrounds. Recent incidence reports suggest an increasing rate of MS among African Americans compared with whites.[1,2] Despite this recent increase in MS in African Americans, Hispanics and Asians are significantly less likely to develop MS than whites of European background and African Americans.[2-4] MS-specific mortality trends demonstrate distinctive disparities by race/ethnicity and age, suggesting that there is an unequal burden of disease. Although there are many determinants of inequalities in health, the authors

Disclosures: Dr L. Amezcua receives funding from NIH/NINDS (1R01NS096212-01), NMSS (RG 1607-25324), California Community Foundation (BA-17-136264), Guthy-Jackson Foundation (GJCF 001), and Biogen. She serves on advisory boards and is a consultant for Genzyme and Biogen. Dr E. Rivas-Rodríguez has no conflicts of interest to disclose.
Department of Neurology, Keck School of Medicine, University of Southern California (USC), 1520 San Pablo Street, Suite 3000, Los Angeles, CA 90033, USA
* Corresponding author.
E-mail address: lamezcua@usc.edu

Neurol Clin 36 (2018) 151–162
https://doi.org/10.1016/j.ncl.2017.08.007
0733-8619/18/© 2017 Elsevier Inc. All rights reserved.

review clinical characteristics and discuss genetic and health disparities related to ethnicity in African American and Hispanic Americans that may be contributing to disease variability in these 2 large minority populations with MS in the United States.

Prevalence, Incidence, and Mortality

MS as estimated by the World Health Organization shows a global median prevalence of 35 cases and a median incidence of 4 cases per 100,000, with a current total estimate of 2.3 million individuals affected with MS. In the United States, the prevalence indicative of all racial and ethnic background is estimated at 400,000[5] using a nationally representative commercially insured electronic claims database. Although there are regional differences reported by west and east coast, the reporting by specific ethnic and racial groups was not available. Nevertheless, in the last several years, published incident reports from 2 large multiethnic cohorts indicate drastic changes in the demographics of MS in the United States. A retrospective cohort study from the multiethnic, Kaiser Permanente plan in Southern California reported an incidence of 2.9% per 100,000 in Hispanics versus a 6.9% in whites, whereas the incidence for African Americans was almost twice that of whites, 10.2% (**Table 1**).[2] **Table 1** shows the incidence of MS in Hispanics is significantly lower than in non-Hispanic whites, but higher than Asians and Native Americans.[2,4] Furthermore, clinical isolated syndrome is also lower in Hispanics when compared with whites, but significantly higher than blacks.[3] Using the US military Veteran population, Wallin and colleagues[1] reported that the rate was still low for Hispanics when compared with whites and African Americans. The estimated annual age-specific incidence rate for Hispanics was reported at 8.2%, significantly lower than whites (9.3) and blacks (12.1) (see **Table 1**). Interestingly, Langer-Gould and colleagues[3] reported that the risk of MS was found to be 3 times more in African American women than in African American men. Lower risk of MS for Hispanics and Asians was found in both men and women. Although limited, these 2 studies highlight that race and ethnicity are likely to play a larger role in the distribution of MS worldwide. In all studies, MS is predominantly a female disease across ethnic groups.

US population-based mortality studies in MS are limited. Redelings and colleagues,[6] using the national multiple cause of death data, analyzed deaths due to MS by race/ethnicity from 1990 to 2001. They found that the overall age-adjusted mortality from MS was 1.44/100,000 population with mortalities highest among whites followed by blacks, Hispanics, American Indians/Alaska Natives, and Asians and Pacific Islanders. The increased MS mortality was uniform in both sexes, although higher in women than in men. Age-adjusted mortality per 100,000 population was 1.58 in whites, 0.39 (95% confidence interval [CI] 0.23–0.26) in Hispanics, and 1.28 (95% CI 0.78–0.83) in blacks. Mortalities increase with age for all groups and decreae for

Table 1 Incidence of multiple sclerosis in diverse minority populations							
Incidence of MS	Cohort	Period	Whites	African American	Hispanic	Asian	Native American
Langer-Gould	Kaiser Permanente Southern California	2008–2010	6.9	10.2	2.9	1.4	n/a
Wallin	US military-Veteran population	1990–2007, 2000–2007 for Hispanics	9.3	12.1	8.2	3.3	3.1

individuals greater than 85 years.[6] Using the Compressed Mortality data file for 1999 to 2015 in the WONDER (Wide-ranging online Data for Epidemiologic Research) system developed by the Centers for Disease Control and Prevention, the authors reported age-specific MS mortality patterns were highest among blacks younger than age 55, whereas whites had the highest rate after age 55. For these 2 groups, MS mortality increased with age in both sexes and peaked at ages 55 to 64 for blacks and 65 to 74 for non-Hispanic whites before declining substantially, whereas for Hispanic whites and Asian or Pacific Islander groups, the risk plateaued after age 55.[7] The higher incidence of MS in whites and a more severe disease course in blacks and Hispanics could be contributing to this observation. Whether these mortality trends in MS may be explained by racial/ethnic disparities in comorbidities is of future interest.

Clinical Presentation

Multiple cross-sectional observations suggest that African Americans and Hispanics have unique clinical characteristics. African Americans are an ethnic group of Americans with ancestral roots to the original peoples of Africa. Hispanics are also a complex ethnic group, wherein both genetic and cultural admixture derives mostly from the original indigenous inhabitants of America, its European settlers, and to some degree, Africans.[8] Variation in MS clinical or MRI disease presentation, severity, and course could be influenced by environmental and genetic factors.

African Americans with Multiple Sclerosis

African Americans have been reported to develop MS at an earlier[9,10] and at later age[11] compared with whites. Although the discrepancies in age of onset have not been rectified, interestingly the studies appear to differ by region of ascertainment (east vs west of the United States), which could suggest genetic and environmental differences within African American cohorts. Nevertheless, the observation that age of onset differs by geography could also be ascribed to differences in methodology and source population.[9,10]

Clinically, African Americans are reported to suffer from more disabling symptoms, poorer recovery, and shorter time to a second MS attack.[11,12] Relapse characteristics more common in African Americans include cerebellar dysfunction, cognitive dysfunction, and opticospinal manifestations such as transverse myelitis[11–13] (**Table 2**). They also have increased occurrence of multifocal signs and symptoms that could indicate a poor prognosis from the start of disease. Although the cause of this variability from whites is unknown, genetic, environmental, and disparities in care could be acting as risk factors.

MS is also characterized by intrathecal humoral inflammation, which has been shown to be greater in African Americans than in whites with MS,[14] although this was shown to not be a predictor of early disease progression. Elevated cerebrospinal fluid (CSF) immunoglobulin G index was found to negatively correlate with brain gray matter volume in African Americans with MS but not in whites with MS. The possibility of a more pronounced CSF humoral response in African Americans with MS warrants further investigation.

A consistent pattern of greater disability has been observed in African Americans compared with whites.[9,10,15] The greater level of disability seen is in part explained by the higher degree of MRI involvement and clinical presentation.[15] MRI results indicate that African Americans with MS have higher T1- and T2-weighted lesion volumes, lower N-acetylaspartate values, and lower brain magnetization transfer ratios (MTRs). Fisniku and colleagues[16] estimated the rate of T2 lesion volume growth per year is faster in SPMS than in RRMS (2.89 cm^3 compared with 0.80 cm^3, respectively).

Table 2

Characteristics of multiple sclerosis by race/ethnicity

A. Signs and Symptoms of Multiple Sclerosis by Race/Ethnicity

Values in Percentages %	Author: Kaufman			Author: Buchanan			Author: Naismith			Author: Amezcua			Author: Hadjixenofontos		
	Caucasian n = 172	Hispanic/ Latino	African American n = 79	Caucasian n = 26,967	Hispanic/ Latino n = 715	African American n = 1,313	Caucasian n = 80	Hispanic/ Latino	African American n = 79	Caucasian n = 76	Hispanic/ Latino n = 119	African American	Caucasian n = 312	Hispanic/ Latino n = 312	African American
Vision	17	NR	19	73.1	69.4	75.9	62	NR	58	NR	NR	NR	15–20	12–15	NR
Vestibular/ brainstem	13	NR	16	NR	NR	NR	59	NR	64	NR	NR	NR	10–15	12–15	NR
Motor abnormalities	20	NR	40	83.2	80.2	85.2	92	NR	99	14.7	13	NR	15–22	22–25	NR
Sensory abnormalities	44	NR	21	NR	NR	NR	95	NR	86	27.9	13.9	NR	15–21	47	NR
Bladder/bowel	NR	NR	NR	82.1	74.9	82	52	NR	72	NR	NR	NR	NR	NR	NR
Gait	NR	NR	NR	80.5	71.4	83.2	NR	NR	NR	NR	NR	NR	NR	NR	NR
Cognitive	NR	NR	NR	79.2	77.4	78.6	18	NR	37	NR	NR	NR	1–5	1–5	NR
Mood	NR	NR	NR	75.3	76	74	56	NR	38	NR	NR	NR	NR	NR	NR
Fatigue	NR	NR	NR	93.1	90	91.9	NR	NR	NR	NR	NR	NR	NR	NR	NR
Pain	NR	NR	NR	75.9	78.8	79.8	NR	NR	NR	NR	NR	NR	NR	NR	NR
Cerebral/other	6	NR	5	NR	NR	NR	NR	NR	NR	NR	NR	NR	NR	NR	NR
Ataxia/tremor/ cerebellar	NR	NR	NR	74.3	73.1	77.5	75	NR	89	NR	NR	NR	5–10	5–12	NR
Spinal cord	NR	NR	NR	NR	NR	NR	NR	NR	NR	NR	NR	NR	30–35	35–40	NR

B. Clinical Manifestation of Multiple Sclerosis by Race/Ethnicity

Values in Percentages %	Author: Langer-Gould			Author: Cree			Author: Amezcua		
	Caucasian n = 218	Hispanic/Latino n = 149	African American n = 70	Caucasian n = 427	Hispanic/Latino n = NR	African American n = 375	Caucasian n = 76	Hispanic/Latino n = 119	African American n = NR
Optic neuritis	43	54	30	22–23	NR	22–23	19.7	31.5	NR
Myelitis	37	27	41	39–41	NR	31–41	13.1	25	NR
Monoregional presentation	12	7	17	NR	NR	NR	NR	NR	NR
Polyregional presentation	6	7	9	11–13	NR	17–20	NR	NR	NR
Brainstem/cerebellum	NR	NR	NR	21–23	NR	16–18	NR	NR	NR
Cognitive	NR	NR	NR	0–2	NR	0–2	NR	NR	NR
Other or unknown	2	3	1	27–30	NR	30–33	18	16.7	NR

Values in percentages of patients for each presentation for all eligible Caucasian, Hispanic/Latino, and African American.

Abbreviation: NR, not reported.

African Americans with higher disability have greater T2 and T1 lesion volumes when compared with white Americans (P<.001–.006).[15,17] The proportion of contrast-enhancing lesions has been shown to be similar in both African American and white American groups. In regards to brain atrophy parameters, African Americans appear to suffer more severe diffuse tissue damage as measured by MTR.[15] Greater lesion volume and atrophy may explain the rapid clinical progression in African American patients, but this has not been confirmed.

African Americans with MS with acute optic neuritis have been reported to have more visual loss and poorer recovery and can often involve both optic nerves.[11,18] Studies using optical coherence tomography found that African Americans appear to have faster retinal nerve fiber loss (RNFL) and ganglion cell/inner plexiform layer (GCIP) thinning compared with white Americans.[18] Kimbrough and colleagues[18] additionally found that African American patients trended toward a greater loss of RNFL per year of disease duration (P = .056) and had a significantly greater loss of GCIP per year of disease duration compared with otherwise similar white American patients (P = .015). In a similar study, Seraji-Bozorgzad and colleagues[19] also showed that the RNFL was significantly thinner in African Americans compared with Caucasian American patients (87.2 μm vs 90.0 μm, P = .004). These findings, similar to MRI data and clinical course of disease, support a more aggressive disease progression in the African American population.

Hispanic Americans with Multiple Sclerosis

Hispanics are one of the largest minority ethnic groups in the United States, and Mexican Americans make up the largest subgroup followed by Puerto Ricans and Cubans. However, most studies to date in Hispanics have relied on self-reported ethnicity, which may not be sufficient to describe the underlying characteristics or to control for the potential confounding effects that stem from this ethnic and cultural variability. Nevertheless, studies on self-reported Hispanics with MS support that there are clinical characteristics that potentially stem from that diversity.

Similar to African Americans, Hispanics are reported to present with MS at a younger age compared with whites either at first symptom or at diagnosis.[9,20,21] A study of 125 Hispanics with MS compared with 100 non-Hispanic whites reported that Hispanics developed their first symptoms earlier (28.4 ± 0.97 years) in contrast to whites (32.5 ± 1.37 years). The difference was significantly younger (P>.001) for those who were US born compared with immigrant Hispanics arriving to the United States at adolescent age or older, with 74% developing MS in the United States. An incident and population-based study from the Kaiser Permanente Group also observed that Hispanics were significantly younger at MS diagnosis than whites or African Americans.[2] This observation continues to be consistent even across other regions of the United States. In a study where predominantly Hispanics of Caribbean background were included, Hispanics compared with whites had younger age at diagnosis and age at examination.[20] However, age at first symptom did not differ significantly between the 2 groups but did find that the US born were significantly younger than the immigrant counterpart. More recently, a study of Hispanics in the Eastern part of the United States suggests that age of onset for Hispanic is younger not only compared with whites but also with African Americans.[10]

Despite most studies thus far being cross-sectional, the clinical presentation difference in Hispanics compared with whites appears to be in the proportion of cases per category described (see **Table 2**). Hispanics with MS from western parts of the United States are more frequently reported to present with optic neuritis compared with whites.[3,21,22] In the southeastern part of the United States, Hispanics appear to present very similar to non-Hispanic whites with primarily sensory symptoms.[20] These differences could be related to genetic ancestral differences within group of Hispanics, such that the Western US Hispanics are predominantly Mexican in origin and have been reported to have a greater proportion of non-European background, which could suggest Native American influence in the disease compared with Hispanics in the southeastern United States, where this proportion may be lower.

Disability in Hispanics has been reported to be comparable to that in whites,[23] but recently rapid disability accumulation (age- and disease duration–adjusted) was found in Hispanics from the southeastern United States compared with whites, primarily among those with relapsing MS.[10] The dissimilarities were reported to not be driven by socioeconomic differences; however, 2 studies support that determinants of ambulatory disability in the Hispanics may be driven by place of birth differences supporting that Hispanics with MS that are not US born may be at a greater disadvantage.[20,24] In addition, access to care has been reported to be a significant factor in disability, highlighting potential health care disparities in disease severity outcomes.[10]

Of interest, the observation that African Americans and Asians are at risk of opticospinal MS is a feature that is also seen in Hispanics. The term opticospinal MS is defined by recurrent optic neuritis and myelitis attacks with minimal brain involvement that is now classified under the new diagnostic criteria of neuromyelitis optica spectrum disorders (NMOSD).[25] Intriguingly, in a cohort of Hispanics with a diagnosis of MS and aquaporin-negative antibody, about 20% were found to have spinal cord MRI features that are associated with opticospinal MS or NMOSD.[26] Those with longitudinal extensive spinal cord lesions (LESCLs) were 7 times more likely to have ambulatory disability compared with "no spinal cord lesions," highlighting the importance of spinal cord imaging and aquaporin antibody assessment in this population, which could be necessary to help guide treatment decisions.[27] Brain MRI lesion burden and visual outcomes are not available in Hispanics.

Genetic Underpinnings in African American and Hispanics with Multiple Sclerosis

Although there is considerable genetic heterogeneity within African Americans[28] and Hispanics, it is the European genetic ancestry that is thought to contribute to the risk of MS in this population.[29–32] The HLA region is the most important MS susceptibility locus genome wide, with a primary signal arising from DRB1*15 alleles.[30,33] Genome-wide association studies done in African Americans have been able to show that known MS genetic risk variants in whites partially overlap with that of African Americans.[31,32] In a study performed by Johnson and colleagues,[34] they analyzed 1574 African American individuals, including 918 MS cases and 656 unrelated control individuals. Seven single-nucleotide polymorphisms in 5 genes of interest (CD6, CLEC16a, EV15, GPC5, TYK2) were found to be significantly associated with MS in this African American dataset. In addition, correlations in HLA genotypes with MS phenotypes in African Americans with MS reported carriers for DRB1*15 alleles were twice more likely to have classic MS and have an earlier age of onset, whereas those following an opticospinal MS were less likely to carry DRB1*15.[35] Efforts in determining other susceptible genes that may be unique to African Americans and Hispanics and better understand phenotypic variability within and from whites are underway.

Potential Health Disparities and Access to Care

The burden of MS may weigh heavier on minorities in the United States compared with whites because of differences in sociocultural factors, such as acculturation, perceptions, income, access, and utilization, which are negatively disproportionate factors affecting these 2 populations compared with whites (**Box 1**). African Americans and

Box 1
Factors that may influence access and utilization of care among minority US groups

Acculturation

Illness perceptions

Socioeconomic status

Education

Community

Religious belief

Hispanics are overrepresented in groups that are socioeconomically disadvantaged by poverty and less education and are disproportionately affected by poor mental health, face barriers to care, and receive lower quality mental health care.[36]

In a survey of individuals with MS using the Independence Care System, a Medicaid long-term managed care plan in New York, specialty contact, disease-modifying therapies (DMT), and preventative care such as osteoporosis were negatively impacted.[23] More than 30% had never seen an MS specialist, and most had a poor understanding of the DMT. A general lack of adequate education and understanding about treatment, known resources, and realistic expectations about treatments were seen in both Hispanics and African Americans with MS.[23] Other major areas of concern were osteoporosis screening and participation in fall-prevention programs.

Although biological differences could be responsible for the clinical differences between whites and these 2 minority populations affected with MS, there are clear observations that MS can also differ by sociocultural factors. Hispanics in the United States represent a complex population of US-born and foreign-born immigrants, whereby immigration patterns have been noted to be influential in chronic inflammatory diseases.[37] Data indicate that these changing patterns among Hispanics may be related to acculturation, the process of cultural and psychological change that results following meeting between cultures.[38] Immigration can come at the expense of health concerns and proper care that could play a role in MS disease progression. In a cross-sectional assessment of Hispanics with MS, increased ambulatory disability was observed to be more common among the late immigrant compared with the US born (28% vs 18%, $P = .04$).[24] Being late-immigrant was independently associated with increased disability (adjusted odds ratio [OR] 2.3 95% CI 1.07–4.82; $P = .03$) compared with US born. Immigrant health-related outcomes are expected to continue.

Racial and ethnic disparities in access to care have been well documented among minority groups in the United States. Lack of access to specialty care has also been associated with development of preventable secondary conditions that are difficult and can have economic ramifications.[39] A study of disability in MS found that about half of the patients had difficulty receiving specialty care because of low income and poor health status.[40] Patients with low socioeconomic status often have difficulty accessing appropriate health care, and some are never treated by an MS specialist.[41] In a study of MS in African American patients in the New York State Multiple Sclerosis Consortium, a greater proportion of African American patients were unemployed compared with non-African American (13.7% vs 8.3%) and were enrolled in social security disability (31.9% vs 25.7%) before age 60.[13] More recent studies have suggested that being African American and living in rural regions is also a disadvantage.[42,43] A national sample (n = 2156) using mailings examined access to and use of neurologists and other specialists for MS and found that lack of health insurance (OR = 0.38), lower income, rural living, and being African American (OR = 0.52) were significantly associated with a lower probability of being under the care of an MS specialist.[44]

Several studies using the North American Research Committee on Multiple Sclerosis have also reported racial and ethnic disadvantages related to access. A study that incorporated more than 21,000 participants with MS found African Americans more likely to have severe disability, and they were also more likely to be in the lowest income and education levels and less likely to have private insurance compared with whites.[45] Buchanan and colleagues[46,47] noted that Hispanics versus whites had never received rehabilitation or support services. In addition, a larger number of Hispanics and African Americans reported mild depression (44%-46% compared with 39% whites with MS) and had never received mental health services. Understanding the level of interaction between these disparities in care and MS may provide avenues that could directly modify MS disease severity and progression. Future research is needed to determine if these significant differences in socioeconomic status, access to care, education level, and other demographic information can explain variations in MS disability in these groups.

Creating Awareness Among Minorities and Increasing Participation in Multiple Sclerosis

Ethnic minorities are known to have lower participation in health research.[48] Some of the common barriers to participation include the delivery of culturally sensitive and competent care to the underserved, lower income, and the less acculturated.[49] In addition, deficiency in the patient-physician relationship and mistrust of the medical community have been reported as barriers.[50] By developing patient navigation and educational opportunities that merge the patients and caregivers, the community, policymakers, health care professionals, and researchers participation of minorities in MS projects might be increased.[49,51] Nevertheless, focusing on clinicians and researchers to help increase their awareness about the barriers to minority participation may prove to also be helpful. Continued research is needed to understand how best to tackle and overcome low participation that could represent a bioethical concern in the care and treatment of MS. Perhaps an integrated care may be one approach to increase participation and access to care.

SUMMARY

African Americans and Hispanics could be at risk of greater MS disease burden early on in the disease course. The higher percent presenting at a younger age, the higher degree of lesion burden, greater disability at an early age, and personal challenges all have the capacity to contribute to health disparities. Although it is considered that the most sensitive of the determinants in MS are biology and genetics, disparities in overall health among different racial and ethnic groups in the United States are a real phenomenon that inarguably needs to be considered in MS if it can be modified. With an increasing understanding of the relationship between these genetics factors and health outcomes, greater opportunities to intervene can be seen. As we move toward personalized health care, health disparities will continue to increase in importance in the management of MS.

REFERENCES

1. Wallin MT, Culpepper WJ, Coffman P, et al. The Gulf War era multiple sclerosis cohort: age and incidence rates by race, sex and service. Brain 2012;135(Pt 6): 1778–85.

2. Langer-Gould A, Brara SM, Beaber BE, et al. Incidence of multiple sclerosis in multiple racial and ethnic groups. Neurology 2013;80(19):1734–9.
3. Langer-Gould A, Brara SM, Beaber BE, et al. The incidence of clinically isolated syndrome in a multi-ethnic cohort. J Neurol 2014;261(7):1349–55.
4. Wallin MT, Kurtzke JF, Culpepper WJ, et al. Multiple sclerosis in Gulf War era veterans. 2. Military deployment and risk of multiple sclerosis in the first Gulf War. Neuroepidemiology 2014;42(4):226–34.
5. Dilokthornsakul P, Valuck RJ, Nair KV, et al. Multiple sclerosis prevalence in the United States commercially insured population. Neurology 2016;86(11):1014–21.
6. Redelings MD, McCoy L, Sorvillo F. Multiple sclerosis mortality and patterns of co-morbidity in the United States from 1990 to 2001. Neuroepidemiology 2006;26(2): 102–7.
7. Amezcua L, Rivas E, Joseph S, et al. Higher age-specific cause mortality among younger blacks with multiple sclerosis in the United States, 1999-2014; ACTRIMS Forum 2017. Multiple Sclerosis Journal 2017;23(1_Suppl):2–90. P082.
8. Millstein J, Conti DV, Gilliland FD, et al. A testing framework for identifying susceptibility genes in the presence of epistasis. Am J Hum Genet 2006;78(1): 15–27.
9. Ventura RE, Antezana AO, Bacon T, et al. Hispanic Americans and African Americans with multiple sclerosis have more severe disease course than Caucasian Americans. Must Scler 2017;23(11):1554–7.
10. Kister I, Chamot E, Bacon JH, et al. Rapid disease course in African Americans with multiple sclerosis. Neurology 2010;75(3):217–23.
11. Cree BA, Khan O, Bourdette D, et al. Clinical characteristics of African Americans vs Caucasian Americans with multiple sclerosis. Neurology 2004;63(11): 2039–45.
12. Naismith RT, Trinkaus K, Cross AH. Phenotype and prognosis in African-Americans with multiple sclerosis: a retrospective chart review. Mult Scler 2006;12(6):775–81.
13. Weinstock-Guttman B, Jacobs LD, Brownscheidle CM, et al. Multiple sclerosis characteristics in African American patients in the New York State multiple sclerosis consortium. Mult Scler 2003;9(3):293–8.
14. Rinker JR 2nd, Trinkaus K, Naismith RT, et al. Higher IgG index found in African Americans versus Caucasians with multiple sclerosis. Neurology 2007;69(1): 68–72.
15. Weinstock-Guttman B, Ramanathan M, Hashmi K, et al. Increased tissue damage and lesion volumes in African Americans with multiple sclerosis. Neurology 2010; 74(7):538–44.
16. Fisniku LK, Brex PA, Altmann DR, et al. Disability and T2 MRI lesions: a 20-year follow-up of patients with relapse onset of multiple sclerosis. Brain 2008;131(Pt 3):808–17.
17. Howard J, Battaglini M, Babb JS, et al. MRI correlates of disability in African-Americans with multiple sclerosis. PLoS One 2012;7(8):e43061.
18. Kimbrough DJ, Sotirchos ES, Wilson JA, et al. Retinal damage and vision loss in African American multiple sclerosis patients. Ann Neurol 2015;77(2):228–36.
19. Seraji-Bozorgzad N, Reed S, Bao F, et al. Characterizing retinal structure injury in African-Americans with multiple sclerosis. Mult Scler Relat Disord 2016;7:16–20.
20. Hadjixenofontos A, Beecham AH, Manrique CP, et al. Clinical expression of multiple sclerosis in Hispanic whites of primarily Caribbean ancestry. Neuroepidemiology 2015;44(4):262–8.

21. Amezcua L, Lund BT, Weiner LP, et al. Multiple sclerosis in Hispanics: a study of clinical disease expression. Mult Scler 2011;17(8):1010–6.
22. Langille MM, Islam T, Burnett M, et al. Clinical characteristics of pediatric-onset and adult-onset multiple sclerosis in Hispanic Americans. J Child Neurol 2016; 31(8):1068–73.
23. Shabas D, Heffner M. Multiple sclerosis management for low-income minorities. Mult Scler 2005;11(6):635–40.
24. Amezcua L, Conti DV, Liu L, et al. Place of birth,age of immigration,and disability in Hispanics with multiple sclerosis. Mult Scler Relat Disord 2015;4(1):25–30.
25. Wingerchuk DM, Banwell B, Bennett JL, et al. International consensus diagnostic criteria for neuromyelitis optica spectrum disorders. Neurology 2015;85(2): 177–89.
26. Amezcua L, Lerner A, Ledezma K, et al. Spinal cord lesions and disability in Hispanics with multiple sclerosis. J Neurol 2013;260(11):2770–6.
27. Trebst C, Jarius S, Berthele A, et al. Update on the diagnosis and treatment of neuromyelitis optica: recommendations of the Neuromyelitis Optica Study Group (NEMOS). J Neurol 2014;261(1):1–16.
28. Tishkoff SA, Reed FA, Friedlaender FR, et al. The genetic structure and history of Africans and African Americans. Science 2009;324(5930):1035–44.
29. Ordonez G, Romero S, Orozco L, et al. Genomewide admixture study in Mexican Mestizos with multiple sclerosis. Clin Neurol Neurosurg 2015;130:55–60.
30. Oksenberg JR, Barcellos LF, Cree BA, et al. Mapping multiple sclerosis susceptibility to the HLA-DR locus in African Americans. Am J Hum Genet 2004;74(1): 160–7.
31. Isobe N, Madireddy L, Khankhanian P, et al. An immunochip study of multiple sclerosis risk in African Americans. Brain 2015;138(Pt 6):1518–30.
32. Isobe N, Gourraud PA, Harbo HF, et al. Genetic risk variants in African Americans with multiple sclerosis. Neurology 2013;81(3):219–27.
33. Hafler DA, Compston A, Sawcer S, et al. Risk alleles for multiple sclerosis identified by a genomewide study. N Engl J Med 2007;357(9):851–62.
34. Johnson BA, Wang J, Taylor EM, et al. Multiple sclerosis susceptibility alleles in African Americans. Genes Immun 2010;11(4):343–50.
35. Cree BA, Reich DE, Khan O, et al. Modification of multiple sclerosis phenotypes by African ancestry at HLA. Arch Neurol 2009;66(2):226–33.
36. Mallinger JB, Lamberti JS. Psychiatrists' attitudes toward and awareness about racial disparities in mental health care. Psychiatr Serv 2010;61(2):173–9.
37. Torres JM, Wallace SP. Migration circumstances, psychological distress, and self-rated physical health for Latino immigrants in the United States. Am J Public Health 2013;103(9):1619–27.
38. Lara M, Gamboa C, Kahramanian MI, et al. Acculturation and Latino health in the United States: a review of the literature and its sociopolitical context. Annu Rev Public Health 2005;26:367–97.
39. Lawthers AG, Pransky GS, Peterson LE, et al. Rethinking quality in the context of persons with disability. Int J Qual Health Care 2003;15(4):287–99.
40. Beatty PW, Hagglund KJ, Neri MT, et al. Access to health care services among people with chronic or disabling conditions: patterns and predictors. Arch Phys Med Rehabil 2003;84(10):1417–25.
41. Buchanan RJ, Zuniga MA, Carrillo-Zuniga G, et al. Comparisons of Latinos, African Americans, and Caucasians with multiple sclerosis. Ethn Dis 2010;20(4): 451–7.

42. Buchanan RJ, Stuifbergen A, Chakravorty BJ, et al. Urban/rural differences in access and barriers to health care for people with multiple sclerosis. J Health Hum Serv Adm 2006;29(3):360–75.
43. Minden SL, Frankel D, Hadden L, et al. Access to health care for people with multiple sclerosis. Mult Scler 2007;13(4):547–58.
44. Minden SL, Hoaglin DC, Hadden L, et al. Access to and utilization of neurologists by people with multiple sclerosis. Neurology 2008;70(13 Pt 2):1141–9.
45. Marrie RA, Cutter G, Tyry T, et al. Does multiple sclerosis-associated disability differ between races? Neurology 2006;66(8):1235–40.
46. Buchanan RJ, Johnson O, Zuniga MA, et al. Health-related quality of life among Latinos with multiple sclerosis. J Soc Work Disabil Rehabil 2012;11(4):240–57.
47. Buchanan RJ, Zuniga MA, Carrillo-Zuniga G, et al. A pilot study of Latinos with multiple sclerosis: demographic, disease, mental health, and psychosocial characteristics. J Soc Work Disabil Rehabil 2011;10(4):211–31.
48. Heller C, Balls-Berry JE, Nery JD, et al. Strategies addressing barriers to clinical trial enrollment of underrepresented populations: a systematic review. Contemp Clin Trials 2014;39(2):169–82.
49. Salman A, Nguyen C, Lee YH, et al. A review of barriers to minorities' participation in cancer clinical trials: implications for future cancer research. J Immigr Minor Health 2016;18(2):447–53.
50. Schmotzer GL. Barriers and facilitators to participation of minorities in clinical trials. Ethn Dis 2012;22(2):226–30.
51. Jandorf L, Fatone A, Borker PV, et al. Creating alliances to improve cancer prevention and detection among urban medically underserved minority groups. The East Harlem Partnership for Cancer Awareness. Cancer 2006;107(8 Suppl):2043–51.

Progressive Forms of Multiple Sclerosis

Distinct Entity or Age-Dependent Phenomena

Burcu Zeydan, MD[a,b], Orhun H. Kantarci, MD[a,*]

KEYWORDS

- Aging • Multiple sclerosis • Progression • Smoldering plaque

KEY POINTS

- Multiple sclerosis (MS) disease course is defined by a subclinical or clinical relapsing-remitting phase, a progressive phase, and the overlapping phase in-between.
- Each phase can have intermittently active or inactive periods.
- The onset of progressive phase of MS is age-dependent but time and pre-progressive phase agnostic.
- Pathologic hallmarks of progressive MS onset are age-dependent but pre-progressive phase agnostic.
- Subclinical activity behavior in patients with radiologically isolated syndrome evolving to primary progressive MS are mostly indistinguishable from patients with relapsing-remitting MS evolving to secondary progressive MS.

DEFINITIONS OF PHENOMENOLOGY IN MULTIPLE SCLEROSIS

Disease course in multiple sclerosis (MS) is defined by the interaction of 2 distinct phenomena: relapses and progression. A "relapse" can present either clinically as new central nervous system (CNS)-related neurologic symptom(s) evolving over hours to days, or subclinically as new MRI lesions without symptoms. Pathologically, an MS relapse is an acute inflammatory demyelination with or without axonal injury. When symptomatic, a relapse is generally expected to plateau over days to weeks, followed by a partial or complete recovery period. In some patients, there may be no recovery at all.

"Clinical recovery" is the maximum improvement attained after the peak deficit related to a relapse. In our experience, stabilization of clinical recovery usually occurs within the first 3 months and rarely continues beyond 6 months following a relapse.[1]

The authors report no disclosures.

[a] Department of Neurology, Mayo Clinic and Foundation, 200 First Street, Southwest, Rochester, MN 55905, USA; [b] Department of Radiology, Mayo Clinic and Foundation, 200 First Street, Southwest, Rochester, MN 55905, USA

* Corresponding author.

E-mail address: kantarci.orhun@mayo.edu

Neurol Clin 36 (2018) 163–171
https://doi.org/10.1016/j.ncl.2017.08.006
0733-8619/18/© 2017 Elsevier Inc. All rights reserved.

"Subclinical recovery" can be seen as resolution of enhancement, changes in diffusion characteristics, and/or shrinkage in size of the MS lesion(s) in MRI. The period through which recovery continues is referred to as the "remission" period, with the pathologic hallmark of remyelination with or without restoration of axonal integrity.

A "pseudo-relapse" is characterized by the emergence of symptoms in the setting of a previous clinical or subclinical relapse and is triggered by factors such as heat, infection, exercise, and fatigue. In our current understanding, this phenomenon appears when the symptomatic threshold is exceeded due to higher demand than the damaged nervous system can deliver. Symptomatic improvement follows swiftly with elimination of the specific trigger. When short-lived (<24 hours), it is easy to distinguish a pseudo-relapse from a relapse, but beyond that time point, it may be necessary to use imaging to rule out a new lesion as the cause of ongoing symptom(s).

"Progression" is the insidious and irreversible worsening of neurologic function due to MS with the pathologic hallmark of progressive axonal injury or loss. Progression can happen without ongoing clinical or subclinical relapses. To avoid confusion, the term "disability progression" should be changed to "disability worsening."[2] Disability worsening can be directly due to MS biology or can be due to other non–MS-related factors. MS-related disability worsening can result from stepwise accumulation of neurologic deficit from relapses, insidious accumulation of neurologic deficit from progressive disease course, or a combination of both. In our clinical practice, we also frequently use the term "pseudo-progression" to describe the disability worsening due to other non–MS-attributable factors, such as being deconditioned or degenerative hip disease.

MS activity is assessed both clinically and by MRI. "Active disease" is defined as new clinical or subclinical relapses (contrast-enhancing T1 hyperintense lesions or new T2 hyperintense lesions or enlarging T2 hyperintense lesions).[2] "Inactive disease" is defined as the absence of clinical events and MRI activity for ≥1 year[2] also known as "no evidence of disease activity."[3]

Based on these definitions, modern disease course classification in MS consists of 2 phases: the "relapsing-remitting phase" and the "progressive phase" (**Fig. 1**). Approximately 4 in 5 patients are expected to evolve from relapsing-remitting to progressive phase of the disease in their lifetime.[4] Each phase is then further defined as active or inactive at any given time.

RELAPSING-REMITTING PHASE OF MULTIPLE SCLEROSIS

Patients can present as asymptomatic or symptomatic during the relapsing-remitting phase of MS. The asymptomatic phase is incidentally discovered when MRIs are obtained in individuals due to reasons unrelated to typical MS symptoms. When the MRI findings fulfill ≥3 of the 4 imaging criteria,[5] a diagnosis of radiologically isolated syndrome (RIS) is established.[6–8] Many asymptomatic individuals also present with typical lesions suggestive of demyelinating disease, but fulfill fewer than 3 of the 4 imaging criteria. In our practice, we refer to these cases as pre-RIS. It is unclear how many of these individuals will evolve to RIS.

Clinically isolated syndrome (CIS) refers to the first symptomatic encounter in the relapsing-remitting phase of MS. This definition has evolved over time due to the changing dissemination in time and space criteria application in MS diagnosis. Originally defined as a single clinical relapse without any weight on MRI findings, CIS can evolve into clinically definite MS[9] when patients experience a second clinical relapse.[10] According to the most recent updates, subclinical relapses also fulfill dissemination in time and space criteria leading, therefore, to a diagnosis of MS

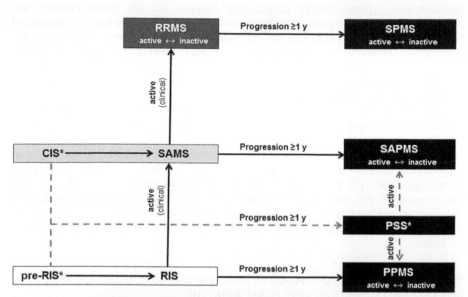

Fig. 1. Phases and disease course evolution in MS. Evolution between relapsing-remitting and progressive phases requires establishment of clinical progression of ≥1 year and is marked by an arrow. Evolution from one diagnostic group to other within a phase requires presence of active disease (dissemination in time) and is also marked by an arrow. When an evolution is likely but yet to be proven, a dashed arrow is used. When subclinical (MRI) activity is insufficient for a phase switch, it is marked by mentioning the need for clinical active status. When a diagnostic group is shown that does not fulfill dissemination in space criteria for MS, it is marked with an asterisk. All other groups need to fulfill dissemination in space criteria for MS. When switching back and forth between active and inactive status does not change the diagnostic group, it is also shown within that group box. CIS, clinically isolated syndrome; PPMS, primary progressive MS; PSS, progressive solitary sclerosis; RIS, radiologically isolated syndrome; RRMS, relapsing-remitting MS; SAMS, single attack MS; SAPMS, single attack progressive MS; SPMS, secondary progressive MS.

without the need for another clinical relapse.[11,12] We refer to patients with CIS who fulfill the current MS diagnostic criteria without a second clinical relapse as single-attack MS (SAMS). Relapsing-remitting MS (RRMS) evolves from CIS or SAMS when recurrent clinical relapses (with or without subclinical relapses) are present.

PROGRESSIVE PHASE OF MULTIPLE SCLEROSIS

Patients are diagnosed as having the clinical progressive phase of the disease if there has been sustained progression for a minimum of 1 year that cannot be explained by relapses or non–MS-related factors. Subgroup classification of the progressive phase is based on the presence or absence of preceding clinical relapses before the onset of progressive disease course. Therefore, primary progressive MS (PPMS) refers to RIS followed by progressive phase[13]; single-attack progressive MS (SAPMS) refers to SAMS followed by progressive phase[4,14]; and secondary progressive MS (SPMS) refers to RRMS followed by progressive phase. SAPMS and

SPMS are also grouped as bout-onset progressive MS. If a single but typical demyelinating lesion with (CIS) or without associated acute symptoms (pre-RIS) leads to an otherwise typical chronic progressive disease course, these patients are described as having progressive solitary sclerosis (PSS)[15,16] (see **Fig. 1**). The natural history and evolution of PSS has not yet been studied extensively. "Progressive-relapsing MS" refers to the active progressive phase with ongoing clinical or subclinical relapses, but this terminology is outdated. However, this category and the current description of active progressive MS highlight the overlap in relapsing-remitting and progressive phases of MS.

We believe that these operational terms (PPMS, PSS, SAPMS, and SPMS) do not relate to specific differences in progressive MS mechanisms but rather to yet-to-be-defined biological mechanisms that explain why relapses remain subclinical in some individuals. The reasons for this assertion are threefold: (1) the onset of progressive phase of MS is age-dependent but time and pre-progressive phase agnostic; (2) pathologic hallmarks of progressive MS onset are also age-dependent but pre-progressive phase agnostic; and (3) subclinical activity behavior in patients with RIS who evolve to PPMS is mostly indistinguishable from patients with RRMS who evolve to SPMS. We discuss these arguments further as follows.

THE ONSET OF PROGRESSIVE PHASE OF MULTIPLE SCLEROSIS IS AGE-DEPENDENT BUT TIME AND PRE-PROGRESSIVE PHASE AGNOSTIC

In contemporary studies, all subtypes of progressive MS are shown to start at an almost identical age.[4,13,17,18] We have shown that 99% of patients with established progressive MS developed progressive disease before the age of 75 with a mean age at progressive MS onset of 45 ± 10 years.[4]

Although time from first clinical relapse to progressive MS onset is shorter for patients with SAPMS compared with patients with SPMS, age at progressive MS onset was indistinguishable between these groups.[4] Because patients with PPMS do not have a preceding clinical relapse, one cannot reliably analyze the time factor (eg, clinical disease duration) before the onset of PPMS. However, patients with PPMS also have the same age at onset of progressive MS as patients with SAPMS or SPMS.[4] Clearly, the duration of a preceding clinically relapsing phase and whether a patient has none, 1, or multiple clinical relapses before the onset of progressive MS do not seem to alter the age when clinically obvious progression ensues.[4,14,17–19]

However, subclinical progression (eg, whole brain, thalamic, or spinal cord atrophy) likely starts long before clinical progression. Indeed, limited recovery from the first 5-year clinical relapse(s) seems to accelerate the progressive MS evolution regardless of later disease course,[1] and deep or cortical gray matter atrophy can present as early as the RIS phase.[20] Patients with PPMS are also likely to do worse in the setting of poor recovery of subclinical relapses, but this cannot be assessed directly because they usually present after symptom onset. RIS offers the only period to study this hypothesis.[13] There certainly needs to be more work in this area to elucidate the imaging biomarkers of subclinical progression.

Predictors of evolution to progressive MS, other than age, with varying levels of supportive evidence are male sex, the presence of spinal cord lesions, tobacco use, low serum 25-hydroxyvitamin D levels, high salt intake, and obesity.[13,21–24] Many of these factors could also interact with the aging process of the nervous system, requiring further study in the setting of MS.

PATHOLOGIC HALLMARKS OF PROGRESSIVE MULTIPLE SCLEROSIS ONSET ARE AGE-DEPENDENT BUT PRE-PROGRESSIVE PHASE AGNOSTIC

Inflammation and oxidative stress are 2 essential mechanisms underlying MS disease pathology. Inflammation in MS is driven by T cells, B cells, activated microglia, and macrophages.[25] It results in active tissue injury and is associated with active demyelination and neurodegeneration independent of clinical phase.[25,26] Oxidative stress is mediated by inflammation and the oxidative burst of microglia. It results in mitochondrial injury and is also associated with demyelination and neurodegeneration independent of the clinical phase.[25] Mitochondrial dysfunction also contributes to oligodendrocyte apoptosis and poor or nonexistent remyelination in MS.[25,27,28] The main mechanisms of disease pathophysiology and basic pathologic premises appear similar in different phases of MS. However, the disease mechanisms vary in severity and quantity, which leads to more intensified effects observed in the progressive phase.

In the relapsing-remitting phase of MS, episodic inflammation, demyelination, and remyelination predominate, whereas progressive axonal dysfunction/loss and limited inflammation predominate in the progressive phase of MS. The sequence of the tissue injury cascade in progressive MS is demyelination, oligodendrocyte loss, a higher predilection for thin axonal damage, astrocytic gliosis, and absence of re-myelination.[26,29] Once the axonal damage/loss threshold is exceeded, the progressive phase of MS ensues.[30–32]

Aging leads to decreased trophic support from the peri-plaque environment, which contributes to the neurodegeneration process.[33] Because remyelinating capacity also declines with age, this lack of remyelination contributes to the progressive MS phase by limiting functional recovery or compensatory myelin maintenance.[34,35]

The possibility of trapped, "compartmentalized inflammation" in the progressive phase of MS leading to limited anti-inflammatory treatment access has also been postulated.[25] Similarly, oxidative stress followed by mitochondrial injury seems to affect progressive MS more intensely. This may be due to higher levels of iron in the older human brain, which accumulates in oligodendrocytes in an age-dependent manner.[25] Mitochondrial aging, therefore, could easily contribute to progressive MS onset.

MS plaques are classified as active, inactive, shadow, and smoldering.[26,36] "Active" plaques show macrophage infiltrates with myelin-degradation products (and reveal gadolinium enhancement). They are described as the pathologic correlates of clinical or subclinical relapses[37] in the relapsing phases of MS, including overlapping relapsing and progressive phases. In contrast, "inactive" plaques, with no or a very limited number of macrophages and activated microglia, are frequently seen in SPMS without relapses. "Shadow" plaques have the ability to remyelinate fully,[38] and are usually seen across the MS continuum.[39]

"Smoldering" plaques with a rim of activated microglia and inactive center expand slowly over time.[26] They are typically associated with both SPMS and PPMS, but they predominate over active plaques in PPMS.[39] As neurodegeneration in progressive MS continues, preexisting chronic plaques may increase in size, resulting in slowly expanding, "smoldering" plaques.[39,40] These plaques show constant neurodegeneration and axonal injury as well as microglia activation, which support "a slow but active" demyelination process in progressive MS.[26]

We refer to the process described previously as the "rise of the smoldering plaque," a seemingly pathologic hallmark of progressive MS[39] peaking at approximately age 47, mirroring the independent epidemiologic observation of established mean age of progressive MS onset of 45.[4] A balance between active and inactive plaques also becomes apparent around the same time.[39] Recent imaging data on the loss of white-matter reserve support this specific age window as well. The compact white-matter myelination in human brain terminates by the fourth decade, and white-matter tracts start to degenerate slowly in the following years.[41,42]

SUBCLINICAL ACTIVITY BEHAVIOR IN PATIENTS WITH RADIOLOGICALLY ISOLATED SYNDROME EVOLVING TO PRIMARY PROGRESSIVE MULTIPLE SCLEROSIS ARE MOSTLY INDISTINGUISHABLE FROM PATIENTS WITH RELAPSING-REMITTING MULTIPLE SCLEROSIS EVOLVING TO SECONDARY PROGRESSIVE MULTIPLE SCLEROSIS

Besides age at progressive MS onset and the pathologic hallmark, "rise of the smoldering plaque," PPMS and bout-onset progressive MS (SPMS and SAPMS) also have almost identical brain imaging features before progressive MS onset and the same female-to-male ratio.[4,17,18] Indeed, the presymptomatic RIS phase of PPMS is indistinguishable from the RRMS phase of SPMS.[13]

Although they share the same biology, these clinical subtypes of the progressive MS phase are still distinct from each other. The main distinction is presence or absence of resistance to acute symptom manifestations of relapses. The biologic mechanism underlying this difference is yet to be fully discovered. Another difference is the long-term disability accrual. The effect of progressive disease course onset on disability accumulation is the same for both subtypes, but the relapse-based disability accumulation gives bout-onset progressive MS a head start at the time of progressive MS onset.[18,43] Also reflecting the pre-progressive phase, patients with BOPMS have a higher tendency for ongoing clinical relapse after progression ensues, leading to further disability accumulation.[43]

SUMMARY

In recent years we have confirmed that the onset of the clinical progressive phase in MS is dependent on aging rather than on the duration of preceding symptomatic disease. In epidemiology studies, age at progression onset in primary progressive MS (mid-fifth decade) is the same as age at progression onset in secondary progressive MS. The imaging findings in the subclinical pre-progression phase of primary progressive MS are largely indistinguishable from the symptomatic relapsing-remitting phase preceding SPMS. Pathologically, all progressive MS subgroups are characterized by the presence of smoldering plaques that also peak in the mid-fifth decade. In imaging studies, the mid-fifth decade marks the end of a plateau and the beginning of a decline in white-matter integrity in normal-aging individuals. Therefore, 2 major conclusions can be reached about progressive MS. Degenerative processes, with or without compartmentalized inflammatory mechanisms leading to white-matter aging, are predominantly responsible for the progressive MS phenotype. Differences between PPMS and SPMS seem to be driven more by the mechanisms leading to subclinical versus clinical presentation of relapses rather than by mechanisms inherent to progression itself. Further study of both these points will elicit a deeper understanding of the biology of progressive MS, which will lead, in turn, to the development of more meaningful treatment interventions.

ACKNOWLEDGMENTS

The authors thank Lea Dacy for help with editing, proofreading, and formatting.

REFERENCES

1. Novotna M, Paz Soldan MM, Abou Zeid N, et al. Poor early relapse recovery affects onset of progressive disease course in multiple sclerosis. Neurology 2015; 85:722–9.
2. Lublin FD, Reingold SC, Cohen JA, et al. Defining the clinical course of multiple sclerosis: the 2013 revisions. Neurology 2014;83:278–86.
3. Rotstein DL, Healy BC, Malik MT, et al. Evaluation of no evidence of disease activity in a 7-year longitudinal multiple sclerosis cohort. JAMA Neurol 2015;72: 152–8.
4. Tutuncu M, Tang J, Zeid NA, et al. Onset of progressive phase is an age-dependent clinical milestone in multiple sclerosis. Mult Scler 2013;19:188–98.
5. Tintore M, Rovira A, Rio J, et al. New diagnostic criteria for multiple sclerosis: application in first demyelinating episode. Neurology 2003;60:27–30.
6. Siva A, Saip S, Altintas A, et al. Multiple sclerosis risk in radiologically uncovered asymptomatic possible inflammatory-demyelinating disease. Mult Scler 2009;15: 918–27.
7. Lebrun C, Bensa C, Debouverie M, et al. Unexpected multiple sclerosis: follow-up of 30 patients with magnetic resonance imaging and clinical conversion profile. J Neurol Neurosurg Psychiatry 2008;79:195–8.
8. Okuda DT, Mowry EM, Beheshtian A, et al. Incidental MRI anomalies suggestive of multiple sclerosis: the radiologically isolated syndrome. Neurology 2009;72: 800–5.
9. Poser CM, Paty DW, Scheinberg L, et al. New diagnostic criteria for multiple sclerosis: guidelines for research protocols. Ann Neurol 1983;13:227–31.
10. Brex PA, Ciccarelli O, O'Riordan JI, et al. A longitudinal study of abnormalities on MRI and disability from multiple sclerosis. N Engl J Med 2002;346:158–64.
11. Polman CH, Reingold SC, Banwell B, et al. Diagnostic criteria for multiple sclerosis: 2010 revisions to the McDonald criteria. Ann Neurol 2011;69:292–302.
12. Filippi M, Rocca MA, Ciccarelli O, et al. MRI criteria for the diagnosis of multiple sclerosis: MAGNIMS consensus guidelines. Lancet Neurol 2016;15:292–303.
13. Kantarci OH, Lebrun C, Siva A, et al. Primary progressive multiple sclerosis evolving from radiologically isolated syndrome. Ann Neurol 2016;79:288–94.
14. Kremenchutzky M, Rice GP, Baskerville J, et al. The natural history of multiple sclerosis: a geographically based study 9: observations on the progressive phase of the disease. Brain 2006;129:584–94.
15. Schmalstieg WF, Keegan BM, Weinshenker BG. Solitary sclerosis: progressive myelopathy from solitary demyelinating lesion. Neurology 2012;78:540–4.
16. Keegan BM, Kaufmann TJ, Weinshenker BG, et al. Progressive solitary sclerosis: gradual motor impairment from a single CNS demyelinating lesion. Neurology 2016;87:1713–9.
17. Koch M, Mostert J, Heersema D, et al. Progression in multiple sclerosis: further evidence of an age dependent process. J Neurol Sci 2007;255:35–41.
18. Confavreux C, Vukusic S. Natural history of multiple sclerosis: a unifying concept. Brain 2006;129:606–16.
19. Scalfari A, Neuhaus A, Daumer M, et al. Age and disability accumulation in multiple sclerosis. Neurology 2011;77:1246–52.
20. Azevedo CJ, Overton E, Khadka S, et al. Early CNS neurodegeneration in radiologically isolated syndrome. Neurol Neuroimmunol Neuroinflamm 2015;2:e102.
21. Okuda DT, Siva A, Kantarci O, et al. Radiologically isolated syndrome: 5-year risk for an initial clinical event. PLoS One 2014;9:e90509.

22. Ascherio A, Munger KL, White R, et al. Vitamin D as an early predictor of multiple sclerosis activity and progression. JAMA Neurol 2014;71:306–14.
23. Healy BC, Ali EN, Guttmann CR, et al. Smoking and disease progression in multiple sclerosis. Arch Neurol 2009;66:858–64.
24. Hernan MA, Jick SS, Logroscino G, et al. Cigarette smoking and the progression of multiple sclerosis. Brain 2005;128:1461–5.
25. Lassmann H, van Horssen J, Mahad D. Progressive multiple sclerosis: pathology and pathogenesis. Nat Rev Neurol 2012;8:647–56.
26. Frischer JM, Bramow S, Dal-Bianco A, et al. The relation between inflammation and neurodegeneration in multiple sclerosis brains. Brain 2009;132:1175–89.
27. Trapp BD, Stys PK. Virtual hypoxia and chronic necrosis of demyelinated axons in multiple sclerosis. Lancet Neurol 2009;8:280–91.
28. Witte ME, Geurts JJ, de Vries HE, et al. Mitochondrial dysfunction: a potential link between neuroinflammation and neurodegeneration? Mitochondrion 2010;10:411–8.
29. Lassmann H. Review: the architecture of inflammatory demyelinating lesions: implications for studies on pathogenesis. Neuropathol Appl Neurobiol 2011;37:698–710.
30. Trapp BD, Peterson J, Ransohoff RM, et al. Axonal transection in the lesions of multiple sclerosis. N Engl J Med 1998;338:278–85.
31. Bjartmar C, Wujek JR, Trapp BD. Axonal loss in the pathology of MS: consequences for understanding the progressive phase of the disease. J Neurol Sci 2003;206:165–71.
32. Confavreux C, Vukusic S, Adeleine P. Early clinical predictors and progression of irreversible disability in multiple sclerosis: an amnesic process. Brain 2003;126:770–82.
33. Rist JM, Franklin RJ. Taking ageing into account in remyelination-based therapies for multiple sclerosis. J Neurol Sci 2008;274:64–7.
34. Hinks GL, Franklin RJ. Delayed changes in growth factor gene expression during slow remyelination in the CNS of aged rats. Mol Cell Neurosci 2000;16:542–56.
35. Zhao C, Li WW, Franklin RJ. Differences in the early inflammatory responses to toxin-induced demyelination are associated with the age-related decline in CNS remyelination. Neurobiol Aging 2006;27:1298–307.
36. Bruck W, Porada P, Poser S, et al. Monocyte/macrophage differentiation in early multiple sclerosis lesions. Ann Neurol 1995;38:788–96.
37. Filippi M, Rocca MA, Barkhof F, et al. Association between pathological and MRI findings in multiple sclerosis. Lancet Neurol 2012;11:349–60.
38. Barkhof F, Bruck W, De Groot CJ, et al. Remyelinated lesions in multiple sclerosis: magnetic resonance image appearance. Arch Neurol 2003;60:1073–81.
39. Frischer JM, Weigand SD, Guo Y, et al. Clinical and pathological insights into the dynamic nature of the white matter multiple sclerosis plaque. Ann Neurol 2015;78:710–21.
40. Rovaris M, Barkhof F, Bastianello S, et al. Multiple sclerosis: interobserver agreement in reporting active lesions on serial brain MRI using conventional spin echo, fast spin echo, fast fluid-attenuated inversion recovery and post-contrast T1-weighted images. J Neurol 1999;246:920–5.
41. Westlye LT, Walhovd KB, Dale AM, et al. Life-span changes of the human brain white matter: diffusion tensor imaging (DTI) and volumetry. Cereb Cortex 2010;20:2055–68.

42. Hasan KM, Kamali A, Abid H, et al. Quantification of the spatiotemporal micro-structural organization of the human brain association, projection and commis-sural pathways across the lifespan using diffusion tensor tractography. Brain Struct Funct 2010;214:361–73.
43. Paz Soldan MM, Novotna M, Abou Zeid N, et al. Relapses and disability accumu-lation in progressive multiple sclerosis. Neurology 2015;84:81–8.

New Advances in Disease-Modifying Therapies for Relapsing and Progressive Forms of Multiple Sclerosis

Angela Vidal-Jordana, MD, PhD

KEYWORDS

- Multiple sclerosis • Treatment • Management • Neuroprotection • Myelin repair

KEY POINTS

- Treatment development in past years has been extremely active and a great number of disease-modifying treatments have emerged for treating multiple sclerosis (MS) patients.
- Newer drugs, some of them with newer mechanisms of action, are still being developed for treating MS patients.
- There is a growing interest in developing new drugs that will promote neuroprotection and/ or myelin repair that may target the most degenerative component of the disease.

INTRODUCTION

Multiple sclerosis (MS) is a chronic autoimmune disease of the central nervous system (CNS) in which inflammation, demyelination, and axonal loss occurs from very early stages of the disease. It mainly affects young people, between 20 and 40 years old, with a female predominance.[1,2]

Treatment development in the past years has been extremely active and a great number of disease-modifying treatments have emerged for treating patients with MS. For the purpose of this review, the Food and Drug Administration (FDA) and the European Medicines Agency (EMA) Web pages were consulted; the ClinicalTrial.gov database was also searched using the following criteria: multiple sclerosis, interventional, with results, and first received from 2010 to March 2017. In this article, we

Conflicts of Interest: A. Vidal-Jordana has received honoraria as speaker and/or for participation in Advisory Boards from Novartis, Roche, Sanofi-Genzyme, and Biogen.
Department of Neurology-Neuroimmunology, Multiple Sclerosis Centre of Catalonia (Edifici Cemcat), Hospital Universitari Vall d'Hebron, Universitat Autònoma de Barcelona, P. Vall d'Hebron 119-129, Barcelona 08035, Spain
E-mail address: avidal@cem-cat.org

Neurol Clin 36 (2018) 173–183
http://dx.doi.org/10.1016/j.ncl.2017.08.011
0733-8619/18/© 2017 Elsevier Inc. All rights reserved.

discuss the newest drugs that, as of March 1, 2017, (1) are currently being evaluated by the FDA or the EMA or have been recently approved by these governmental agencies, and (2) are under development and have completed at least 1 phase 2 clinical trial with published results in the past 3 years (2014).

NEWLY RELEASED AND FORTHCOMING DRUGS

In recent years, a wealth of new therapies have been approved for the treatment of MS (**Table 1**). It is beyond the scope of this article to address them; instead, I discuss the newest drugs that, as of March 1, 2017, were currently being evaluated by the FDA or the EMA or that were approved by these governmental agencies during 2016.

Table 1
Current and forthcoming drugs for the treatment of multiple sclerosis

Drug	Posology	FDA/EMA Approval
Interferon beta 1b	Subcutaneous per 48 h	1993/1995
Interferon beta 1a	Intramuscular per 1 wk	1996/1997
Interferon beta 1b	Subcutaneous 3 times per week	2002/1998
Pegylated interferon beta	Subcutaneous per 2 wk	2014/2014
Glatiramer acetate	Subcutaneous per 24 h per 48 h	1996/2001 2014/2014
Natalizumab	Intravenous per 4 wk	2006/2006
Fingolimod	Oral per 24 h	2010/2011
Teriflunomide	Oral per 24 h	2012/2013
Alemtuzumab	Intravenous per 1 y[a]	2014/2013
Dimethyl fumarate	Oral per 12 h	2013/2014
Daclizumab	Subcutaneous per 4 wk	2016/2016
Ocrelizumab	Intravenous per 6 mo	2017/awaiting
Cladribine	Oral per 1 y[b]	Under EMA review

Abbreviations: EMA, European Medicines Agency; FDA, US Food and Drug Administration.
[a] Alemtuzumab is administered in 2 treatment courses: in the first course, alemtuzumab is administered on 5 consecutive days; in the second course, alemtuzumab is administered on 5 consecutive days.
[b] The recommended treatment schedule has not been confirmed. In clinical trials, cladribine was administered in 2 treatment courses: in the first course, cladribine is taken for 5 consecutive days in the first month and for 5 consecutive days in the second month, this same treatment course is repeated a second time 12 months later.

Daclizumab

Daclizumab is a humanized monoclonal antibody that binds to the α-chain of the high-affinity interleukin (IL)-2 receptor blocking its binding. This leads to an endogenous increase of free available IL-2 that will bind to the intermediate-affinity IL-2 receptor producing different immunologic effects, such as expansion of the regulatory CD56 natural killer cells, inhibition of T-cell activation, and a reduction in lymphoid tissue inducer.[3]

Efficacy

Two clinical trials demonstrated that daclizumab was superior than placebo[4] and intramuscular interferon beta (IM IFN-β)[5] to treat patients with relapsing-remitting MS (RRMS). Daclizumab, administered subcutaneously at a dosage of 150 mg every 4 weeks, was associated with a 54% and 45% reduction in the annualized relapse rate (ARR) compared with placebo and to IM IFN-β treatment, respectively.[4,5] Daclizumab treatment also reduced the risk of 3-month confirmed disability progression, but only in the placebo-controlled trial.[4,5] Regarding MRI disease activity, daclizumab treatment significantly reduced the number of new T2 lesions and the number of gadolinium (Gd)-enhancing lesions both compared with placebo (70% and 85% reduction, respectively) as well as with IM IFNβ (54% and 65% reduction, respectively).

Safety

The most common adverse events reported under daclizumab treatment include nonopportunistic infections, cutaneous events, and hepatic disorders.[3–5] Hepatic disorders were reported in approximately 16% of daclizumab-treated patients, and serious hepatic adverse events were observed in 1% of daclizumab-treated patients.[3] Thus, liver enzyme monitoring should be conducted monthly while on daclizumab, and at least up to 4 months after the last dose of daclizumab.[6,7] One-third of patients reported cutaneous adverse events, with rash, dermatitis, and eczema the most frequent skin reactions. Serious cutaneous adverse events (such as toxic skin eruption or exfoliative rash) were experienced by 2% of daclizumab-treated patients.[3] Referral to a dermatologist is recommended in cases of severe or diffuse skin reaction[6,7]; management of these cutaneous adverse events may need topic or systemic corticosteroid treatment.

Ocrelizumab

Ocrelizumab is a humanized monoclonal antibody that selectively binds to the B-cell-surface CD20 antigen.[8] The adhesion of ocrelizumab to its target produces a selective depletion of B cells presenting with the antigen: pre-B cells, mature B cells, and memory B cells, but it will not affect lymphoid stem cells and plasma cells.[8]

Efficacy

Ocrelizumab has demonstrated to be more effective than IFN-β thrice weekly to treat RRMS in 1 phase 2[9] and 2 phase 3 clinical trials.[8] The results of the 2 phase 3 clinical trials demonstrated that, compared with subcutaneous IFN-β, ocrelizumab significantly reduced by 46% to 47% the ARR after 2 years of treatment.[8] Patients receiving ocrelizumab had a 40% lower risk of presenting 12-week confirmed disability progression than IFN-β–treated patients. Regarding MRI parameters, ocrelizumab treatment reduced by 77% to 83% the mean number of new T2 lesions and by 94% to 95% the mean number of Gd-enhancing lesions. These results were consistent with the results reported in the phase 2 trial.[9] Of note, most of the MRI disease activity occurred during the first 6 months after treatment onset,[8] and was detectable as early as 8 weeks.[9] Ocrelizumab efficacy was also evaluated in patients with primary progressive MS yielding, for the first time in this disease phenotype, positive results.[10] Thus, compared with placebo, ocrelizumab significantly reduced by 24% and 25% the risk of presenting

12-week and 24-week confirmed disability progression, respectively.[10] Brain MRI endpoints, such as volume of hyperintense T2-weighted lesions, brain volume change, and mean number of new T2 lesions, also favored ocrelizumab over placebo.[10]

Safety

Similar rates of adverse events, including serious adverse events, were reported in the ocrelizumab group as well as in the IFN-β or placebo groups.[8,10] The most common adverse event reported in the ocrelizumab group was infusion-related reactions that occurred in approximately 35% to 40%.[8,10] Other common adverse events were nasopharyngitis, upper respiratory tract infection, and urinary tract infections.[8,10] It is worth mentioning that an imbalance in the incidence of neoplasms was observed in the ocrelizumab groups that warrants further investigation.[8,10]

Cladribine

Cladribine is a synthetic purine analog that enters the cell via the purine nucleoside transporters and is subsequently phosphorylated. The accumulation of the active metabolite, 2-chlorodeoxyadenosine triphosphate, disrupts cellular metabolism and damages DNA, causing cell death. This process ultimately leads to lymphocyte depletions and long-lasting lymphopenia.

Efficacy

Cladribine has demonstrated to be effective in treating RRMS in 1 phase 3 clinical trial,[11] as well as to delay conversion to MS after presenting a clinically isolated syndrome (CIS).[12] Compared with placebo, oral treatment with cladribine reduced in approximately 56% the ARR (57.6% reduction for the 3.5-mg/kg dose, and 54.5% reduction for the 5.25-mg/kg dose) and in approximately 32% the risk of presenting 3-month confirmed disability progression (33% reduction for the 3.5-mg/kg dose, and 31% reduction for the 5.25-mg/kg dose).[11] Regarding MRI parameters, cladribine reduced in approximately 75% the risk of presenting new T2 lesions (73.4% and 76.9% reduction for the 3.5-mg/kg and 5.25-mg/kg dose, respectively), and in approximately 86% the risk of presenting Gd-enhancing lesions (85.7% and 87.9% reduction for the 3.5-mg/kg and 5.25-mg/kg dose, respectively).[11] After a CIS, cladribine treatment significantly delayed the time to conversion to clinically definite MS, with 62% to 67% risk reduction in time to conversion to MS for the 5.25-mg/kg and 3.5-mg/kg doses, respectively.[12]

Safety

The most common adverse event was lymphocytopenia, which is in line with the drug's mechanism of action.[11,12] Infections, and especially opportunistic infections (such as activation of herpes virus, activation of latent tuberculosis or fungal infections), were also more commonly reported in the cladribine-treatment arm.[11,12] Because of a suspected increase in cancer risk under cladribine treatment, in 2011 the application for marketing authorization was withdrawn.[13] This association could not be confirmed in the long-term safety monitoring of the clinical trials,[14] and the drug is currently under review in the EMA.

DRUGS UNDER DEVELOPMENT

Newer drugs, some of them with novel mechanisms of action, are still being developed for treating patients with MS. This section focuses on the new drugs that are under development and have completed at least 1 phase 2 clinical trial with published results in the past 3 years (**Table 2**).

Table 2
New drugs under development for treating multiple sclerosis

Drug	Design	Randomization	Primary Outcome
Secukinumab	Phase 2, 73 active MS, 24 wk (NCT01874340)	Placebo vs secukinumab 10 mg/kg	Cumulative number of CUAL[a] observed on brain MRI scans from week 4 to week 24
Ponesimod	Phase 2b, 464 RRMS, 24 wk (NCT01006265)	Placebo vs ponesimod 10, 20, or 40 mg (up-titration for the 20-mg and 40-mg doses)	Cumulative number of new Gd-enhancing lesions from weeks 12–24
Siponimod	Phase 3, 1651 SPMS, 2 y (NCT01665144)	Placebo vs siponimod 2 mg (up-titration)	Delay in time to confirmed disability progression as measured by EDSS
Ozanimod	Phase 2, 258 RRMS, 24 wk (NCT01628393)	Placebo vs ozanimod 0.5, 1 mg (up-titration for both doses)	Cumulative number of new Gd-enhancing lesions from weeks 12–24
Amiselimod	Phase 2, 415 RRMS, 24 wk (NCT01742052)	Placebo vs amiselimod 0.1, 0.2, or 0.4 mg	Total number of Gd-enhancing lesions from weeks 8–24
MD1003 or high-dose biotin	Phase 3, 154 progressive MS, 1 y (NCT02220933)	Placebo vs MD1003 (300 mg biotine) as add-on therapy if needed	Proportion of patients with improvement of MS-related disability at month 9, confirmed at month 12
Opicinumab	Phase 2, 82 first ON, 32 wk (NCT01721161)	Placebo vs opicinumab	Optic nerve conduction velocity measured by FF-VEP
	Phase 2b, RR or SPMS, 84 wk (NCT01864148)	Placebo vs opicinumab 3, 10, 30, or 100 mg/kg as add-on therapy to IM IFN	Percentage of patients experiencing confirmed improvement of neurophysical and/or cognitive function over 72 wk
GSK239512	Phase 2, 131 RRMS, 1 y (NCT01772199)	Placebo vs GSK239512 as add-on therapy to IFN or GA	Mean changes in MTR post-lesion compared with pre-lesion in newly developed lesions

Abbreviations: CUAL, combined unique active lesions; EDSS, Expanded Disability Status Scale; FF-VEP, full-field visual evoked potentials; Gd, gadolinium; IFN, interferon beta; IM, intramuscular; MS, multiple sclerosis; MTR, magnetization transfer ratio; ON, optic neuritis; RRMS, relapsing-remitting multiple sclerosis; SPMS, secondary progressive multiple sclerosis.
[a] CUAL was defined as new gadolinium-enhancing lesions on T1-weighted scans and new or enlarging lesions on T2-weighted scans (without double counting).

Secukinumab

Secukinumab is a fully human monoclonal antibody that selectively binds to human IL-17A, a proinflammatory cytokine involved in MS pathogenesis, neutralizing its bioactivity.[15]

Efficacy

The efficacy of secukinumab has been recently evaluated in a 6-month, placebo-controlled, phase 2 clinical trial. At the end of the study, patients receiving secukinumab presented with a lower cumulative number of combined unique active lesions (CUAL) on brain MRI. More specifically, secukinumab reduced the mean cumulative CUAL by almost 50%; however, this difference was not statistically significant ($P = .087$), and therefore the primary outcome was not met.[15] When analyzing radiological outcomes separately (a prespecified secondary endpoint), secukinumab reduced the mean cumulative number of new Gd-enhancing lesions at each monthly visit starting at week 16. As for new or enlarging T2 lesions, secukinumab reduced the mean cumulative number at the end of the study but not before.[15]

Safety

The overall incidence of adverse events was similar between both treatment arms, although infections were more frequently reported in patients receiving secukinumab.[15]

Sphingosine 1-Phosphate Receptor Modulators

Sphingosine 1-phosphate (S1P) is a signaling molecule involved in a wide range of immunologic, cardiovascular, and neurologic processes through interaction with 5 members of the transmembrane receptor family. Each of the S1P receptors are differently expressed in the following cell structures: $S1P_1$ receptor is mainly expressed in lymphocytes, neural cells, endothelial cells, atrial myocytes, and smooth muscle cells; $S1P_2$ receptor is expressed in the CNS, endothelial cells, and smooth muscle cells; $S1P_3$ receptor is expressed in neural cells, endothelial cells, and smooth muscle cells; $S1P_4$ receptor is expressed in lymphocytes; and $S1P_5$ receptor is expressed in the CNS, oligodendrocytes, and natural killer cells.

The S1P receptor modulators mechanism of action in MS is through binding of the S1P receptors on the lymphocytes ($S1P_1$ or $S1P_4$). Initial agonist actions between S1P with the S1P receptor in the lymphocytes are followed by an internalization and degradation of the receptor leading to a functional antagonism that will prevent lymphocyte egression from the lymph nodes. When the modulation is not restricted to these receptors (as is the case for instance of fingolimod) serious adverse events may appear. Thus, S1P receptor modulators with an improved safety profile and shorter half-lives are being pursued.

Ponesimod

Ponesimod is a selective $S1P_1$ receptor modulator.

Efficacy The efficacy of ponesimod has been recently tested in a double-blind, placebo-controlled, dose-finding phase 2b study. In this study, all 3 doses of ponesimod significantly reduced the cumulative number of new T1 Gd-enhancing lesions with a greater reduction seen in the highest doses (43%, 83%, and 77% reduction for the 10-mg, 20-mg, and 40-mg doses, respectively). The ARR, as well as other radiological secondary efficacy endpoints, were also significantly reduced in the ponesimod-treatment arms.

Safety Anxiety, dizziness, dyspnea, insomnia, peripheral edema, and elevated hepatic enzymes were more frequently reported in the ponesimod-treatment arms as compared with placebo. During treatment initiation, bradycardia was observed in 2% of the patients, as well as first-degree (1.2%) and second-degree (0.9%) atrioventricular block. These cardiac events occurred during the first 3 hours after treatment intake and returned to predose levels 6 hours after treatment onset. As expected, lymphocyte counts were reduced after treatment onset but were rapidly reversed after treatment withdrawal, reaching levels close to baseline within 1 week.

A phase 3 clinical trial comparing ponesimod (at the 20-mg dose) versus teriflunomide is currently being conducted (NCT02425644).

Siponimod

Siponimod is a selective $S1P_1$ and $S1P_5$ receptor modulator.[16]

Efficacy In a phase 2 placebo-controlled clinical trial, siponimod significantly reduced CUAL by 72% in patients with RRMS.[16] Siponimod's efficacy has been tested also in patients with secondary progressive MS (SPMS) in whom the drug also met the primary outcome: compared with placebo, siponimod significantly delayed the time of presenting confirmed disability progression.[17]

Safety The detailed safety reports come from the phase 2 trial in RRMS,[16] as the SPMS clinical trial has not been published yet.[17] Bradycardia occurred more frequently in the siponimod high-dose treatment arms (10 and 2 mg), as well as the occurrence of first-degree and second-degree atrioventricular blocks. Specifically, at the 2-mg dose (the dose that has been used in the SPMS clinical trial), bradycardia was reported in 6% of the patients, and also 6% of the patients presented a second-degree atrioventricular block.[16] Lymphopenia and liver enzyme abnormalities were also more frequently reported in the siponimod-treatment arms.[16]

Ozanimod

Ozanimod selectively modulates $S1P_1$ and $S1P_5$ receptors.[18]

Efficacy A phase-2 double-blind, placebo-controlled clinical trial tested the superiority of ozanimod as compared with placebo[18] in reducing radiological disease activity. In this study, both doses of ozanimod significantly reduced the cumulative number of Gd-enhancing lesions from week 12 to 24 (84% and 89% reduction for the 0.5-mg and 1-mg dose, respectively).[18] Other radiological secondary outcomes, such as the number of Gd-enhancing lesions at week 24, and the cumulative number of new T2 lesions, were also significantly lower in both ozanimod arms compared with placebo.[18]

Safety Similar proportions of adverse events occurred in the active and placebo arms.[18] The most common cardiovascular event reported was orthostatic hypotension, which usually occurred the first day after treatment onset while being under cardiac monitoring, and resolved without intervention. The cardiac monitoring performed the first 24 hours after treatment onset revealed a minimum heart rate oscillation of less than 2 beats per minute. No cases of bradycardia were reported in the ozanimod treatment arm, and the proportion of patients presenting a second-degree atrioventricular block type 1 was similar in the placebo and ozanimod arms.[18]

Two phase-3 clinical trials, comparing both doses of ozanimod against intramuscular IFN-β-1a are currently ongoing (NCT02047734 and NCT02294058).

Amiselimod

Amiselimod is another S1P receptor modulator with high affinity for $S1P_1$ receptor.[19]

Efficacy In the recently published phase-2 placebo-controlled clinical trial, amiselimod proved to be more effective than placebo in reducing radiological disease activity.[19] Specifically, the number of Gd-enhancing lesions from week 8 to 24 was dose-dependently reduced by ozanimod treatment, with significant reductions observed in the 0.2-mg and 0.4-mg treatment arms (estimated incident rate ratio reduction of 61% and 77% for the 0.2 and 0.4 mg, respectively). Accordingly, both amiselimod doses (0.2 and 0.4 mg) reached statistical significance in other secondary outcomes, such as the number of new T2 lesions between weeks 4 to 24 and the reduction of gray matter volume loss from baseline to week 24.[19]

Safety Treatment-related adverse events were similar in all treatment arms, except for headache, liver enzyme abnormalities, and lymphopenia being more frequently reported in the amiselimod-treated patients. The cardiac and Holter monitoring provided no evidence of any cardiac adverse event except for 1 case of second-degree atrioventricular block and 1 episode of nonsustained ventricular tachycardia in the amiselimod 0.1 and 0.2 treatment arms, respectively.

DRUGS UNDER DEVELOPMENT WITH NEWER GOALS

In the future, a wealth of additional treatment options will be available to patients with both relapsing and progressive forms of MS. Most of these treatments target the immune system and are very effective in reducing disease activity with little impact on the more degenerative component of the disease. Notwithstanding, it seems that there is also an increasing interest in developing new drugs that will promote neuroprotection and/or myelin repair through different mechanisms of action.[20] Here new drugs are discussed with a specific focus on promoting neuroprotection or remyelination that, as of March 1, 2017, have completed at least 1 phase 2 clinical trial with published results in the past 3 years (see **Table 2**).

MD1003 or High-Dose Biotin

MD1003 is an oral formulation of high-dose biotin, an oral ubiquitous vitamin also known as vitamin H.[21,22] In patients with MS, biotin may exert its effect by enhancing fatty acid synthesis, through the activation of carboxylases, that ultimately will support myelin repair. Also, biotin may enhance energy production in neurons, protecting against hypoxia-driven axonal degeneration.[21,22]

Efficacy
Biotin has been recently tested in patients with progressive MS, yielding very encouraging results. High-dose biotin has demonstrated to be able to reverse MS-related disability[21,22]: almost 13% of the patients allocated to the biotin treatment arm presented a disability improvement (measured either with Expanded Disability Status Scale scale or timed 25-foot walk) at month 9 that was confirmed at month 12.[22] This was significantly different from the placebo treatment arm in which none of the patients reached this outcome. The results in other secondary outcomes were consistent with the main results of the trial, except for a greater proportion of patients presenting with new T2 lesions in the biotin-treated patients.[22] We should wait for the complete MRI analysis to be published to better understand these results.[23]

Safety
The proportion of patients reporting adverse events, and severe adverse events, were similar across active and placebo arms.[22] There were no special adverse events related to biotin intake, but it is important to take into consideration that biotin may alter blood test results (especially thyroid function), which may hamper patients' care.[24]

Opicinumab

Leucine-rich repeat and immunoglobulinlike domain-containing neurite outgrowth inhibitor receptor protein 1 (LINGO-1) is expressed exclusively on oligodendrocytes and neurons of the CNS.[25,26] LINGO-1 is a negative regulator of oligodendrocyte differentiation and remyelination. LINGO-1 antagonism has proved to be beneficial to enhance remyelination and axonal regeneration.[25,26] Opicinumab is a human monoclonal antibody targeting LINGO-1 that has been recently tested in patients with MS in 2 phase 2 clinical trials.[26,27]

Efficacy

The first phase 2 clinical trial tested opicinumab in acute optic neuritis. Unfortunately, the study did not reach its primary endpoint, as opicinumab failed to demonstrate an improvement in optic nerve conduction velocity measured with full-field visual evoked potentials.[26] No treatment effect was proved for other secondary outcomes, such as preserving the thickness of the retinal nerve fiber layer or the retinal ganglion cell layer.[26] The second phase 2b clinical trial was conducted as an add-on therapy to IM IFN-β in patients with RRMS. Again, the study failed to prove a linear dose response of opicinumab in improving disease disability, as higher opicinumab doses were not associated with higher proportion of patients presenting neurologic improvement.[27] Despite the negative results on the primary outcomes, the results obtained in these 2 phase 2 clinical trials suggest that remyelination improvement in the human CNS might be possible and provide important information about the design of future studies.

Safety

The overall incidence of adverse events was similar between both treatment arms (opicinumab and placebo), although, as expected, hypersensitivity reactions occurred with a higher frequency in the opicinumab-treated patients.[26,27] Of note, weight gain of more than 7% was also more frequent with opicinumab than with placebo.[26,27]

GSK239512

Histamine H3 receptors are expressed by neurons and oligodendrocyte precursor cells (OPC) and have a role in controlling OPC differentiation. GSK239512 is an oral selective H3 receptor antagonist/inverse agonist drug that has demonstrated to promote OPC differentiation in vitro and to enhance remyelination in the cuprizone mouse model of remyelination.

Efficacy

GSK239512 has been recently tested as add-on therapy to IFN-β or glatiramer acetate in a phase 2 clinical trial. Lesion remyelination was assessed by analyzing changes in magnetization transfer ratio (MTR) as a surrogate marker of in vivo myelin content. Compared with placebo, GSK239512 had a small positive effect (effect size between 0.243 and 0.344) on lesion MTR, indicating a relative increase in lesion remyelination. This positive effect on lesion remyelination did not have an impact into conventional MRI or clinical assessments. Nevertheless, the results of this study provide not only new insights in lesion remyelination, but also validate the approach of MTR lesion assessment for future multicenter clinical trials.

Safety

The incidence of adverse events was similar in the whole duration of the study. However, during the titration phase, more adverse events, particularly insomnia and sleep-related disorders were reported in the GSK239512 arm.

SUMMARY

Over the past years an increasing number of disease-modifying treatments have emerged for treating patients with MS. All of these therapies have demonstrated to be effective in reducing clinical and radiological disease activity, and therefore modifying the natural history of MS. This new treatment scenario is still constantly changing, as newer drugs are being developed that may be available in the near future. It is encouraging to notice that newer goals, such as neuroprotection and myelin repair that may in some way help us to treat the degenerative component of the disease, are also being pursued.

REFERENCES

1. Noseworthy JH, Lucchinetti C, Rodriguez M, et al. Medical progress: multiple sclerosis. New Englan J Med 2000;343:938–52.
2. Compston A, Coles A. Multiple sclerosis. Lancet 2008;372(9648):1502–17.
3. Shirley M. Daclizumab: a review in relapsing multiple sclerosis. Drugs 2017;77(4): 447–58.
4. Gold R, Giovannoni G, Selmaj K, et al. Daclizumab high-yield process in relapsing-remitting multiple sclerosis (SELECT): a randomised, double-blind, placebo-controlled trial. Lancet 2013;381(9884):2167–75.
5. Kappos L, Wiendl H, Selmaj K, et al. Daclizumab HYP versus Interferon Beta-1a in relapsing multiple sclerosis. N Engl J Med 2015;373(15):1418–28.
6. US Food and Drug Administration. Zinbryta (daclizumab) injection: US prescribing information. 2017. Available at: https://www.accessdata.fda.gov/drugsatfda_docs/label/2016/761029s000lbl.pdf. Accessed March 30, 2017.
7. European Medicines Agency. Zinbryta: summary of product characteristics. 2017. Available at: http://www.ema.europa.eu/docs/en_GB/document_library/EPAR_-_Product_Information/human/003862/WC500210598.pdf. Accessed March 30, 2017.
8. Hauser Stephen L, Bar-Or A, Comi G, et al. Ocrelizumab versus interferon beta-1a in relapsing multiple sclerosis. N Engl J Med 2017;376(3):221–34.
9. Kappos L, Li D, Calabresi PA, et al. Ocrelizumab in relapsing-remitting multiple sclerosis: a phase 2, randomised, placebo-controlled, multicentre trial. The Lancet 2011;378(9805):1779–87.
10. Montalban X, Hauser SL, Kappos L, et al. Ocrelizumab versus placebo in primary progressive multiple sclerosis. N Engl J Med 2017;376(3):209–20.
11. Giovannoni G, Comi G, Cook S, et al. A placebo-controlled trial of oral cladribine for relapsing multiple sclerosis. N Engl J Med 2010;362(5):416–26.
12. Leist TP, Comi G, Cree BA, et al. Effect of oral cladribine on time to conversion to clinically definite multiple sclerosis in patients with a first demyelinating event (ORACLE MS): a phase 3 randomised trial. Lancet Neurol 2014;13(3):257–67.
13. European Medicines Agency. Refusal of the marketing authorization for Movectro (cladribine): outcome of re-examination. 2011. Available at: http://www.ema.europa.eu/docs/en_GB/document_library/Medicine_QA/2011/02/WC500102304.pdf. Accessed March 30, 2017.
14. Pakpoor J, Disanto G, Altmann DR, et al. No evidence for higher risk of cancer in patients with multiple sclerosis taking cladribine. Neurol Neuroimmunol Neuroinflamm 2015;2(6):e158.
15. Havrdová E, Belova A, Goloborodko A, et al. Activity of secukinumab, an anti-IL-17A antibody, on brain lesions in RRMS: results from a randomized, proof-of-concept study. J Neurol 2016;263(7):1287–95.

16. Selmaj K, Li DK, Hartung HP, et al. Siponimod for patients with relapsing-remitting multiple sclerosis (BOLD): an adaptive, dose-ranging, randomised, phase 2 study. Lancet Neurol 2013;12(8):756–67.
17. Kappos L, Bar-Or A, Cree B, et al. Efficacy and safety of siponimod in secondary progressive multiple sclerosis. Results of the placebo controlled, double-blind, Phase III EXPAND study. Oral presentation. Mult Scler J., vol. 22. London (UK); 2016. p. 828–883.
18. Cohen Jeffrey A, Arnold Douglas L, Comi G, et al. Safety and efficacy of the selective sphingosine 1-phosphate receptor modulator ozanimod in relapsing multiple sclerosis (RADIANCE): a randomised, placebo-controlled, phase 2 trial. Lancet Neurol 2016;15(4):373–81.
19. Kappos L, Arnold Douglas L, Bar-Or A, et al. Safety and efficacy of amiselimod in relapsing multiple sclerosis (MOMENTUM): a randomised, double-blind, placebo-controlled phase 2 trial. Lancet Neurol 2016;15(11):1148–59.
20. Kremer D, Göttle P, Hartung HP, et al. Pushing forward: remyelination as the new frontier in CNS diseases. Trends Neurosci 2016;39(4):246–63.
21. Sedel F, Papeix C, Bellanger A, et al. High doses of biotin in chronic progressive multiple sclerosis: a pilot study. Mult Scler Relat Disord 2015;4(2):159–69.
22. Tourbah A, Lebrun-Frenay C, Edan G, et al. MD1003 (high-dose biotin) for the treatment of progressive multiple sclerosis: a randomised, double-blind, placebo-controlled study. Mult Scler J 2016;22(13):1719–31.
23. Chataway J. Biotin in progressive multiple sclerosis: a new lead? Mult Scler 2016; 22(13):1640–1.
24. Siddiqui U, Egnor E, Sloane JA. Biotin supplementation in MS clinically valuable but can alter multiple blood test results. Mult Scler J 2016;23(4):619–20.
25. Ineichen BV, Plattner PS, Good N, et al. Nogo-A antibodies for progressive multiple sclerosis. CNS Drugs 2017;31(3):187–98.
26. Cadavid D, Balcer L, Galetta S, et al. Safety and efficacy of opicinumab in acute optic neuritis (RENEW): a randomised, placebo-controlled, phase 2 trial. Lancet Neurol 2017;16(3):189–99.
27. Cadavid D, Edwards KR, Hupperts R, et al. Efficacy analysis of opicinumab in relapsing multiple sclerosis: the Phase 2b SYNERGY trial. Oral Presentation. Mult. Scler. J., vol. 22. London, UK; 2016. p. 7–87.

The Dynamics of the Gut Microbiome in Multiple Sclerosis in Relation to Disease

Ellen M. Mowry, MD, MCR[a], Justin D. Glenn, PhD[b],*

KEYWORDS

- Gut microbiome • Multiple sclerosis • Neuroinflammation • Gut bacteria
- Experimental autoimmune encephalomyelitis

KEY POINTS

- Preclinical and clinical case-control studies indicate that multiple sclerosis (MS) is associated with gut microbial dysbiosis, although its role in MS development is unknown.
- Alterations of the MS gut microbiota may include reduction of bacteria species that generate immune-modulatory molecules, including short-chain fatty acids, and increases in some immune-stimulatory and neurotoxic species.
- Preliminary studies suggest that gut immunity could be biased toward inflammation in MS and may promote immune responses targeting central nervous system tissue.
- There is no current established therapy for targeting the gut microbiome for MS therapy, but several lines of intervention are under investigation, including vitamin D supplementation, probiotic consumption, and diet modification.

INTRODUCTION

Multiple sclerosis is a chronic, inflammatory autoimmune disease of the central nervous system characterized by attacks on and degradation of myelin sheaths, axonal dropout, and gradual neuron loss. Its pathogenesis has been extrapolated mainly through the understanding of disease-causing mechanisms comprising its classical mouse model, experimental autoimmune encephalomyelitis (EAE).[1] EAE induction involves subcutaneous immunization of mice with an emulsion composed of a myelin component, such as myelin oligodendrocyte glycoprotein (MOG) peptide/protein or proteolipoprotein (PLP) peptide and complete Freund adjuvant in addition to pertussis toxin administration. In response, myelin peptide-specific T cells become activated as

Disclosure: The authors have nothing to disclose.
[a] Department of Neurology, Johns Hopkins School of Medicine, 600 North Wolfe Street, Pathology 627, Baltimore, MD 21287, USA; [b] Department of Neurology, Johns Hopkins School of Medicine, 600 North Wolfe Street, Meyer Building, Room 6-138, Baltimore, MD 21287, USA
* Corresponding author.
E-mail address: jglenn7@jhmi.edu

proinflammatory T cells (including T_H1 and T_H17) and attack once in the CNS. EAE immunization results in a reliable and reproducible ascending paralysis that can be evaluated with a well-defined severity score point-based system. EAE can also be induced by adoptively transferring activated $CD4^+$ T cells from EAE-immunized mouse donors into naïve recipients.

Although EAE gives insight into the possible cellular and molecular mechanisms that underlie MS pathogenesis, it does not reflect MS etiology, which is only partially understood. As is the case with many autoimmune diseases, heritable, genetic components and environmental factors are thought to contribute to MS development. In addition to sex differences, smoking, viral infection (with Epstein-Barr virus), lower vitamin D levels, and obesity, particularly in adolescence, appear to increase MS risk.[2–5] A growing body of studies and literature is centered on the association of gut microbial dysbiosis and the development of MS, and this topic will be the remaining focus of this article.

NORMAL COMPOSITION OF THE HUMAN GUT MICROBIOTA

The gut microbiota refers to the total number and composition of microbes that inhabit the gut, while the microbiome comprises the total genetic makeup of the microbiota. Its bacterial component has received the most attention and study due in part to its great density within the gut. The adult human intestine contains over 70% of the body's microbes, up to 100 trillion, and the microbiome number is 10 times larger than that of somatic and germ cells.[6,7] Gut commensal bacteria perform a large range of indispensable tasks for the promotion of human health, beginning with energy extraction.[7] The gut sits as an anaerobic bioreactor in which bacteria break down complex, otherwise indigestible, polysaccharides into monosaccharides and eventually fatty acids. Moreover, gut bacteria play integral roles in other forms of nutrient and xenobiotic metabolism; normal development of intestinal stroma, parenchyma, and the immune system; and the steady-state release of antimicrobial and immune-modulatory molecules.

Of the 55 known bacterial divisions, only 8 have been identified in the gut, 5 of which are rare.[7,8] The remaining 3 divisions include cytophaga-flavobacterium-bacteroides, firmicutes, and proteobacteria, with the former two composing around 30% each of bacteria isolated from feces and the mucus covering intestinal epithelium. Proteobacteria is present but not as prominent. The composition of a healthy gut contains large fractions of the phyla Firmicutes and Bacteroidetes, including the genera *Bacteroides*, *Prevotella*, and *Ruminococcus*, followed by Actinobacteria and Verrucomicrobia, but low in Proteobacteria phyla members.[9,10]

Factors that contribute to the formation and stable establishment of the normal human gut microbiota include mode of delivery in parturition, type of infant feeding (breast vs bottle), and diet.[11] Going into adulthood, diet is arguably the primary determinant of gut microbial composition and shapes the prospective interactions between the host and microbiota. Diets rich in fruits, vegetables, and fibers promote gut bacterial diversity and enrich for phyla involved in insoluble carbohydrate metabolism such as Firmicutes, while diets heavy in meat consumption are enriched for bile-metabolizing bacteria.[12,13]

EVIDENCE LINKING GUT DYSBIOSIS AND MODELS OF MULTIPLE SCLEROSIS

First, gut bacteria are required for induction of EAE. Mice housed in germ-free facility conditions, in which the gut is devoid of bacterial pathogens, developed a significantly less severe course of EAE compared with those in specific pathogen-free (SPF) conditions.[14] This was supported by a decrease in the proinflammatory cytokines interferon (IFN)γ and interleukin (IL)-17A and a concomitant increase in the abundance of immunosuppressive Foxp3$^+$ regulatory T cells (Tregs). Only when segmented filamentous bacteria (SFB), a *Clostridium*-related bacterium known to promote IL-17A-producing T$_H$17 differentiation, was allowed to colonize the intestines of germ-free mice were proinflammatory T cell development and optimal EAE restored.[14–16] In a transgenic mouse model of spontaneous EAE, germ-free mice maintained an extremely low disease incidence compared with SPF counterparts throughout rearing.[17] Subsequent experiments demonstrated that gut bacterial presence leads to gut T$_H$17 induction and cooperation with myelin-reactive B cells to initiate autoimmune demyelination and disease. A recent finding revealed the presence of a regulatory population of gut intraepithelial autoantigen-specific CD4$^+$ T cells in mice transgenic for a myelin-specific CD4$^+$ T cell clone.[18] These cells were induced by nonself-antigens derived from gut microbiota and suppressed proinflammatory T cell responses via their expression of the immune-suppressive molecule Lag-3.

Beyond the general gut bacterial requirement for EAE induction, studies have also attempted to determine the role of specific bacterial species in the disease. The species *Bacteroides fragilis* produces the capsular molecule polysaccharide A (PSA), which significantly reduces EAE severity by reducing IL-17A and IFNγ expression in T cells and inducing an IL-10-producing Foxp3$^+$ Treg population.[19] Oral treatment of mice with the lactic acid bacterial species *Pediococcus acidilactici* ameliorated clinical EAE.[20] The authors found lower expression of IFNγ and IL-17A but a significant increase in the number of IL-10-producing Treg cells; they also speculate that this bacterial infection could induce a population of IL-10-producing Foxp3$^-$ T regulatory cells (Tr1). Furthermore, a combination of lactobacilli strains reduced CNS inflammation and MOG-reactive T cell responses in EAE.[21] The strains *Lactobacillus paracasei* and *L plantarum* DSM 15312 induced Foxp3$^+$ Tregs and increased serum TGF-β1 concentrations, while the strain *L plantarum* DSM 15313 increased serum IL-27 levels. The cytokine IL-27 can suppress T$_H$1 and T$_H$17 responses but enhance Tr1 expression of IL-10. A probiotic combination of 5 strains-*L casei*, *L acidophilus*, *L reuteni*, *Bifidobacterium bifidum*, and *Streptococcus thermophilus*-known as IRT5, also ameliorated EAE prophylactically and therapeutically via decreased T$_H$1 and T$_H$17 but increased IL-4 and IL-10 from CD4$^+$ T cells.[22]

These studies indicate a major immune-modulatory bacterial mechanism of improving preclinical neuroinflammatory autoimmune disease by suppressing proinflammatory T$_H$1 and T$_H$17 responses and inducing/enhancing the formation of IL-10-producing Tr1 and Foxp3$^+$ Treg cells. Importantly, the bacterial species administered were largely gut commensals derived from the major phyla Bacteroidetes, Firmicutes, and to a smaller extent Actinobacteria, which again are implicated as crucial for healthy gut function in people. However, it should be known that particular species within these phyla could also promote disease, as in the case of SFB.

EVIDENCE LINKING GUT DYSBIOSIS AND MULTIPLE SCLEROSIS

A recent string of highly informative studies probing the bacterial microbiota of people with and without MS shows striking similarities and some differences in overall findings (**Table 1**).

Cantarel and colleagues[23] embarked on a small-scale study to determine potential effects of glatiramer acetate (GA) and vitamin D treatment on the gut microbiome of people with MS and how they compared with non-MS persons. Compared with non-MS persons, those with MS exhibited no whole bacterial community differences

Table 1
Major notable differences in abundance of gut bacterial and other phyla members derived from MS persons in relation to healthy controls

	Bacteroidetes	Firmicutes	Actinobacteria	Proteobacteria	Euryarchaeota	Verrucomicrobia
Cantarel et al,[23] 2015	↓ Bacteroidaceae	↓ Fecalibacterium ↑ Ruminococcus				
Miyake et al,[24] 2015	↓ Bacteroides ↓ Prevotella ↓ Anaerostipes	↓ Clostridia ↓ Faecalibacterium ↓ S. thermophilus	↑ Eggerthella lenta (Bifidobacterium)			
Chen et al,[25] 2016	↓ Pedobacter ↓ Flavobacterium ↓ Anaerostipes ↑ Parabacteroides	↓ Blausia ↓ Dorea ↓ Erysipelotrichaceae ↓ Lachnospiraceae ↑ Veillonellaceae ↑ Lactobacillus ↑ Coprobacillus	↓ Adlercreutzia ↓ Collinsella	↑ Pseudomonas ↑ Mycoplana ↑ Haemophilas		
Tremlett et al,[26] 2016	↓ Bacteroidales ↓ Bacteroides ↑ Parabacteroides	↓ Lachnospiraceae ↓ Ruminococcaceae ↓ Clostridiales ↑ Christensenellaceae	↑ Bifidobacterium	↑ Desulfovibrio	↑ Methanobrevibacter	↑ Akkermansia
Jangi et al,[27] 2016	↓ Butyricimonas ↓ Prevotella		↓ Collinsella ↓ Slackia		↑ Methanobrevibacter	↑ Akkermansia

For MS values compared to control values, ↓ = relative decrease and ↑ = relative increase.

but harbored different levels of some operational taxonomic units (OTUs). These consisted of fewer Bacteroidaceae, *Faecalibacterium* but higher *Ruminococcus*. OTUs from Rickenellaeae II, Lachnospiraceae, Porphyromonadaceae, *Bacteroides*, and *Oscillobacter* were sufficiently different to potentially have predictive ability in MS versus non-MS persons. GA treatment was associated with a whole-community shift before and after vitamin D, with differences in OTUs belonging to Bacteroidaceae, *Faecalibacterium, Ruminococcus,* Lactobacillaceae, *Clostridium*, and other Clostridiales. Vitamin D supplementation trended for a whole-community shift in which *Faecalibacterium* and Enterobacteriaceae OTUs increased while those of *Ruminococcus* decreased.

Miyake and colleagues[24] also noted no significant difference in bacterial species number, richness, or the Shannon index, a measure of bacterial diversity, in the guts of MS individuals relative to those without MS. MS individuals had less abundant *Firmicutes* and *Bacteroidetes* but more prevalent *Actinobacterial* species, although phyla representation was not significantly different. At the genus level, *Bacteroides, Faecalibacterium, Prevotella,* and *Anaerostipes* were decreased, and those of *Bifidobacterium* and *Streptococcus* were increased relative to non-MS persons. The researchers drilled down to identify 21 species that showed differential abundances in MS versus non-MS individuals. Within the 19 less-abundant species, 14 were of the Clostridial clade (n = 12 Clostridia cluster XIVa, n = 2 Clostridia cluster IV), and the other 5 less abundant were in the *Bacteroides, Prevotella,* and *Sutterella* genera. *Eggerthella lenta* and *S thermophilus* were the increased species in the MS group.

Chen and colleagues[25] reported no overall difference in gut bacterial species richness between healthy controls and patients with relapsing-remitting MS (RRMS), although there was a trend toward decreased richness in active versus inactive RRMS disease. Similar to findings by Miyake and colleagues, this study did observe a difference in microbiota structure between RRMS patients and non-MS persons. Going further, they identified differential abundance in 35 taxa in the 4 most abundant phyla. The genera *Adlercreutzia* and *Collinsella* of Actinobacteria were decreased in those with MS. Within Proteobacteria, RRMS patients had higher *Pseudomonas* and *Mycoplana* levels but less *Haemophilus* compared with healthy controls. In RRMS Bacteroidetes phylum, *Pedobacter* and *Flavobacterium* were lower and *Parabacteroides* was at higher abundance than healthy controls. Finally in Firmicutes, the genera *Blausia* and *Dorea* were both decreased, while some members of the genera *Lactobacillus* and *Coprobacillus* were decreased in RRMS relative to their healthy controls. Families of *Erysipelotrichaceae, Lachnospiraceae, Veillonellaceae* in Firmicutes were also lower in RRMS persons.

A unique study probing potential differences in gut bacteria between early onset pediatric MS and control children by Tremlett and colleagues[26] concluded no significant difference in gut bacterial beta diversity between controls and patients naïve to immune-modulatory drugs (IMD); however, there was a difference with exposure to the drugs within the patient population. Patients exposed to IMD had alpha diversity higher richness and gut microbiota that were more similar to controls in comparison to IMD-naïve MS patients. The researchers noted a relative increase in abundance of *Desulfovibrio, Bifidobacterium,* and *Christensenellaceae* family, with relative decrease in *Clostridiales* order members such as *Lachnospiraceae* and *Rumniococcaceae*, among others, in MS versus non-MS. Functional pathway analyses showed enrichment of those involved in glutathione metabolism and lipopolysaccharide biosynthesis in MS patients.

In the largest and one of the most recent studies yet, Jangi and colleagues[27] investigated the gut microbial composition of 60 MS individuals and also performed serologic analysis, profiled cytokine proliferation and gene expression from mononuclear cells and evaluated methane concentrations from the breath. Again, this research team found similar microbial within-sample richness and evenness but found similar community structures between MS and non-MS guts. MS persons had a significantly greater abundance of phyla members Euryarchaeota and Verrucomicrobia compared to controls. At the genus level, *Methanobrevibacter* and *Akkermansia* were increased in MS persons compared to controls, which belong to the phyla Euryarchaeota and Verrucomicrobia, respectively. On the contrary, the genera *Butyricimonas* and *Prevotella*, within phylum Bacteroidetes, and those of *Collinsella* and *Slackia* of the phylum Actinobacteria were significantly decreased in the MS guts. No serum anti-*Methanobrevibacter* antibody differences were found between the two groups. Interestingly, of all subjects with detectable methane in the breath, those of MS patients were at a significantly higher level than those without MS, thus validating the increased abundance of methanogens in the guts of MS individuals. It is notable, however, that methanogens are greater in those with constipation, and since this symptom is common in people with MS, it can't be excluded that the findings are due to, rather than caused by, MS.[27,28]

Clinical Study Interpretation

Most of the studies found no significant differences in the overall bacterial richness and diversity between MS and non-MS guts but did observe disparities in the gut microbial structures. These conclusions suggest potential group-wise differences in bacterial abundance at the sub-phylum levels. As mentioned, a healthy gut is thought to consist mostly of Firmicutes and Bacteroidetes phyla followed by Actinobacteria, Verrucomicrobia, and Proteobacteria. The teams that tested for Bacteroidetes and Firmicutes abundance saw substantial reductions in certain members associated with the MS status.

Bacteroidetes members including *Bacteroides*, *Butyricimonas*, and *Prevotella* are involved in metabolism of large, complex polysaccharides otherwise indigestible, into short-chain fatty acids (SCFAs), including butyrate. Fatty acid chain length is known to greatly influence immune responses. Long-chain fatty acids (LCFAs) promote CD4$^+$ T cell differentiation toward T_H1 and T_H17, worsen EAE and decrease Treg differentiation while SCFAs promote Treg differentiation and ameliorate EAE.[29] PSA from *B fragilis* should also be kept in mind for its immunosuppressive properties mainly through enhancing Treg differentiation.

Firmicutes phylum members in the gut are crucial with Bacteroidetes members in also generating butyrate and other SCFAs, and many were commonly shown to be reduced in MS guts, and included species in *Faecalibacterium*, *Blausia*, Dorea; of the families such as Lachnospiraceae, Ruminococcaceae, Erysipelotrichaceae, and Veillonellaceae and multiple Clostridial clade members.

The Verrucomicrobial genus *Akkermansia* was reported as increased in MS guts relative to controls, and this mucin degrader is known to generate SCFAs, which could again siphon into immunosuppression.[27,30] However, it also has been reported to promote inflammation by up-regulating genes in both the innate and adaptive immune responses, including antigen presentation, adaptive cell adhesion molecules, and T cell proliferation.[30] The archaeon *Methanobrevibacter* identified as increased in MS guts is thought to promote inflammatory responses via recruitment of immune cells and activation of dendritic cells.[27,31] Intriguingly both *Akkermansia* and *Methanobrevibacter* were enriched in pediatric and general MS cases along with decreased abundance of Lachnospiraceae and some members from Bacteroidetes.[23,24,26,27] Future studies with pediatric cases could enlighten on the timing of this gut microbiome structural alteration in relation to MS development.

The culmination of these studies suggest that the intestinal immune response in MS persons, just as in pre-clinical rodent models, could be skewed toward that of inflammation, such as one conducive for T_H17 and T_H1 development, and less so for Treg differentiation. Importantly, a recent study concluded that patients with RRMS were found to have activated IL-17A$^+$IL-22$^+$ CD4$^+$ T cells in the gut, but not in peripheral blood mononuclear cells.[32] They also had a higher T_H17/Treg ratio in the gut mucosa compared to controls.

Gut bacterial products may also contribute to MS development. Rumah and colleagues[33] published isolation of the bacillus *Clostridium perfringens* type B from a young woman's fecal samples presenting with MS, which was the first time this bacterium has been isolated from humans. It is especially provocative as having a possible role in MS in that its toxin, epsilon toxin, has tropism for the BBB and has been shown to preferentially bind to and induce death of oligodendrocytes and lead to CNS demyelination.[34] Sera and cerebrospinal fluid (CSF) from MS patients and those without the disease found immunoreactivity ten times higher in those with MS than controls, indicating prior exposure to the toxin. Another study for the first time linked *C perfringens* to neuromyelitis optica (NMO), a CNS autoimmune disease thought to be mediated against the water channel aquaporin-4 (AQP4).[35] T_H17 cells specific for AQP4 cross-react with a homologous sequence of *C. perfrigens* adenosine triphosphate-binding cassette transporter and exhibit a more vigorous proliferation from NMO patients compared to controls.[36] Importantly, the researchers found over-representation of this bacterium in MS versus healthy control guts.[35]

POTENTIAL INTERVENTION
Vitamin D Supplementation

Untreated MS persons under vitamin D supplementation increased their gut *Akkermansia*, *Faecalibacterium*, and *Coprococcus* genera OTUs, and these bacteria are associated with reduced inflammation through SCFA, such as butyrate, production and potential promotion of immune tolerance.[23] It was shown that people with MS exhibited a lowered serologic increase in vitamin D after administration compared to healthy controls.[37] However, when given cholecalciferol at high doses, there was a significant reduction of T_H17, CD161$^+$ CD4$^+$ T cells and effector memory cells and an increase in naïve and central memory CD4$^+$ T cell frequencies.[38] Cholecalciferol studies in human MS trials have provided mixed results but importantly, some had substantial limitations in design that limit interpretability. Positive outcomes included lowered gadolinium-enhancing lesion number, lower end-study number of persons with increased expanded disability status scale,[2] trend to reduced relapse rate, and reduced risk to MS progression.[39–42] Others found no effect on EDSS, lesion number, relapse rate, function or fatigue.[39,43,44] None evaluated the gut microbiota.

Probiotics

Probiotics are live organisms that exert beneficial health on the host and are a key therapeutic for intestinal illness.[9] Bacterial probiotic administration in pre-clinical MS disease models show mixed results, including EAE disease still occurring though no worse than control animals and disease reduction when treated prophylactically or during disease.[21,22,45] Amelioration of disease, when achieved, was attributed to lower T_H1/T_H17 frequencies and higher IL-10$^+$ and Foxp3$^+$ Treg cell frequencies. Disease outcome differences among these studies could be due to a range of variables, including administered bacterial species, amount given, mode of delivery and frequency. In 2016, Kouchaki and colleagues[46] published a study in which they undertook a double-blind placebo-controlled clinical trial to evaluate the effects of probiotic administration on MS patient disease. Patients received a probiotic capsule containing *L acidophilus*, *L casei*, *B bifidum*, and *Lactobacillus fermentum*, or a starch placebo for 12 weeks. Probiotic intake resulted in a statistically significant, though not clinically significant, decrease in EDSS (probiotic v. placebo = −0.3 ± 0.6 v. +0.1 ± 0.3, P = .001) and had favorable impacts on mental health, inflammatory factors, and markers of insulin resistance. However, short-term reductions in EDSS in this small trial may suggest more of imbalanced randomization with respect to disease features and should be interpreted with caution.

Diet

Diet type is a known and heavily investigated risk factor in autoimmune diseases such as MS.[47] The Western diet is typified as rich in salt, saturated fat, protein, sugar, increased calorie load, and is associated with increasing autoimmune disease prevalence.[47–49] The Western diet is linked to increased inflammation and its components, such as LCFAs and high salt amounts, have been shown to increase gut inflammatory cell abundance, which may include decreased SCFA output from beneficial gut bacterial species.[29,50,51] On the other hand, low-calorie diets rich in fruits, vegetables, and fish decrease inflammation and have a restorative effect on gut microbiota.[47,52] Ketogenic diets, intermittent fasting, and calorie-restriction diets have interestingly shown reduced inflammation, increased neuroprotection, and EAE prevention when administered prior to EAE disease and give hope for intervention in human studies.[53–56] A recent very-low-calorie, low-protein fast-mimicking diet (FMD) in mice dramatically reduced EAE severity and was more effective than a ketogenic diet.[57] These diets were then moved to a randomized, parallel-group pilot trial in MS patients for a 6 month period.[57] Those on the diet reported meaningful improvements on health-related quality of life, had slight reductions in lymphocytes and white blood cell count, and a mild reduction in EDSS scores compared to those on control diet. More clinical trials for evaluating the effects of calorie restriction on MS are in process.[58–60]

SUMMARY

MS, like most other autoimmune diseases, is a multi-faceted disease thought to involve heritable and non-heritable, environmental components that contribute to its as-of-yet unknown etiology. Over time, knowledge of genetic and lifestyle variants associated with the disease, including the importance of the gut microbiota to neuro-inflammatory autoimmune disease, has increased. Preliminary studies for altering the gut microbiota in MS patients have largely been small in subject number and had mixed results dependent upon intervention type. Active areas of interventional studies assessing the microbiota as an endpoint include probiotic administration, and diet alteration studies, among others.

Considering the large number of genetic variants and environmental factors associated with MS, more precise, future individualized testing may aid to tailor a specific bacterial concoction per MS subject for better disease prognosis. To this end, more research may be done to determine if there is an association of abundance of certain gut bacterial strains in the MS gut with specific sets of MS genetic variants and/or lifestyle habits within the MS pool, as a general bacterial regimen may not cover all MS individuals. Moreover, variation of the bacterial load given, route of administration, and frequency may be considered. Though much work lies ahead for better understanding the links between MS development and prognosis and the gut microbiota, promising clinical trials for gut microbial manipulation for therapy are underway.

REFERENCES

1. Pierson E, Simmons SB, Castelli L, et al. Mechanisms regulating regional localization of inflammation during CNS autoimmunity. Immunol Rev 2012;248(1): 205–15.
2. Olsson T, Barcellos LF, Alfredsson L. Interactions between genetic, lifestyle and environmental risk factors for multiple sclerosis. Nat Rev Neurol 2017;13(1): 25–36.
3. Munger KL, Levin LI, Hollis BW, et al. Serum 25-hydroxyvitamin D levels and risk of multiple sclerosis. JAMA 2006;296(23):2832–8.
4. Langer-Gould A, Brara SM, Beaber BE, et al. Childhood obesity and risk of pediatric multiple sclerosis and clinically isolated syndrome. Neurology 2013;80(6): 548–52.
5. Munger KL, Bentzen J, Laursen B, et al. Childhood body mass index and multiple sclerosis risk: a long-term cohort study. Mult Scler 2013;19(10):1323–9.
6. Savage DC. Microbial ecology of the gastrointestinal tract. Annu Rev Microbiol 1977;31:107–33.
7. Backhed F, Ley RE, Sonnenburg JL, et al. Host-bacterial mutualism in the human intestine. Science 2005;307(5717):1915–20.
8. Hugenholtz P, Goebel BM, Pace NR. Impact of culture-independent studies on the emerging phylogenetic view of bacterial diversity. J Bacteriol 1998;180(18): 4765–74.
9. Jandhyala SM, Talukdar R, Subramanyam C, et al. Role of the normal gut microbiota. World J Gastroenterol 2015;21(29):8787–803.
10. Hollister EB, Gao C, Versalovic J. Compositional and functional features of the gastrointestinal microbiome and their effects on human health. Gastroenterology 2014;146(6):1449–58.
11. Mueller NT, Bakacs E, Combellick J, et al. The infant microbiome development: mom matters. Trends Mol Med 2015;21(2):109–17.
12. Lynch SV, Pedersen O. The human intestinal microbiome in health and disease. N Engl J Med 2016;375(24):2369–79.
13. David LA, Maurice CF, Carmody RN, et al. Diet rapidly and reproducibly alters the human gut microbiome. Nature 2014;505(7484):559–63.
14. Lee YK, Menezes JS, Umesaki Y, et al. Proinflammatory T-cell responses to gut microbiota promote experimental autoimmune encephalomyelitis. Proc Natl Acad Sci U S A 2011;108(Suppl 1):4615–22.
15. Snel J, Blok HJ, Kengen HMP, et al. Phylogenetic characterization of Clostridium related segmented filamentous bacteria in mice based on 16S ribosomal RNA analysis. Syst Appl Microbiol 1994;17(2):172–9.
16. Ivanov II, Atarashi K, Manel N, et al. Induction of intestinal Th17 cells by segmented filamentous bacteria. Cell 2009;139(3):485–98.
17. Berer K, Mues M, Koutrolos M, et al. Commensal microbiota and myelin autoantigen cooperate to trigger autoimmune demyelination. Nature 2011;479(7374): 538–41.
18. Kadowaki A, Miyake S, Saga R, et al. Gut environment-induced intraepithelial autoreactive CD4(+) T cells suppress central nervous system autoimmunity via LAG-3. Nat Commun 2016;7:11639.

19. Ochoa-Reparaz J, Mielcarz DW, Ditrio LE, et al. Central nervous system demyelinating disease protection by the human commensal Bacteroides fragilis depends on polysaccharide A expression. J Immunol 2010;185(7):4101–8.

20. Takata K, Kinoshita M, Okuno T, et al. The lactic acid bacterium Pediococcus acidilactici suppresses autoimmune encephalomyelitis by inducing IL-10-producing regulatory T cells. PLoS One 2011;6(11):e27644.

21. Lavasani S, Dzhambazov B, Nouri M, et al. A novel probiotic mixture exerts a therapeutic effect on experimental autoimmune encephalomyelitis mediated by IL-10 producing regulatory T cells. PLoS One 2010;5(2):e9009.

22. Kwon HK, Kim GC, Kim Y, et al. Amelioration of experimental autoimmune encephalomyelitis by probiotic mixture is mediated by a shift in T helper cell immune response. Clin Immunol 2013;146(3):217–27.

23. Cantarel BL, Waubant E, Chehoud C, et al. Gut microbiota in multiple sclerosis: possible influence of immunomodulators. J Investig Med 2015;63(5):729–34.

24. Miyake S, Kim S, Suda W, et al. Dysbiosis in the gut microbiota of patients with multiple sclerosis, with a striking depletion of species belonging to clostridia XIVa and IV clusters. PLoS One 2015;10(9):e0137429.

25. Chen J, Chia N, Kalari KR, et al. Multiple sclerosis patients have a distinct gut microbiota compared to healthy controls. Sci Rep 2016;6:28484.

26. Tremlett H, Fadrosh DW, Faruqi AA, et al. Gut microbiota in early pediatric multiple sclerosis: a case-control study. Eur J Neurol 2016;23(8):1308–21.

27. Jangi S, Gandhi R, Cox LM, et al. Alterations of the human gut microbiome in multiple sclerosis. Nat Commun 2016;7:12015.

28. Kim G, Deepinder F, Morales W, et al. Methanobrevibacter smithii is the predominant methanogen in patients with constipation-predominant IBS and methane on breath. Dig Dis Sci 2012;57(12):3213–8.

29. Haghikia A, Jorg S, Duscha A, et al. Dietary fatty acids directly impact central nervous system autoimmunity via the small intestine. Immunity 2015;43(4):817–29.

30. Derrien M, Van Baarlen P, Hooiveld G, et al. Modulation of mucosal immune response, tolerance, and proliferation in mice colonized by the mucin-degrader Akkermansia muciniphila. Front Microbiol 2011;2:166.

31. Bang C, Weidenbach K, Gutsmann T, et al. The intestinal archaea Methanosphaera stadtmanae and Methanobrevibacter smithii activate human dendritic cells. PLoS One 2014;9(6):e99411.

32. Martinelli V, Messina MJ, Alberto M, et al. The role of gut immunity in multiple sclerosis patients [Abstract]. Neurology 2016;86(16).

33. Rumah KR, Linden J, Fischetti VA, et al. Isolation of Clostridium perfringens type B in an individual at first clinical presentation of multiple sclerosis provides clues for environmental triggers of the disease. PLoS One 2013;8(10):e76359.

34. Linden JR, Ma Y, Zhao B, et al. Clostridium perfringens epsilon toxin causes selective death of mature oligodendrocytes and central nervous system demyelination. MBio 2015;6(3):e02513.

35. Cree BA, Spencer CM, Varrin-Doyer M, et al. Gut microbiome analysis in neuromyelitis optica reveals overabundance of Clostridium perfringens. Ann Neurol 2016;80(3):443–7.

36. Varrin-Doyer M, Spencer CM, Schulze-Topphoff U, et al. Aquaporin 4-specific T cells in neuromyelitis optica exhibit a Th17 bias and recognize Clostridium ABC transporter. Ann Neurol 2012;72(1):53–64.

37. Bhargava P, Steele SU, Waubant E, et al. Multiple sclerosis patients have a diminished serologic response to vitamin D supplementation compared to healthy controls. Mult Scler 2016;22(6):753–60.

38. Sotirchos ES, Bhargava P, Eckstein C, et al. Safety and immunologic effects of high- vs low-dose cholecalciferol in multiple sclerosis. Neurology 2016;86(4): 382–90.
39. Dankers W, Colin EM, van Hamburg JP, et al. Vitamin D in autoimmunity: molecular mechanisms and therapeutic potential. Front Immunol 2016;7:697.
40. Burton JM, Kimball S, Vieth R, et al. A phase I/II dose-escalation trial of vitamin D3 and calcium in multiple sclerosis. Neurology 2010;74(23):1852–9.
41. Soilu-Hanninen M, Aivo J, Lindstrom BM, et al. A randomised, double blind, placebo controlled trial with vitamin D3 as an add on treatment to interferon beta-1b in patients with multiple sclerosis. J Neurol Neurosurg Psychiatry 2012;83(5): 565–71.
42. Derakhshandi H, Etemadifar M, Feizi A, et al. Preventive effect of vitamin D3 supplementation on conversion of optic neuritis to clinically definite multiple sclerosis: a double blind, randomized, placebo-controlled pilot clinical trial. Acta Neurol Belg 2013;113(3):257–63.
43. Mosayebi G, Ghazavi A, Ghasami K, et al. Therapeutic effect of vitamin D3 in multiple sclerosis patients. Immunol Invest 2011;40(6):627–39.
44. Kampman MT, Steffensen LH, Mellgren SI, et al. Effect of vitamin D3 supplementation on relapses, disease progression, and measures of function in persons with multiple sclerosis: exploratory outcomes from a double-blind randomised controlled trial. Mult Scler 2012;18(8):1144–51.
45. Kobayashi T, Suzuki T, Kaji R, et al. Probiotic upregulation of peripheral IL-17 responses does not exacerbate neurological symptoms in experimental autoimmune encephalomyelitis mouse models. Immunopharmacol Immunotoxicol 2012;34(3):423–33.
46. Kouchaki E, Tamtaji OR, Salami M, et al. Clinical and metabolic response to probiotic supplementation in patients with multiple sclerosis: a randomized, double-blind, placebo-controlled trial. Clin Nutr 2017;36(5):1245–9.
47. Jorg S, Grohme DA, Erzler M, et al. Environmental factors in autoimmune diseases and their role in multiple sclerosis. Cell Mol Life Sci 2016;73(24):4611–22.
48. Thorburn AN, Macia L, Mackay CR. Diet, metabolites, and "western-lifestyle" inflammatory diseases. Immunity 2014;40(6):833–42.
49. Odegaard AO, Koh WP, Yuan JM, et al. Western-style fast food intake and cardiometabolic risk in an Eastern country. Circulation 2012;126(2):182–8.
50. Kleinewietfeld M, Manzel A, Titze J, et al. Sodium chloride drives autoimmune disease by the induction of pathogenic TH17 cells. Nature 2013;496(7446):518–22.
51. Wu C, Yosef N, Thalhamer T, et al. Induction of pathogenic TH17 cells by inducible salt-sensing kinase SGK1. Nature 2013;496(7446):513–7.
52. De Filippo C, Cavalieri D, Di Paola M, et al. Impact of diet in shaping gut microbiota revealed by a comparative study in children from Europe and rural Africa. Proc Natl Acad Sci U S A 2010;107(33):14691–6.
53. Esquifino AI, Cano P, Jimenez-Ortega V, et al. Immune response after experimental allergic encephalomyelitis in rats subjected to calorie restriction. J Neuroinflammation 2007;4:6.
54. Kafami L, Raza M, Razavi A, et al. Intermittent feeding attenuates clinical course of experimental autoimmune encephalomyelitis in C57BL/6 mice. Avicenna J Med Biotechnol 2010;2(1):47–52.
55. Kim DY, Hao J, Liu R, et al. Inflammation-mediated memory dysfunction and effects of a ketogenic diet in a murine model of multiple sclerosis. PLoS One 2012; 7(5):e35476.

56. Piccio L, Stark JL, Cross AH. Chronic calorie restriction attenuates experimental autoimmune encephalomyelitis. J Leukoc Biol 2008;84(4):940–8.
57. Choi IY, Piccio L, Childress P, et al. A diet mimicking fasting promotes regeneration and reduces autoimmunity and multiple sclerosis symptoms. Cell Rep 2016; 15(10):2136–46.
58. Mowry EM, University JH. A pilot study of intermittent calorie restriction in multiple sclerosis. In: ClinicalTrials.gov. Bethesda (MD): National Library of Medicine (US); 2000. Available at: https://clinicaltrials.gov/ct2/show/NCT02647502 NLM Identifier: NCT02647502. Accessed March 15, 2017.
59. Piccio L, Medicine. WUSo. Calorie restriction in multiple sclerosis patients. In: ClinicalTrials.gov. National Library of Medicine (US). Bethesda (MD): National Libray of Medicine (US); 2000. Available at: https://clinicaltrials.gov/ct2/show/NCT02411838?term=calorie+and+multiple+sclerosis&rank=1 NLM Identifier: NCT02411838. Accessed March 15, 2017.
60. Mowry EM, University JH. A pragmatic trial of dietary programs in people with multiple sclerosis (MS). In: ClinicalTrials.gov. Bethesda (MD): National Library of Medicine (US); 2000. Available at: https://clinicaltrials.gov/ct2/show/NCT02846558 NLM Identifier: NCT02846558. Accessed April 3, 2017.

Advanced Symptom Management in Multiple Sclerosis

Elizabeth Crabtree-Hartman, MD

KEYWORDS

- Symptom management • Quality of life • Pseudoexacerbation
- Nonpharmacologic treatment • Spasticity • Neuropathic pain • Neurogenic bladder
- Neurogenic bowel

KEY POINTS

- Symptom management can have a profound impact on quality of life.
- Symptom management should always begin with respectful listening and appropriate counseling/validation.
- Meaningful symptom management is time consuming, and it is imperative to develop tools and resources to maximize efficiency in the clinic.
- An increase in baseline symptoms is often a pseudoexacerbation caused by a physiologic stressor such as an infection (urologically silent urinary tract infection) or emotional stress.

INTRODUCTION

Although the armamentarium of disease-modifying therapies has expanded greatly, a more significant impact on quality of life for patients with multiple sclerosis (MS) remains via meaningful symptom management. Disease-modifying therapies have had a positive impact on disability and the neurologic symptoms therein. Historically, in the pretreatment era, longitudinal data disclosed that one-third to one-half of patients showed progressive decline 15 years after onset, with up to 54% transitioning to secondary progressive MS (SPMS) after 19 years.[1,2] More recently, longitudinal data showed only 11.3% of patients transitioning to SPMS after a median of 16.8 years.[3] Therefore, patients are incurring less disability and, by definition, fewer symptoms caused by MS. However, current disease-modifying therapies are preventive, and decrease the risk for incurring new symptoms/disability; they do not, with few exceptions, improve ongoing

Disclosure: The author has received honoraria from Genzyme, Biogen, Novartis and Teva Neuroscience.
Department of Neurology, Tulane University School of Medicine, 131 S. Robertson Street, Suite 1300, New Orleans, LA 70112, USA
E-mail address: crabtreehartman@gmail.com

symptoms. In this setting, most patients have 1 or more active symptoms caused by MS, and most are undermanaged. Thus, meaningful symptom management is one of the major means by which quality of life can be improved for patients with MS.

There are challenges to comprehensive symptom management to consider and target. Time is one of the major hurdles. Some thought can be given to who should undertake symptom management. Should this responsibility be managed by a specialist in MS, nurse practitioner [NP] MS specialist, general neurologist, and so forth, or combinations of these? Regardless of who is in charge, certain strategies can improve clinical efficiency. Predating the clinic visit, patients could respond to questionnaires on paper or digitally, and this information can be organized for the care provider before the clinic encounter and/or uploaded into the clinic note. Within the clinic visit, establish the patient's priorities and apprise the patient of reasonable expectations for the current visit, as well as the plan for continuity to address remaining items of concern. Maximize templates/smart sets/dot phrases for the electronic medical record. Internet-based visits can serve as a convenient and effective tool for symptom management follow-up visits. In addition, providing a road map for the patient regarding symptom management can reduce anxiety and interpersonal viscosity.

Other challenges to symptom management include communication barriers, polypharmacy, and the partial efficacy of many medications. Lack of access to prescribed medications caused by insurance denial occurs with regularity. Without a means for close follow-up, care providers may not learn of insurance denials for months, during which time the patients have gone undertreated. Some thought can be given to which tools may assuage these challenges in a particular practice environment.

Understanding patients' expectations is crucial for time management. It is common for patients to want to avoid medications. For any given symptom, nonpharmacologic and pharmacologic interventions can be offered, but time should be budgeted differently if the patient does not want to consider medications.

GENERAL GUIDELINES

Evaluation of an initial presentation of a neurologic symptom generates a broad differential diagnosis regarding the origin of the patient's clinical complaints: exacerbation versus pseudoexacerbation versus unrelated to MS. If the symptoms may be caused by a relapse, a distinct approach to management ensues. A pseudoexacerbation is characterized by an escalation of baseline symptoms, most frequently including, but not limited to, fatigue and spasticity. Common causes for pseudoexacerbation include urinary tract infection (UTI) (symptomatic or urologically silent), physiologic stressor caused by a medical condition (eg, thyroid, anemia, diabetes), dehydration, emotional stress, and changes in temperature/barometric pressure fronts. Appropriate history taking and laboratory inquiry can guide management of a pseudoexacerbation. Treatment of a urologically silent UTI can result in resolution of neurologic symptoms or a return to baseline severity. A presenting symptom also can be either directly MS related or indirectly MS related. For instance, low back pain or hip pain is common among patients who have experienced a partial myelitis with incomplete recovery. Because of the use of accessory muscles for ambulation, a musculoskeletal pain syndrome can develop. During history taking, it is important to consider secondary syndromes and counsel patients accordingly; avoid assuming that the condition is not caused by MS.

Multiple Sclerosis Symptoms

MS symptoms can present in well-recognized constellations, as interrelated symptoms, or as individual symptoms (**Table 1**). MS symptoms often occur in constellations because of shared localization, are interrelated functionally, and/or are poorly understood. A more detailed discussion of underlying pathophysiology is provided later. Symptoms can also occur individually or have less consistent interrelated symptoms.

A common constellation of symptoms presents because of partial myelitis with incomplete recovery. Patients may experience all of the following symptoms or a combination therein: spasticity, bladder symptoms (frequency/urgency most commonly), bowel symptoms (constipation most commonly), sexual dysfunction, and Lhermitte phenomenon are the clinical features of this constellation. Gait disturbance or imbalance is also often associated. Secondary symptoms include lower back pain and hip pain. It is important to recognize this relationship because female patients may report tightness in the legs but may assume that the bladder frequency is caused by age and therefore not report it if unprompted. Guided history taking allows care providers to offer a more comprehensive approach to symptom management.

Another common constellation of symptoms comprises fatigue, mood, and cognition. Localization is less well understood for these symptoms, and their concomitance may be caused by functional impact rather than shared localization. For instance, undermanaged fatigue can slow processing speed and thereby manifest as cognitive challenges as well. Often treatment of one of these features benefits the others, such as mood improvement positively affecting fatigue and/or cognition.

Autonomic dysregulation can include cardiovascular changes, autonomic dysreflexia, and sudomotor changes. Thermal dysregulation or heat sensitivity may be secondary to sudomotor changes. Fatigue and sexual dysfunction are sometimes thought to be part of the constellation of autonomic dysregulation sequelae.

MANAGEMENT STEPS

For any patient with MS with a neurologic symptom, thoughtful listening, informed history taking, and appropriate validation of experience serve as part of the treatment

Table 1
Multiple sclerosis symptoms

Common Constellations	Interrelated Symptoms	Additional Symptoms
• Leg weakness • Gait imbalance • Spasticity • Bladder and bowel • Sexual dysfunction	• Bladder → fatigue	• Visual: • Blurred vision • Diplopia • Nystagmus
• Fatigue • Depression • Cognitive challenges	• Pain → mood	• Trigeminal neuralgia
	• Pain → fatigue	• Tremor
• Cardiovascular changes • Autonomic dysreflexia • Sudomotor changes • Thermal dysregulation	• Pain → cognition	
	• Pain → sexual dysfunction	

MS symptoms may occur as complete or partial constellations, as interrelated symptoms, or as individual entities.

regimen. History regarding symptom management may occur organically during the patient interview or using digital tools before or during clinic. A comprehensive treatment approach can include:

1. Informed history taking and query of patient expectations
2. Diagnostics may be indicated to clarify alternative/contributing medical conditions or medications
3. Consideration of other contributing MS symptoms
4. Maximization of building blocks: disease-modifying therapy, vitamin D status, nutrition, exercise/physical therapy (PT), stress management
5. Nonpharmacologic address: behavior modification, complementary medicine modalities
6. Pharmacologic address: medications and/or supplements

Clearly this list can be too time consuming to execute during a 30-minute follow-up visit without extending care beyond the clinic. **Table 2** shows time management strategies for the steps listed here. Addressing other contributing medical conditions may obviate, or at least streamline, medications. For instance, diagnosing and treating hypothyroidism may ameliorate fatigue. The patient's medication list should be evaluated for potential involvement, such as pain medication with constipation as a side effect. Consideration of other contributing MS symptoms can affect sequencing or the so-called road map for symptom management. Fatigue may be the chief complaint, but management may begin by addressing undertreated neurogenic bladder, thereby improving sleep and/or daytime energy use. Maximizing the building blocks of MS care is essential at any visit but is particularly germane for symptom management. Disease-modifying therapies should be considered as potential contributors to symptoms (fatigue, headache, leg pain) or potential positive effects (fatigue, cognition).

Table 2	
Time management strategies in multiple sclerosis symptom management	
Steps for Symptom Management	**Time Management Strategies**
1. Informed history taking and query of patient expectations	• Online survey before visit, at home • Online survey in waiting room • Dot phrases for common responses
2. Clarify alternative or contributing medical conditions and/or medications	• Smart sets with prepopulated orders for any given symptom
3. Consideration of other contributing MS symptoms	• Red cap surveys or dot phrases or part of a progress note in smart sets
4. Maximization of the building blocks: disease-modifying therapy, vitamin D status, nutrition, and exercise/PT	• Dot phrases or part of a smart set with progress note, diagnostics, and referrals prepopulated
5. Nonpharmacologic address: behavior modification, complementary medicine modalities	• Dot phrases or part of a smart set for typical instructions, such as for fatigue or bladder
6. Pharmacologic address: medications and/or supplements	• Dot phrases or part of a smart set for typical starting doses and instructions for the after-visit summary

Stepwise meaningful symptomatic address is challenging in a 30-minute to 45-minute follow-up visit. Time management strategies extending the encounter beyond the clinic can maximize efficiency and improve care.

Patients may or may not be interested in starting a new medication for symptom management. Many patients are not seeking medication but wish to understand their symptoms and receive guidance regarding behavioral strategies and/or complementary modalities. Specific strategies for nonpharmacologic address are discussed later.

If a patient is interested in pharmacologic agents, a few principles apply (**Box 1**). It is advisable to initiate medication changes sequentially rather than in parallel. This approach helps to discern which medications confer a therapeutic effect or undesirable side effects. Whenever possible, seek a 2-for-1, wherein a medication confers benefit on more than 1 symptom. This benefit may occur as a direct benefit, such as an improvement in fatigue with treatment of depression with bupropion, or may be conferred when a side effect proves beneficial, such as improvement of nocturnal urinary frequency caused by the anticholinergic side effects of tricyclic antidepressants (TCAs) at bedtime for neuropathic pain. Patients with MS may be more sensitive to medications' therapeutic effects and untoward side effects. Therefore, it is recommended to start medications at a low dose and titrate doses slowly. In addition, have a means for medication follow-up to ensure that the medication was covered by insurance and that the patient is tolerating the medication and titrating as directed. This event can be billable with an Internet-based medicine visit by an NP or neurologist, or a nonbillable phone call by nursing staff.

Management of Specific Symptoms

Fatigue

Fatigue is one of the most common symptoms in MS and can present early in the disease course. At some point it affects more than 30% to 80% of patients, and is a major symptom in 50% to 60%.[4] In the absence of focal symptoms, it is often misdiagnosed as chronic fatigue syndrome.

Fatigue can be associated with activity, be an exacerbation, or be unprecipitated. Treatment of fatigue in patients with MS should begin with a thoughtful analysis of potential contributing factors. General medical conditions, such as anemia, hypothyroidism, and B_{12} deficiency, can add to or masquerade as MS-associated fatigue. Recommended laboratory evaluation is shown in **Box 2**. Separate MS symptoms may also affect fatigue. For instance, patients with lower extremity motor involvement and urinary frequency are at risk for fatigue caused by overexertion and inefficient energy use. Their fatigue may benefit from a bladder agent that decreases the number of trips to the restroom per day and number of awakenings at night. Treatment of certain MS symptoms, including sleep disorder, pain, anxiety, and depression, improves fatigue. In contrast, some medications used for other indications may also contribute

---

Box 1
Starting medications for symptom management

- Start or dose adjust 1 medication at a time
- Target more than 1 symptom whenever possible
- Start at low doses
- Advance or titrate slowly
- Have a clear follow-up plan in place for medication check

Following these guidelines facilitates effective symptom management and potentially streamlines medications/dosages.

Box 2
Recommended laboratory investigation for new or escalating fatigue

- Diagnostics:
  - Urinalysis/urine culture
  - 25-Hydroxyvitamin D
  - Thyroid panel
  - Testosterone
  - Complete blood count/liver function tests
  - Vitamin B_{12}

These diagnostics are recommended for new or escalating fatigue and can be tailored to the individual; for instance, checking levels if the person is taking antiepileptic drugs.

---

negatively. Common offenders are antispasmodic agents, some antidepressants, opiate pain medications, some bladder agents, and memantine.[5] Some patients report worsening fatigue associated with interferon therapy. Liver transaminase levels and liver function tests can be evaluated if fatigue is temporally related to starting, or changing the dose of, an interferon. Fatigue may improve with other disease-modifying therapies, such as natalizumab, fingolimod, and alemtuzumab.

Once contributing clinical factors have been addressed, and if fatigue persists, management includes nonpharmacologic address and/or pharmacologic address. Patients can be advised to plan their activities and take regular rests from activity to maximize energy conservation. **Box 3** shows nonpharmacologic address and energy conservation tips. Many patients with MS are heat sensitive and some experience an increase in fatigue associated with increased core body temperature. Although patients can be assured that they are not making their MS worse by getting warm, they may experience less fatigue by avoiding heat. Home cooling devices, such as air conditioners and fans, and personal cooling devices, such as cooling collars/belts/vests, can be of benefit.

Because deconditioning can add to fatigue, an appropriate, regular exercise program can be of benefit. Patients of more than ideal body weight may expend more energy throughout the day than is necessary, and they too can benefit from an exercise

---

Box 3
Nonpharmacologic address of fatigue

- Energy conservation
  - Set reasonable expectations
  - Planning rest periods
  - Set priorities
  - Perform heavy tasks early in the day
  - Rearrange workspace ergonomically

- Exercise regularly
  - Pool exercise for the heat-sensitive patients
  - Yoga

- Plan social calendar with appropriate time to rest

- Be mindful of hydration and nutrition

Maximizing behavioral strategies as described here can avoid the need for medication, or decrease the dose and/or frequency with which medications are used.

regimen and a modified diet. For those who are heat sensitive, low-impact exercise regimens such as pool therapy or yoga (except for Bikram) can be explored. Adherence to a diet and/or exercise regimen is increased when the plan is formalized. Merely advising patients to exercise and lose weight is likely less effective than referring them to PT and for a nutrition consult. Other lifestyle modifications that can benefit fatigue include limiting alcohol intake and maximizing sleep hygiene.

Positive data exist for complementary medicine modalities in the treatment of fatigue, including yoga and exercise,[6] acupressure,[7] mindfulness-based training,[8] and certain supplements/herbal therapy. The supplement L-carnitine (1 g orally twice a day) was shown to be as effective as amantadine in treating MS-associated fatigue,[9] and coenzyme Q10 at a dose of 500 mg/d was shown to benefit fatigue and depression.[10] Recent data on a derivative of vitamin D, alfacalcidol, are promising,[11] as are data on vitamin A.[12] Data regarding American ginseng (100–400 mg) were negative in a 6-week placebo-controlled crossover design.[13] However, more recently, ginseng 250 mg twice a day was shown to have a significant impact on fatigue scores compared with placebo.[14]

Once all of these modalities have been maximized, patients with MS may continue to have fatigue that affects their quality of life. There are medications that may benefit fatigue as a side effect, and therefore target more than 1 MS symptom. Dalfampridine is US Food and Drug Administration (FDA) approved to improve walking, but may also benefit fatigue and motor endurance. 4-Aminopyridine (4-AP) has a shared mechanism of action with dalfampridine, and can be compounded as immediate release (for more frequent dosing) or extended release (for cost when dalfampridine is not covered). 4-AP may also benefit fatigue, motor performance, and spasticity, but remains controversial because of inconsistent data regarding efficacy and untoward side effects.[15] Clinicians should ensure that the compounding pharmacy is accredited. Selective serotonin reuptake inhibitors (SSRIs) and bupropion are sometimes used to improve fatigue because of their common side effect of stimulation. Bupropion can increase anxiety and fractionate rapid eye movement (REM) sleep, and should be avoided in patients with anxiety and/or insomnia. SSRIs are notorious for conferring sexual dysfunction and should be avoided in patients already experiencing sexual dysfunction. A pilot study with low-dose naltrexone (LDN) in MS of 4.5 mg taken at bedtime did not find benefit on fatigue, although patients reported a marginal improvement of their quality of life,[16] whereas a more recent chart review of more than 200 patients disclosed greater than 50% reporting an improvement in fatigue.[17] Anecdotally, for patients who experience LDN as too activating for bedtime dosing, LDN can be taken after breakfast and may improve fatigue in that setting.

Agents specifically targeting fatigue include amantadine, modafinil, armodafinil, and the amphetamine/amphetaminelike agents (**Box 4**). Amantadine is an antiviral agent that likely has activity at the dopamine receptor and the N-methyl-D-aspartate (NMDA) receptor and is partially effective in treating fatigue. Aspirin (500 mg/d) was compared with amantadine (100 mg twice a day) in a crossover trial design and was of equal efficacy to amantadine.[18] Modafinil is a stimulant that is FDA approved for narcolepsy and has shown promise in 2 pilot studies, but it subsequently did not improve scores on the Modified Fatigue Impact Scale compared with placebo in a large, randomized study.[19] The dose of modafinil is 100 mg after breakfast, before 11 AM, and can be increased to a maximum of 400 mg/d. Patients may be tempted to take a second dose in the afternoon, but this should be discouraged because insomnia is likely to ensue. Armodafinil was also designed for narcolepsy and work-shift sleep disorder (so-called graveyard shift) and may benefit MS-related fatigue. It is not a time-release version of modafinil, contrary to popular belief, but it does

---

Box 4
Recommended dosing for fatigue supplements/medications

- Supplements:
  - L-Carnitine 1000 mg by mouth twice a day
  - Coenzyme Q10 500 mg/d
- Medications:
  - Amantadine 100 mg by mouth twice a day
  - Modafinil(Provigil) 100 to 400 mg by mouth after breakfast, before 11 AM
  - Armodafinil (Nuvigil) 150 to 250 mg by mouth after breakfast, before 11 AM
  - Methylphenidate (Ritalin) 20 mg by mouth after breakfast, before 11 AM
  - Amphetamine/dexamphetamine (Adderall) 10 mg after food twice a day, can increase up to 30 mg twice a day
  - Lisdexamphetamine diesylate (Vyvanse) 20 mg after breakfast, before 11 AM; can increase up to lowest effective dose, maximum 70 mg

---

have a delayed peak of action. Armodafinil can be started at 150 mg and increased to 250 mg as needed; it is also dosed after breakfast and before 11 AM Anecdotally, patients are less likely to report an abrupt afternoon wearing off, or crash, with armodafinil compared with modafinil.

The stimulants used in treating attention deficit/hyperactivity disorder (ADHD) are also options. These stimulants are off-label, controlled substances, with the potential for abuse and therefore their use should be minimized. Agents commonly used for MS-related fatigue include methylphenidate (Ritalin), amphetamine/dexamphetamine, and lisdexamphetamine dimesylate (see **Box 4**). Of note, lisdexamphetamine may have a positive impact on cognitive function as well as fatigue.[20] However, the choice of agent is often dictated by insurance coverage or lack thereof because none of the agents discussed earlier are FDA approved for MS-related fatigue.

Antidepressants, supplements, and herbal therapies are prescribed to be taken daily. However, it is important to apprise patients that many of the fatigue agents can be taken as needed rather than every day. Some patients benefit from having a fatigue medication as a tool in the tool kit when they have a pronounced need for pharmacologic intervention. If a patient is navigating options for treating fatigue for an upcoming event, such as a professional conference or a family gathering, recommend test driving the medication before the event. The patient can then anticipate the therapeutic effect and/or side effects.

Depression
Depression in MS is frequent among patients with MS, with lifetime prevalence of up to 50%. In a recent evaluation of depression in the BEYOND (Betaferon Efficacy Yielding Outcomes of a New Dose) trial, depression was found to occur in 24.4% to 24.7% of patients exposed to the interferon beta-1b arm (500 mg and 250 mg respectively) and in 32.4% exposed to glatiramer acetate. This analysis did not find increased depression among the patients treated with interferon beta-1b.[21] As with other symptoms in MS, depression is likely multifactorial. Depression can present early in MS, and identifying a reactive component versus depression caused by underlying MS disorder is challenging. Recognition and treatment of depression is often inadequate, and recent data highlight that untreated depression in MS is likely to worsen over time, thus emphasizing the importance of recognizing depression and treating early. Further highlighting the need to treat early is the high risk for suicide in MS. In combined data from 2 Canadian MS clinics, suicide was the cause of death in 28.6% of patients, which is 7.5

times that for the age-matched general population.[22] A Danish study found the suicide risk to be higher among younger, male patients,[23] whereas a Canadian study identified suicide risk factors of living alone, severe depression, and alcohol abuse.[24]

The data are mixed regarding clinical and radiologic correlates for depression in MS. Certain clinical features, such as disability status, fatigue, and cognitive impairment, correlate with depression in MS in some studies but not in others. Radiologically, data are similarly divergent. Correlation has been found with disorders in the right hemisphere and in the left hemisphere. Lesion load in the right frontal white matter or in the left inferior medial frontal region, and/or atrophy of the right temporal lobe or the left anterior temporal lobe, may be of relevance. Neuroimaging studies have been plagued by small sample sizes and inconsistent methods of evaluation for depression.[25]

Treatment of depression in MS begins with evaluating for possible untoward contribution from general medical conditions and/or medication profiles. Formal neurocognitive testing can delineate potential contribution from other symptoms, such as fatigue, and can identify whether a patient's depression follows an expected pattern on testing for MS. Nonpharmacologic and pharmacologic address may be used. Both psychotherapy and cognitive behavior therapy have been helpful in treating depression in MS. Tai chi was shown to improve depression in patients with MS.[26] A pilot study is underway evaluating cost-effectiveness of so-called can-do treatment, wherein the multidisciplinary team includes a psychiatrist, psychiatric nurse, specialized MS nurse, physiotherapist, and dance therapist. In addition to standard medical care the study arm patients will be offered group sessions and group social activities, and each morning will participate in a joint activity.[27] Exercise can have a positive impact on mood and fatigue.[28] Other nonpharmacologic modalities with positive data in treating depression, although not specifically studies in patients with MS, include spending time outdoors in the morning and blue light therapy.

Various supplements have been studied for a potential role in treating MS-related depression. Recently, high-dose vitamin A was shown to benefit depression and fatigue compared with placebo.[12] Patients received 25,000 IU/d of retinyl palmitate (RP) for 6 months followed by 10,000 IU/d of RP for 6 months. Fatigue and depression scores were obtained at baseline and at 12 months, so it is unclear whether the therapeutic effect was apparent more quickly than 12 months. Zinc sulfate may also confer a therapeutic effect on depression. A pilot study showed a significant improvement in depression among patients receiving zinc sulfate (220 mg containing 50 mg of zinc element per day) compared with placebo.[29] Other outcome measures did not improve, such as gait and strength. As mentioned previously, coenzyme Q10 at a dose of 500 mg/d was shown to benefit fatigue and depression.[10] A pilot study of omega-3 fatty acids (6 g/d) versus placebo failed to show a significant impact on depression.[30] It is important to be familiar with this literature, because many patients are drawn to maximizing address outside of prescription antidepressants.

Supportive data regarding specific antidepressant therapy for patients with MS, such as TCAs (desipramine, moclobemide) and SSRIs (sertraline, fluvoxamine), are based on small numbers of patients, often no control group, and differing rating scales for depression. A study of paroxetine did not show a statistically significant difference versus the control group, despite a 57% response rate in the treatment group. The placebo group showed an impressive 40% response rate, as defined by a 50% decrease in the Hamilton Rating Scale for Depression.[31] The serotonin-norepinephrine reuptake inhibitors (SNRIs), duloxetine and venlafaxine (Effexor), are effective in treating depression and neuropathic pain in patients without MS. Duloxetine has shown a positive effect on depression outcome measures in patients with MS.[32] Many pharmacologic options for the treatment of depression exist but have not been studied specifically in the setting of MS.

Cognition
Cognitive impairment occurs in 40% to 65% of patients with MS and can be seen at any point in the timeline of the demyelinating disorder spectrum. It is seen in radiologically isolated syndrome, clinically isolated syndrome, all phases of clinical MS, and in pediatric-onset MS. A collection of imaging correlates in the adult population have been identified, including T2 lesion volume and regional atrophy on traditional MRI. Experimental MRI (higher Tesla or functional imaging) has disclosed (focal) cortical lesions and atrophy, abnormal cortical integrity, and early changes in normal-appearing brain tissue. A recent study of newly diagnosed patients with relapsing-remitting MS (RRMS) disclosed that higher levels of nitrite/nitrate (NOx), metabolites of NO, in cerebrospinal fluid correlated with impaired processing speed but failed to detect a statistically significant impact on other domains, such as verbal intelligence quotient, working memory, and perceptual orientation.[33] This trial was a small study of 23 patients but may suggest a role of NOx in neurodegenerative processes that contribute to cognitive impairment.

Cognitive challenges can co-occur or be compounded by depression, anxiety, and fatigue. Indirectly, symptoms that disrupt sleep, such as bladder frequency, spasticity, or pain, can also heighten cognitive dysfunction. Medications for other MS symptoms can affect cognition negatively, especially antispasmodics, opioids, and some agents for neuropathic pain. Systematic address of potential contributors should be undertaken.

Cognitive challenges are common in the general population with senescence and with hormonal states such as perimenopause/menopause and andropause. Thus it is common for patients to wonder whether their challenges are caused by MS. Domains typically affected in MS-related cognitive dysfunction are:

- Information processing speed
- Complex attention
- Executive function
- Memory (episodic)

However, there is considerable overlap with other causes of cognitive decline, and the threshold should be low for referral to neuropsychology for formal cognitive testing.

In addition, evaluation of cognitive dysfunction should query for hormonal dysfunction (thyroid panel, testosterone, growth hormone), metabolic abnormalities (comprehensive metabolic panel), anemia (complete blood count [CBC] with differential), vitamin deficiency (B_{12}, 25-hydroxyvitamin D, folate), and infectious contributors (urinalysis [UA]/urine culture [UC]).

Cognition in MS can improve with treating contributing MS symptoms such as fatigue and depression. Regarding nonpharmacologic avenues of approach, there is substantial evidence for regular exercise benefiting cognitive function in patients with MS.[34] There are also data supporting computer-based cognitive rehabilitation.[35] Anecdotally, many patients report improvement in mood and cognition with yoga, but it has generated mixed data when evaluated systematically.[36] Practical application of this information would be to validate patients who undertake yoga whether or not they experience benefit cognitively. In addition, there have been 2 negative trials regarding gingko and cognition in MS.[37]

Memantine, a noncompetitive NMDA receptor antagonist, has been studied in the setting of MS-related cognitive dysfunction. This study was predicated by favorable data for patients with Alzheimer disease, and a protective effect observed the mouse model for MS, experimental encephalomyelitis. Studies with patients with MS have been either terminated early because of significant side effects (worsening of baseline symptoms) or have been negative trials.[37,38] There are also negative data for donepezil[39] and rivastigmine.[40] Therefore, thus far Alzheimer disease medications have not shown significant benefit for patients with MS. In contrast, there are some supportive data for medications approved for ADHD/narcolepsy. The positive trials include lisdexamphetamine dimesylate,[20] L-amphetamine,[41] and methylphenidate (Ritalin).[42] Improvements in cognition were not limited to increased processing speed, suggesting that these medications may have benefits beyond improving fatigue or alertness. Patients can be counseled that although there is no single medication that can reverse MS-related cognitive challenges, cognition can improve by addressing the components of care listed earlier.

Bladder dysfunction
Involvement of the central nervous system (CNS) in MS can lead to neurogenic bladder dysfunction (NBD), affecting from 50% to 90% of patients and significantly affecting quality of life. MS NBD increases the risk of UTIs, but there is low risk in terms of developing renal insufficiency. Bladder dysfunction can be divided functionally into a filling phase disorder, a voiding phase disorder, or a combination therein. Filling phase disorders are much more common and are usually caused by detrusor overactivity or spasticity. Urgency, frequency, nocturnal frequency of urine, and/or urge incontinence are common symptoms. When 1 or more of these symptoms is present, the term overactive bladder is used. Voiding phase disorders are typically caused by detrusor-sphincter dyssynergia (DSD), wherein bladder contractility is not appropriately coordinated with sphincter relaxation, and result in hesitancy, slow voiding, and/or retention. Urgency, frequency, nocturnal frequency of urine, and urge incontinence can also be present with voiding phase disorders. Hypocontractile detrusor, or flaccid bladder, leads to incomplete emptying and thus increased residual volume, but is the least common syndrome. All of these increase the risk for UTI.

Management of bladder symptoms begins with history taking and subsequent diagnostics. UA/UC can evaluate for infection and guide antibiotic treatment. Many of the symptoms discussed earlier may be secondary to, or escalated by, UTI and can resolve or improve with simply treating with appropriate antibiotic coverage. UTI does not preclude the existence of one of the underlying disorders of bladder function noted earlier, and UTI may be the presenting feature. Differentiating NBD from bladder dysfunction caused by weakness of the pelvic floor musculature can be challenging. There is overlap clinically in features such as urinary frequency, urgency, and incontinence. However, urinary retention and/or unprecipitated, large-volume incontinence may be more suggestive of CNS involvement. Evaluation by a urologist to guide further diagnostics, such as bladder ultrasonography and urodynamic studies, is helpful. Of note, if ultrasonography reveals a substantial postvoid residual, most bladder medications should be avoided.

Treatment again can be divided into nonpharmacologic and pharmacologic measures. Behavioral measures include limiting irritants such as caffeine, citrus fruits, and carbonated beverages. Individual sensitivity to such agents varies, and patients can be encouraged to keep a bladder diary to evaluate individual sensitivities to irritants. Fluid intake can be limited to 90 to 120 mL (3-4 ounces) per hour during the day and stopping fluids 1 to 2 hours before bedtime. Patients should not discontinue fluids throughout the day because this can increase the risk for UTI and can affect other MS symptoms, such as fatigue. Patients should be counseled that insufficient fluid intake can irritate a neurogenic bladder and cause an escalation of bladder symptoms. Thus, although counterintuitive to many symptomatic patients, they need sufficient hydration for a variety of health reasons and to avoid escalation of baseline bladder symptoms. Symptoms can be worsened by weakness of the pelvic floor muscles, and can therefore benefit from pelvic floor exercises. Planning can also decrease anxiety and accidents. Patients can use the restroom before car trips and can take note of the nearest restroom when in a novel environment.

Hyperreflexic and spastic bladders often respond to treatment with antimuscarinic agents. Oxybutynin (Ditropan) and tolterodine (Detrol) are available in sustained-release formulation. Newer agents, such as solifenacin (VESIcare) and trospium (Sanctura), are also dosed once per day and may have less crossover to the CNS. Failure of one medication does not preclude use of the class of medications, and a patient who does not sustain benefit from one agent may show response to a different agent. All of the antimuscarinic agents have potential side effects of xerostomia, constipation, urinary retention, and light-headedness. Contraindications include significant urinary retention, gastric stasis, and other conditions with severe impairment of intestinal mobility, and uncontrolled narrow-angle glaucoma. Mirabegron, a beta-adrenergic receptor agonist, is another treatment option for neurogenic bladder. It is less likely to cause xerostomia, and can be considered in patients who get benefit from antimuscarinics but cannot tolerate the side effects. **Table 3** provides dosing recommendations.

If refractory to oral agents, patients may benefit from a referral to urology or neuro-urology. There are options for refractory detrusor hyperactivity that are overseen by a urologist, all of which have pros and cons. Intravesical botulinum A toxin can confer benefit lasting for 6 to 9 months[43] and is considered a "game changer" by many patients. However, it can transiently induce reliance on self-catheterization. Sacral neuromodulation (InterStim) is FDA approved for overactive bladder, is well tolerated, and can improve fecal incontinence. Its placement precludes future MRI scans, and therefore it should be reserved for a select patient population. Percutaneous tibial nerve stimulation has shown moderate benefit compared with sham. It requires weekly visits and therefore can be considered for highly motivated patients who are attracted to nonpharmacologic avenues of treatment.

However, disorders of the voiding stage are more difficult to treat and DSD is less amenable to pharmacologic therapy alone. First-line agents are often ineffectual,

Table 3
Antimuscarinic medications for overactive bladder

Generic	Brand	Dose	Frequency
Oxybutynin	Ditropan	2.5–5 mg	Up to 3 times a day
	Ditropan XL	5mg/10 mg/15 mg	Daily
	Oxytrol patch	3.9 mg/d	Patch twice weekly
	Gelnique	10%	1 g applied daily
Tolterodine	Detrol	1–2 mg	Up to twice a day
	Detrol LA	2mg/4 mg	Daily
Solifenacin	Vesicare	5–10 mg	Daily
Trospium chloride	Sanctura	20 mg	Twice a day
	Sanctura XR	60 mg	Daily
Darifenacin	Enablex	7.5–15 mg	Daily
Propiverine	Detrunorm IR	15 mg	Twice a day
	Detrunorm ER	30 mg	Daily

and data regarding intravesical botulinum A toxin are not promising.[44] Behavioral address, such as abdominal massage, can help with urinary hesitancy/retention. Pelvic floor PT also may be of benefit. If postvoid residuals are greater than 150 mL, intermittent catheterization may be the best option. For patients who are refractory to intermittent self-catheterization, an indwelling catheter or suprapubic catheterization may be indicated. Any indwelling device can increase the risk for infection, carries psychological weight for the patient, and therefore should be avoided if possible.

Bowel dysfunction

Neurogenic bowel disorder (NBD) occurs in several neurologic disorders, and bowel dysfunction occurs in more than 50% of patients with MS.[45] Constipation is the most common clinical feature of MS-related NBD, but bowel urgency and frequency, or leakage and incontinence, can occur. Bowel dysfunction can incur/worsen several symptoms, including bladder dysfunction, sexual dysfunction, depression, and fatigue. Bowel dysfunction has a negative impact on social functioning and quality of life, and patients with spinal cord lesions rank bowel dysfunction second in importance only to extremity weakness.[45]

Pathophysiology is usually multifactorial, and includes MS-related contributors as well as indirect contributors. Autonomic dysfunction caused by MS can incur increased colonic transit time, delayed gastric emptying, and/or sphincteric dysregulation. Somatic dysfunction, such as weakened abdominal muscles or decreased sensory feedback, can compound the milieu. Indirect contributors can include decreased activity, decreased fluid intake caused by bladder symptoms, and decreased food/fiber intake. In addition, medications commonly used in symptom management for patients with MS can be constipating (**Box 5**).

Management of bowel symptoms in MS is largely empiric, with few systematic data specifically addressing this patient population. Management of constipation can begin with history taking regarding bowel symptoms, food intake, fiber intake, fluid intake, and medication profile review. First-line diagnostics include UA/UC, thyroid panel, hemoglobin A1c, and vitamin D status. Referral to gastroenterology for diagnostics such as anorectal physiology and colonic transit studies may direct pelvic floor PT and/or biofeedback strategies, although currently there is little evidence that the results improve management/clinical outcomes.[46]

Box 5
Medications commonly used that can negatively affect constipation

Medications:
  Anticholinergics
  Antihypertensives
  Analgesics
  Antidepressants
  Antipsychotics
  Antihistamines
  Tricyclic antidepressants
  Sedatives/anxiolytics
  Antacids
  Diuretics
  Iron supplements

Medications commonly used in symptom management can have an untoward effect on bowel function.

Initial behavioral strategies can include streamlining constipating medications, encouraging adequate fluid intake, and encouraging regular AM bowel movements, 20 to 30 minutes after a warm meal. Regular exercise has shown benefit for other patient populations with neurogenic constipation, and pelvic floor rehabilitation/PT can benefit bowel function in patients with MS. Patients can also be counseled to avoid constipating/gas-producing aliments such as alcohol, caffeine, and the substitutes sorbitol, xylitol, maltitol, and lactitol. Adequate fiber intake should be encouraged. Patients often have hurdles to adequate food/caloric intake for regular bowel movements. Hurdles include fatigue, decreased mobility and/or dexterity, and decreased appetite caused by medications and/or decreased physical activity. Patients may benefit from reminders to eat regularly, such as alerts/alarms on their phones.

Constipation can improve with certain nonpharmacologic interventions as well as pharmacologic interventions. Digital rectal stimulation increases motility in the anorectum and left colon by activating preserved anorectal reflexes.[47] Abdominal massage was shown to improve constipation in a small cohort of patients with MS.[48] Biofeedback increases sensory awareness in patients with incontinence and can be of benefit in patients with less severe symptoms and milder manometry measures. Pharmacologically, bulking agents and/or stool softeners can be of benefit. Chelated magnesium (250–500 mg) taken at bedtime can promote a morning bowel movement and assuage the often concomitant spasticity/nocturnal muscle spasms. Osmotic laxatives or stimulant laxatives also can be helpful. Prokinetic agents can help immensely but, because of the risk of consequent bowel frequency/urgency, their introduction should be done cautiously and with appropriate counseling. Similarly, colonic and rectal stimulants should be overseen by a gastroenterologist.

Treatment options for bowel incontinence similarly include counseling regarding nutrition and avoidance of irritating foods/beverages. Patients can be counseled to prepare a small kit, including wipes and clean underwear, so that episodes of leakage/incontinence when away from the home are less stressful. Other management approaches (anal plug, sphincteric injections) can be considered after evaluation by a gastroenterologist, and appropriate referrals should be placed readily.

Sexual dysfunction

There is a growing appreciation for the incidence of sexual dysfunction among patients with MS, with 50% to 85% of patients reporting at least 1 sexual dysfunction.[49] Some evidence suggests a correlation with disease duration and increased age.[50] However, there is substantial support for early onset, and more than 50% of women report sexual dysfunction 2 to 5 years after diagnosis.[51]

The most common challenge among men and women with MS is decreased libido.[52,53] Other common symptoms among women include decreased vaginal lubrication, difficulty reaching orgasm, and anorgasmia. Men with MS can experience erectile dysfunction, delayed orgasm, and/or anorgasmia. Diminished sensation in erogenous zones may be a complaint specific to the MS population.

Clinically, sexual dysfunction in patients with MS correlates with bladder dysfunction.[50,52] Evidence is less robust for a correlation with pyramidal involvement[53,54] or with cerebellar dysfunction.[53] Other potential clinical correlates are depression, anxiety, and progressive rather than relapsing-remitting symptoms. The data are conflicting regarding disability status, disease duration, and bowel dysfunction. Potential radiologic correlates of T1 lesion load and pontine involvement[55] are based on small numbers.

Sexual function is a complex product of biological, psychological, societal, and interpersonal factors, and MS can affect each of these domains. Also, changes caused by perimenopause, menopause, and andropause are experienced by many patients with MS at some point in their MS diagnosis, and can alter sexual function. Therefore, sexual dysfunction in patients with MS likely represents a multifactorial process. Likely, as with patients without MS, sexual dysfunction may be most appropriately approached with a biopsychosocial construct that addresses the interdependent aspects of sexuality. Streamlining medications with an untoward impact on sexual function; maximizing address of disease activity; and addressing interrelated symptoms, such as depression and fatigue, can summate to a beneficial impact on sexual function. Patients may benefit from individual or couple counseling. In addition, pelvic floor muscle training and electrostimulation, combined or individually, can improve sexual dysfunction in women with MS.[56]

Good data regarding specific pharmacologic treatment of sexual dysfunction in MS are scarce, with only 5 clinical trials since 1996 with a PubMed search of key title words "sexual dysfunction" and "multiple sclerosis". The only study evaluating a pharmacologic agent is a negative trial regarding the efficacy of sildenafil for the treatment of female sexual dysfunction in MS.[57] Flibanserin (Addyi) is a 5-hydroxytryptamine (5HT) (1A) agonist/5HT (2A) antagonist initially investigated as an antidepressant that was shown to have a positive impact on libido. Although it was FDA approved for hypoactive sexual desire disorder in 2015, its use has not been studied in the MS population. Of note, bupropion is an antidepressant that is not associated with sexual dysfunction and may also improve fatigue for patients with MS. Potential side effects include an increase in anxiety and disruption of REM sleep, so not all patients are good candidates, and it has not been studied specifically in sexual dysfunction in patients with MS. Although data for male patients are mixed regarding phosphodiesterase inhibitors, their use is common for patients with MS. Although formal recommendations regarding pharmacologic address of sexual dysfunction specifically in the MS population are lacking, there is a role for neurologists in addressing sexual dysfunction. Starting a dialogue regarding sexual dysfunction and counseling the patient is part of treatment. Streamlining medications and addressing compounding comorbidities can be undertaken by the MS team. In addition, identifying potential contributions from other specialists and generating the appropriate referrals are within the domain of the neurologist/MS team. **Box 6** shows the role of the neurologist.

Spasticity

Spasticity is common in the MS population and is typically the sequela from partial myelitis. Spasticity can be experienced as muscle tightness, muscle spasms or cramping, or pain that is often described as deep or aching. Spasticity is often most challenging during the night or on rising in the morning. An increase in spasticity

---

Box 6
Role of neurologists in the treatment of sexual dysfunction

Open the dialogue/listen/validate

Maximize disease-modifying therapy

Identify/address contributing MS symptoms

Streamline medications with untoward side effects on sexual function

Appropriate referral (urologist, gynecologist, couples counseling)

Neurologists taking care of patients with sexual dysfunction can play a significant role in addressing and treating patients' concerns.

may be the first sign of a systemic infection, and diagnostics should include UA/UC and CBC with differential to evaluate for pseudoexacerbation. Nonpharmacologic approaches to spasticity include stretching of the spastic limbs, which can be repeated several times a day; acupuncture; and massage therapy. However, the benefit from these modalities tends to be transient. For nighttime spasms or spasticity that disrupts sleep, a good initial address can be with chelated magnesium taken at bedtime (250–500 mg). Magnesium taken at bedtime also encourages a morning bowel movement, which tends to be beneficial, because constipation commonly accompanies lower extremity spasticity. Magnesium should be avoided or prescribed cautiously for patients with bowel frequency/urgency.

With any of the antispasmodics, some patients incur gait deterioration with address of spasticity, specifically if very weak in their lower extremities. Thus, treatment should begin with a low dose with subsequent gentle advancement as necessary. Baclofen is a muscle relaxant that is the most common first-line agent. Tizanidine is often used as a second-line agent but is more associated with drowsiness, which may limit daytime use. There are some head-to-head data regarding baclofen and tizanidine,[58] but all of these trials are plagued by small sample size. Most efficacy outcome measures did not clearly disclose superiority regarding spasticity/clonus, although 1 trial showed more consistent improvement in bladder, muscle strength, and activities of daily living in the tizanidine arm. Tizanidine was associated with more sedation and xerostomia, and baclofen is associated with more weakness as a side effect. Cyclobenzaprine and carisoprodol can be explored as well but have not been studied in patients with MS. Because benzodiazepines have activity at the GABA receptor, they are sometimes used as adjunct therapy. Their use should be limited because of their side effect profile and the potential for tolerance and dependence. Gabapentin dosed at 900 mg 3 times per day was shown to significantly improve spasticity in a placebo-controlled clinical trial with patients with MS and may additionally improve neuropathic pain.[59] Because all of the antispasmodics are associated with sedation, it is recommended that dosing starts low and at bedtime. Titration should go slowly, with escalation of evening and bedtime dosages preceding increased morning dosages.

If patients continue to have significant spasticity despite appropriate address with oral agents, they may benefit from a baclofen pump or from botulinum toxin A injections. Botulinum A injections are especially helpful in the setting of spasticity of limited distribution, such as in 1 upper extremity. It is also particularly helpful in wheelchair-bound patients with adductor spasticity who are having difficulty with self-hygiene or intimate relations. Intramuscular botulinum toxin can be administered every 3 months, whereas more frequent dosing may lead to the formation of neutralizing antibodies and decreased efficacy. Intramuscular botulinum toxin administration is not a time-consuming procedure, it works well, and tends to have no significant side effects. Its use is limited when spasticity is widespread and comprehensive address would supersede maximum dosing recommendations. Evaluation for a baclofen pump is indicated when spasticity is refractory to antispasmodics and/or intramuscular botulinum toxin, or if spasticity in the lower extremities involves too many muscle groups for meaningful address with intramuscular injections.

In addition, medical marijuana has been evaluated in the treatment of spasticity for patients with MS. The cannabinoids include delta-9-tetrahydrocannabinol (THC) and cannabidiol (CBD). In 1987, a small trial of a THC-rich strain in 13 patients disclosed significant benefit, and more recent data with 30 patients in a crossover design reported reduction in Ashworth scores and reduced pain associated with smoked cannabis (4% delta-9-THC). There was no difference in timed walk, but a reduction in paced auditory serial addition test (PASAT) scores was seen with cannabis treatment.[60] The large CAMs (Cannabinoids for treatment of spasticity and other symptoms related to multiple sclerosis) study failed to reveal a significant impact on the primary outcome measure of the Ashworth score but did disclose improvement in the patients' perceptions of spasticity and in pain scores.[61] Nabiximols (Sativex) is an oral mucosal spray that contains delta-9-THC and CBD in a 1:1 ratio, and is approved in 16 countries outside the United States for the treatment of spasticity in patients with MS. It can significantly reduce spasticity and is generally well tolerated. The most common side effects are dizziness in up to 24.7% of patients and fatigue in 12.3%.[62,63] These agents are likely to increase in use for refractory spasticity or as adjunct therapy.

Pain
At one time, pain was not recognized as a common component of MS. Patients with MS can experience neuropathic pain, pain associated with spasticity, and secondary musculoskeletal pain syndromes caused by compensatory muscle group use/overuse. Similar to fatigue and spasticity, an escalation of baseline pain should prompt a query for pseudoexacerbation. Treatment of pain associated with spasticity is addressed earlier. Clinical trials to address neuropathic pain specifically in MS are limited and include nabilone as adjunct therapy and nabiximols (Sativex), and these are discussed later. At present, neuropathic pain is approached as in other clinical scenarios. Maximization of nonpharmacologic or complementary modalities may decrease the number and dosage of medications necessary. There are some data to support massage therapy and/or acupuncture for patients who express interest in complementary modalities. Pain meditation podcasts are readily available and are often helpful additions to an otherwise comprehensive plan.

At present, the agents most commonly used for neuropathic pain include antidepressants such as TCAs and selective SNRIs, and antiepileptic drugs such as gabapentin and pregabalin as first-line treatment recommendations. Several societies have generated treatment recommendations based on the Grading of Recommendations Assessment, Development, and Evaluation (GRADE) system with:

- Strong recommendations for TCAs, SNRIs, and the antiepileptic drugs gabapentin and pregabalin as first-line agents
- Weak recommendations for lidocaine patches, capsaicin patches, opioids, and botulinum toxin A
- Strong recommendations against levetiracetam and mexiletine
- Weak recommendations against valproate and cannabinoids

Of note, opioids are recommended as second-line or third-line therapy because of the weak efficacy data and concern regarding the risk for addiction, tolerance, and use/abuse of these medications. In addition, in the setting of trigeminal neuralgia, both carbamazepine and oxcarbazepine can be used, but oxcarbazepine tends to be better tolerated.[64]

A reasonable approach is to consider comorbidities and target a 2-for-1 or even 3-for-1, wherein a single medication may confer benefit on 2 or 3 symptoms. For instance, low-dose TCAs taken at bedtime can target pain and, because of anticholinergic side effects, also benefit insomnia and bladder frequency at night. Thus, although the tertiary amine amitriptyline has more anticholinergic side effects than the secondary amine nortriptyline, this may prove beneficial for patients with overactive bladder and nocturnal frequency of bladder. The most common limiting side effect with amitriptyline is xerostomia, and nortriptyline may be preferable in this setting. The doses used for neuropathic pain (25–75 mg) are lower than those used to treat depression (150–300 mg) so, if targeting depression and pain, an SNRI may be preferred.

Duloxetine (Cymbalta) and venlafaxine (Effexor) can both be considered. Gabapentin may improve spasticity and anxiety in addition to addressing neuropathic pain.

Recent therapeutic advances underdevelopment for neuropathic pain include selective voltage-gated sodium channel antagonists (Nav 1.7, Nav 1.8), peptides isolated from venoms of spiders and snails, and a monoclonal antibody against nerve growth factor, but they have not yet been studied in the MS population. As mentioned earlier, there are supportive clinical trial data for nabilone, an oral synthetic opioid, as combination therapy with gabapentin.[65] There are also supportive data for nabiximols (Sativex). Of note, both of these randomized, placebo-controlled trials took place after the weak recommendations against cannabinoids.

A COMMENT ON AGENTS THAT MAY IMPROVE FUNCTION GLOBALLY: FAMPRIDINE, DALFAMPRIDINE, LOW-DOSE NALTREXONE, HIGH-DOSE BIOTIN

Dalfampridine is FDA approved to improve walking in patients with MS. Dalfampridine and fampridine are both broad-spectrum potassium channel blockers and improve conduction along demyelinated pathways. Because of this generalized effect, both agents may confer benefit on myriad symptoms in patients with MS. Dalfampridine is time release and the maximum dosing and frequency is 10 mg twice per day. Because it is FDA approved, it is more likely to be covered by insurance, so out-of-pocket expense to the patient is potentially low/none. Fampridine is a compounded formula and therefore can be immediate release. Dosing can be tailored to the individual in terms of frequency (up to 4 times a day) but high dosages approaching 0.8 to 1.0 mg/kg/d should be avoided because of increased risk of seizure. Ensure that the compounding pharmacy of choice is certified and check prices, because both can be variable. Anecdotally, these agents have conferred benefit in the setting of diplopia, dysphagia, and motor endurance, among other symptoms, and thus can be considered when other symptomatic therapies are unavailable/ineffective.

LDN has been studied with health-related questionnaires regarding quality of life and with retrospective chart review. Patients report improvement in quality of life when treated with LDN,[16] and retrospective chart review revealed that greater than 50% reported an improvement in fatigue as well as 60% reporting stabilization or improvement while on LDN.[17] Anecdotally, improvement in cognition, mood, diplopia, and bladder symptoms have been reported. LDN is well tolerated, safe, and low cost, and can be considered when other symptomatic therapies are unavailable or ineffective.

High-dose biotin (HDB) was serendipitously noted to benefit patients with progressive MS who had been misdiagnosed with biotin-responsive leukoencephalopathy, which led to a pilot study of 23 consecutive patients with progressive MS. Lacking a placebo arm, 89% of patients reported stabilization/improvement after 3 to 8 months of therapy.[66] A subsequent larger placebo-controlled study disclosed a much lower response rate of 12.7% of patients stabilizing/improving. A variety of symptoms improved in both studies. Compounded biotin at 300 mg/d costs $160 to $400 out of pocket and is unfeasible financially for many patients. For patients who can afford it, HDB can be considered once patients are appropriately counseled regarding the likelihood of response and delay of onset of efficacy.

SUMMARY

Informed care providers with tools to maximize efficiency can impart significant improvement in quality of life for patients living with MS. Symptom management can be time consuming, and thought must be given to the constructs that will allow individual facilities to provide meaningful care. A few general rules:

1. Always be a respectful listener and validate patients when appropriate
2. Do not assume that everything is caused by MS
3. Always evaluate for other contributing health conditions, medications, and other contributing MS symptoms
4. Building blocks such as vitamin D_3 and exercise are essential; nutrition and stress management are often also meaningful in symptom management
5. Do not assume that all patients want a prescription; be knowledgeable about evidence-based options for supplements and complementary modalities
6. With medications:
   a. Target more than 1 symptom when possible
   b. Start low and go slowly
   c. Separate new medications with a sufficient window to discern benefit and/or side effects
   d. Have a system for feedback and feedforward that is preferably not in clinic: phone call to nurse/NP, Internet visit with NP or neurologist

REFERENCES

1. Tremlett H, Zhao Y, Devonshire V. Natural history of secondary progressive multiple sclerosis. Mult Scler 2008;14:314–24.
2. Tedeholm H, Skoog B, Lisovskaja V, et al. The outcome spectrum of multiple sclerosis: disability, mortality, and a cluster of predictors from onset. J Neurol 2015; 262:1148–63.
3. University of California, San Francisco MS-EPIC Team, Cree BA, Gourraud PA, Oksenberg JR, et al. Long-term evolution of multiple sclerosis disability in the treatment era. Ann Neurol 2016;80(4):499–510.
4. Amato MP, Portaccio E. Management options in multiple sclerosis-associated fatigue. Expert Opin Pharmacother 2012;13:207–16.
5. Nourbakhsh B, Revirajan N, Waubant E. Association between glutamate blockade and fatigue in patients with multiple sclerosis. JAMA Neurol 2015; 72(11):1374–5.
6. Hasanpour Dehkordi A. Influence of yoga and aerobics exercise on fatigue, pain and psychosocial status in patients with multiple sclerosis: a randomized trial. J Sports Med Phys Fitness 2016;56(11):1417–22.
7. Bastani F, Sobhani M, Emamzadeh Ghasemi HS. Effect of acupressure on fatigue in women with multiple sclerosis. Glob J Health Sci 2015;7(4):375–81.
8. Grossman P, Kappos L, Gensicke H, et al. MS quality of life, depression, and fatigue improve after mindfulness training: a randomized trial. Neurology 2010; 75(13):1141–9.
9. Tomassini V, Pozzilli C, Onesti E, et al. Comparison of the effects of acetyl L-carnitine and amantadine for the treatment of fatigue in multiple sclerosis: results of a pilot, randomized, double-blind, crossover trial. J Neurol Sci 2004;218(1–2): 103–8.
10. Sanoobar M, Dehghan P, Khalili M, et al. Coenzyme Q10 as a treatment for fatigue and depression in multiple sclerosis patients: a double blind randomized clinical trial. Nutr Neurosci 2016;19(3):138–43.
11. Achiron A, Givon U, Magalashvili D, et al. Effect of alfacalcidol on multiple sclerosis-related fatigue: a randomized, double-blind placebo-controlled study. Mult Scler 2015;21(6):767–75.

12. Bitarafan S, Saboor-Yaraghi A, Sahraian MA, et al. Effect of vitamin A supplementation on fatigue and depression in multiple sclerosis patients: a double-blind placebo-controlled clinical trial. Iran J Allergy Asthma Immunol 2016;15(1):13–9.

13. Kim E, Cameron M, Lovera J, et al. American ginseng does not improve fatigue in multiple sclerosis: a single center randomized double-blind placebo-controlled crossover pilot study. Mult Scler 2011;17(12):1523–6.

14. Etemadifar M, Sayahi F, Abtahi SH, et al. Ginseng in the treatment of fatigue in multiple sclerosis: a randomized, placebo-controlled, double-blind pilot study. Int J Neurosci 2013;123(7):480–6.

15. Rossini PM, Pasqualetti P, Pozzilli C, et al. Fatigue in progressive multiple sclerosis: results of a randomized, double-blind, placebo-controlled, crossover trial of oral 4-aminopyridine. Mult Scler 2001;7(6):354–8.

16. Cree BA, Kornyeyeva E, Goodin DS. Pilot trial of low-dose naltrexone and quality of life in multiple sclerosis. Ann Neurol 2010;68(2):145–50.

17. Turel AP, Oh KH, Zagon IS, et al. Low dose naltrexone for treatment of multiple sclerosis: a retrospective chart review of safety and tolerability. J Clin Psychopharmacol 2015;35(5):609–11.

18. Shaygannejad V, Janghorbani M, Ashtari F, et al. Comparison of the effect of aspirin and amantadine for the treatment of fatigue in multiple sclerosis: a randomized, blinded, crossover study. Neurol Res 2012;34(9):854–8.

19. Stankoff B, Waubant E, Confavreux C, et al, French Modafinil Study Group. Modafinil for fatigue in MS: a randomized placebo-controlled double-blind study. Neurology 2005;64(7):1139–43.

20. Morrow SA, Smerbeck A, Patrick K, et al. Lisdexamfetamine dimesylate improves processing speed and memory in cognitively impaired MS patients: a phase II study. J Neurol 2013;260(2):489–97.

21. Schippling S, O'Connor P, Knappertz V, et al. Incidence and course of depression in multiple sclerosis in the multinational BEYOND trial. J Neurol 2016;263(7):1418–26.

22. Sadovnick AD, Eisen K, Ebers GC, et al. Cause of death in patients attending multiple sclerosis clinics. Neurology 1991;41:1193–6.

23. Stenager EN, Stenager E, Koch-Henricksen N, et al. Suicide and multiple sclerosis: an epidemiologic investigation. J Neurol Neurosurg Psychiatry 1992;55:542–5.

24. Feinstein A. An examination of suicidal intent in patients with multiple sclerosis. Neurology 2002;59(5):674–8.

25. Siegert RJ, Abernethy DA. Depression in multiple sclerosis: a review. J Neurol Neurosurg Psychiatry 2005;76(4):469–75.

26. Burschka JM, Keune PM, Oy UH, et al. Mindfulness-based interventions in multiple sclerosis: beneficial effects of Tai Chi on balance, coordination, fatigue and depression. BMC Neurol 2014;14:165.

27. Jongen PJ, Heerings M, Ruimschotel R, et al. An intensive social cognitive program (can do treatment) in people with relapsing remitting multiple sclerosis and low disability: a randomized controlled trial protocol. BMC Neurol 2016;16:81.

28. Razazian N, Yavari Z, Farnia V, et al. Exercising impacts on fatigue, depression, and paresthesia in female patients with multiple sclerosis. Med Sci Sports Exerc 2016;48(5):796–803.

29. Salari S, Khomand P, Arasteh M, et al. Zinc sulphate: a reasonable choice for depression management in patients with multiple sclerosis: a randomized, double-blind, placebo-controlled clinical trial. Pharmacol Rep 2015;67(3):606–9.

30. Shinto L, Marracci G, Mohr DC, et al. Omega-3 fatty acids for depression in multiple sclerosis: a randomized pilot study. PLoS One 2016;11(1):e0147195.

31. Ehde DM, Kraft GH, Chwastiak L, et al. Efficacy of paroxetine in treating major depressive disorder in persons with multiple sclerosis. Gen Hosp Psychiatry 2008;30(1):40–8.

32. Solaro C, Bergamaschi R, Rezzani C, et al. Duloxetine is effective in treating depression in multiple sclerosis patients: an open-label multicenter study. Clin Neuropharmacol 2013;36(4):114–6.

33. Okada K, Kobata M, Sennari Y, et al. Levels of nitric oxide metabolites in cerebrospinal fluid correlate with cognitive impairment in early stage multiple sclerosis [letter]. J Neurol Neurosurg Psychiatry 2017;88(10):892–3.

34. Motl RW, Sandroff BM, Benedict RH. Cognitive dysfunction and multiple sclerosis: developing a rationale for considering the efficacy of exercise training. Mult Scler 2011;17(9):1034–40.

35. Cerasa A, Gioia MC, Valentino P, et al. Computer-assisted cognitive rehabilitation of attention deficits for multiple sclerosis: a randomized trial with fMRI correlates. Neurorehabil Neural Repair 2013;27(4):284–95.

36. Velikonja O, Curić K, Ozura A, et al. Influence of sports climbing and yoga on spasticity, cognitive function, mood and fatigue in patients with multiple sclerosis. Clin Neurol Neurosurg 2010;112(7):597–601.

37. Lovera JF, Kim E, Heriza E, et al. Ginkgo biloba does not improve cognitive function in MS: a randomized placebo-controlled trial. Neurology 2012;79(12):1278–84.

38. Villoslada P, Arrondo G, Sepulcre J, et al. Memantine induces reversible neurologic impairment in patients with MS. Neurology 2009;72:1630–3.

39. Krupp LB, Christodoulou C, Melville P, et al. Multicenter randomized clinical trial of donepezil for memory impairment in multiple sclerosis. Neurology 2011;76(17):1500–7.

40. Mäurer M, Ortler S, Baier M, et al. Randomised multicentre trial on safety and efficacy of rivastigmine in cognitively impaired multiple sclerosis patients. Mult Scler 2013;19(5):631–8.

41. Sumowski JF, Chiaravalloti N, Erlanger D, et al. L-amphetamine improves memory in MS patients with objective memory impairment. Mult Scler 2011;17(9):1141–5.

42. Harel Y, Appleboim N, Lavie M, et al. Single dose of methylphenidate improves cognitive performance in multiple sclerosis patients with impaired attention process. J Neurol Sci 2009;276(1–2):38–40.

43. MacDonald R, Monga M, Fink HA, et al. Neurotoxin treatments for urinary incontinence in subjects with spinal cord injury or multiple sclerosis: a systematic review of effectiveness and adverse effects [review]. J Spinal Cord Med 2008;31(2):157–65.

44. Gallien P, Reymann J, Amarenco G, et al. Placebo controlled, randomized, double blind study of the effects of botulinum A toxin on detrusor sphincter dyssynergia in multiple sclerosis patients. J Neurol Neurosurg Psychiatry 2005;76(12):1670–6.

45. Worsøe J, Rasmussen M, Christensen P, et al. Neurostimulation for neurogenic bowel dysfunction. Gastroenterol Res Pract 2013;2013:563294.

46. Coggrave M, Wiesel PH, Norton C. Management of faecal incontinence and constipation in adults with central neurological diseases [review]. Cochrane Database Syst Rev 2006;(2):CD002115.

47. Shafik A, El-Sibai O, Shafik IA. Physiologic basis of digital-rectal stimulation for bowel evacuation in patients with spinal cord injury: identification of an anorectal excitatory reflex. J Spinal Cord Med 2000;23(4):270–5.

48. McClurg D, Hagen S, Hawkins S, et al. Abdominal massage for the alleviation of constipation symptoms in people with multiple sclerosis: a randomized controlled feasibility study. Mult Scler 2011;17(2):223–33.

49. Tepavcevic DK, Kostic J, Basuroski ID, et al. The impact of sexual dysfunction on the quality of life measured by MSQoL-54 in patients with multiple sclerosis. Mult Scler 2008;14:1131–6.

50. Zivadinov R, Zorzon M, Bosco A, et al. Sexual dysfunction in multiple sclerosis: II. Correlation analysis. Mult Scler 1999;5(6):428–31.

51. Nortvedt MW, Riise T, Frugård J, et al. Prevalence of bladder, bowel and sexual problems among multiple sclerosis patients two to five years after diagnosis. Mult Scler 2007;13(1):106–12.

52. Demirikiran M, Sarica Y, Uguz S, et al. Multiple sclerosis patients with and without sexual dysfunction: are there any differences? Mult Scler 2006;12:209–14.

53. Hulter BM, Lundberg PO. Sexual function in women with advanced multiple sclerosis. J Neurol Neurosurg Psychiatry 1995;59(1):83–6.

54. Barak Y, Achiron A, Elizur A, et al. Sexual dysfunction in relapsing-remitting multiple sclerosis: magnetic resonance imaging, clinical, and psychological correlates. J Psychiatry Neurosci 1996;21(4):255–8.

55. Zorzon M, Zivadinov R, Locatelli L, et al. Correlation of sexual dysfunction and brain magnetic resonance imaging in multiple sclerosis. Mult Scler 2003;9(1):108–10.

56. Lúcio AC, D'Ancona CA, Lopes MH, et al. The effect of pelvic floor muscle training alone or in combination with electrostimulation in the treatment of sexual dysfunction in women with multiple sclerosis. Mult Scler 2014;20(13):1761–8.

57. Dasgupta R, Wiseman OJ, Kanabar G, et al. Efficacy of sildenafil in the treatment of female sexual dysfunction due to multiple sclerosis. J Urol 2004;171(3):1189–93.

58. Bass B, Weinshenker B, Rice GP, et al. Tizanidine versus baclofen in the treatment of spasticity in patients with multiple sclerosis. Can J Neurol Sci 1988;15(1):15–9.

59. Cutter NC, Scott DD, Johnson JC, et al. Gabapentin effect on spasticity in multiple sclerosis: a placebo-controlled, randomized trial. Arch Phys Med Rehabil 2000;81(2):164–9.

60. Corey-Bloom J, Wolfson T, Gamst A, et al. Smoked cannabis for spasticity in multiple sclerosis: a randomized, placebo-controlled trial. CMAJ 2012;184(10):1143–50.

61. Zajicek J, Fox P, Sanders H, et al, UK MS Research Group. Cannabinoids for treatment of spasticity and other symptoms related to multiple sclerosis (CAMS study): multicentre randomised placebo-controlled trial. Lancet 2003;362(9395):1517–26.

62. Leocani L, Nuara A, Houdayer E, et al. Sativex(®) and clinical-neurophysiological measures of spasticity in progressive multiple sclerosis. J Neurol 2015;262(11):2520–7.

63. Serpell MG, Notcutt W, Collin C. Sativex long-term use: an open-label trial in patients with spasticity due to multiple sclerosis. J Neurol 2013;260(1):285–95.

64. Gilron I, Baron R, Jensen T. Neuropathic pain: principles of diagnosis and treatment [review]. Mayo Clin Proc 2015;90(4):532–45.

65. Turcotte D, Doupe M, Torabi M, et al. Nabilone as an adjunctive to gabapentin for multiple sclerosis-induced neuropathic pain: a randomized controlled trial. Pain Med 2015;16(1):149–59.

66. Sedel F, Papeix C, Bellanger A, et al. High doses of biotin in chronic progressive multiple sclerosis: a pilot study. Mult Scler Relat Disord 2015;4(2):159–69.

Multiple Sclerosis in the Contemporary Age

Understanding the Millennial Patient with Multiple Sclerosis to Create Next-Generation Care

Madison R. Hansen, BA, Darin T. Okuda, MD, MSc*

KEYWORDS

- Multiple sclerosis • Millennials • Generation X • Baby boomers • Telehealth
- Telemedicine • Mobile applications

KEY POINTS

- Most patients diagnosed with MS over the next 10 to 15 years will be from the millennial generation.
- Patients with MS of the millennial generation may be greater challenged by specific health disorders (ie, obesity and mental health disorders) in comparison with other generations.
- The collective millennial personae are more cost conscious, desire more immediate feedback, and are less likely to have a primary care physician compared with the generational cohorts before them.
- Effective care for a millennial patient with MS will require the use of technology to emphasize prevention and provide education, especially within the first year of diagnosis.
- More financial resources and incentives will further help increase the engagement of millennial patients with MS.

BACKGROUND

Millennials, most commonly defined as those born between 1982 and 2000, became America's largest subpopulation in 2015 at 83.1 million, exceeding the baby boomers' generation, those born between 1946 and 1964, for the first time.[1] A wealth of information has been published describing the preferences and characteristics of this new

Disclosure Statement: M.R. Hansen has nothing to disclose. Dr D.T. Okuda received lecture fees from Acorda Therapeutics, Genentech, Genzyme, and Teva, advisory and consulting fees from EMD Serono, Genentech, Genzyme, and Novartis and research support from Biogen.
Neuroinnovation Program, Multiple Sclerosis and Neuroimmunology Imaging Program, Department of Neurology and Neurotherapeutics, UT Southwestern Medical Center, Clinical Center for Multiple Sclerosis, 5959 Harry Hines Boulevard, Suite 920, Dallas, TX 75390-8806, USA
* Corresponding author.
E-mail address: darin.okuda@utsouthwestern.edu

Neurol Clin 36 (2018) 219–230
http://dx.doi.org/10.1016/j.ncl.2017.08.012
0733-8619/18/© 2017 Elsevier Inc. All rights reserved.

neurologic.theclinics.com

dominant generation.[2–5] The term "millennial" dates back to 1991 when Strauss and Howe used the term to label the latest generation at that time.[6] Overall, millennials have been described as sheltered, confident, and team-oriented.[7] The most defining characteristic of the millennial generation is undoubtedly their usage and demand of technology. They are "digital natives": they have grown up with computers and the Internet from an early age and, hence, use technology in almost every aspect of their lives. It has been estimated that 80% of millennials sleep with a cell phone by their bed,[8] 63% feel like they are attached to their phone or tablet, and 36% feel that social media has "helped them find their identity."[9] Even millennials themselves feel this is their most defining characteristic; "technology use" was the most popular answer when millennials were asked what makes their generation unique.[8] Besides being technologically savvy, this generation is also the most ethnically and racially diverse generation in history,[1] and is on track to become the most educated generation, especially among women.[10] Of course, one must be wary of overgeneralization when attributing characteristics to people solely based on their birth year. Acknowledging the potential life cycle effects, period effects, and cohort effects on this generation creates a more mindful understanding of millennials. Life cycle effects refer to how young people may become more like older generations as they age themselves, whereas period effects speak to how individuals are impacted by major events differently depending on where they are in the life cycle. Cohort effects explain how period events may impact millennials more strongly compared with other generations because the events are occurring during a very formative time in their lives.[11] All in all, using a generational approach remains valid because even as a widely heterogeneous group on the individual level, as a cohort, the generation is still unmistakably different from the generations before them.

These stark differences between generations initiate changes in corresponding industries as a new generation comes of age. Common teaching practices have already transformed to account for the millennial generation in the classroom. Around the year 2000, the millennials "went to college," sparking dialogue on the best teaching practices to engage this new millennial learner. In the more recent years, curriculum and educational practices of graduate-level instruction have been the center of educational reform as the millennial generation enters this stage of life. The concept of a "flipped classroom" is gaining momentum as the learning style specifically accounts for millennials' preference of interactive learning.[12] Passive learning is done outside of the classroom where lecture videos are posted online for the student to view on their own time and at their preferred pace. Class time is then reserved for active learning with a focus on critical thinking, teamwork, and collaboration with the instructor. Increasing technology and social media use in multiple aspects of the learning experience was also a common adaptation to the traditional learning experience made by multiple institutions. Displaying a Twitter hashtag on the online learning portal for an especially difficult neuroanatomy module helped raise morale, relieve anxieties, and facilitate communication among second-year medical students.[13] When millennial radiology residents were given iPads to help supplement and facilitate their residency program, 70% reported a preference for reading journals on the iPad.[14] Another medical institution used the push technology of Twitter and Facebook to deliver educational content to their students in a manner more similar to updates or notifications.[15] Incorporating more interactive learning, social media, and online resources into the classroom setting has allowed teachers to more effectively reach the millennial generation. In essence, the education sector has realized that to be an effective teacher, it is imperative to understand the student.

Just as the education system has transformed and adapted to the demands of the millennial generation, so too will the health care system as this generation ages. It is especially imperative for the MS health care system to adapt, and quickly, as most newly diagnosed patients over the next 10 to 15 years will be millennials. MS most commonly affects people in their mid-20s to 30s, with the average age of onset being approximately 30 years of age.[16] In 2017, millennial adults are aged 17 to 35, making them the generation most at risk for developing this enigmatic and heterogeneous condition. A new wave of patients having distinct preferences regarding their approach to acquiring and assimilating information is upon specialists in neuroimmunology, and prior management approaches used in other age demographics may be suboptimal for this contemporary group. Perhaps the same mindset used to spark change in the education system should be applied to the health care system, specifically care in MS. Achieving the best quality of care for the patient comes first with a deep understanding of the patient and the unique challenges they face.

CHALLENGES
Increased Prevalence of Obesity and Mental Health Disorders Among the Millennial Population

Logically, efforts aimed at improving general health will assist with enhancing neurologic health. Obesity and mental health disorders are 2 common general health concerns with significantly higher prevalence within the millennial population compared with the generations before them. These health concerns complicate both symptoms of MS and disease state, further emphasizing their significance to an MS provider.

The millennial generation grew up during a time in which the prevalence of obesity among children and teens skyrocketed. The incidence of obesity in the 1980s and 1990s nearly tripled, rising from approximately 5% in the 1960s to 15% in the 1980s and 1990s.[17] As a result, many millennials have poor health habits marked by unhealthy diets and poor exercise regimens that will substantially increase their risk of obesity as they age. According to a 2007 study of the health behaviors among US high school students, two-thirds did not meet the recommended guidelines for physical activity, and more than 25% of participants reported less than 60 minutes of collective physical activity over the previous week. More than one-third endorsed watching 3 or more hours of television per day and almost 25% reported spending 3 or more hours a day playing computer or video games.[18] As of 2014, approximately one-third of millennials were obese, with a higher prevalence among adult women compared with adult men.[19] Multiple studies have found at least a twofold increased risk of MS in patients with a body mass index ≥ 30 kg/m^2 during their young adult lives,[20,21] especially for female individuals,[22] when compared with healthy-weighted controls. Pairing this with the fact that MS affects women in a 3:1 ratio compared with men,[16] it is more likely that millennial patients diagnosed with MS will be overweight compared with older generations.

Mental health problems are also rising among millennials. The 2 most common are anxiety and depression, which are also commonly identified in patients with MS. One in 5 millennials reports experiencing depression, compared with only 16% in Generation X (those born between 1965 and 1981) and baby boomers.[23] Forty-eight percent of millennials strongly or somewhat agreed with the statement "I worry about the negative effects of social media on my physical and mental health."[9] Much research has shown the complex intermingling of depression and MS.[24] There is a higher likelihood of developing depression if you have MS, proven by the higher incidence rate of depression in the MS population compared with that of the general population.[24] The prevalence of depression, generalized anxiety, and social anxiety among college students has all risen over the past 6 years. In fact, the number of students seeking mental health help increased at 5 times the rate of new students starting college during that time.[25] If a diagnosis of MS puts the patient at greater risk for developing mental health disorders like depression and anxiety, what will the outcome be of the millennial patient who might already be suffering from such a disorder at the time of their MS diagnosis?

The increased prevalence of obesity and mental health disorders among the millennial population will create additional challenges for the millennial patient with MS. The long-term impact these disorders have on MS symptoms and disease state when present at the time of diagnosis should be further studied to help devise effective health solutions. Management of these disorders will have to be prioritized in the plan of care for the millennial patient with MS.

Potential Impacts of Millennials' Extreme Cost Consciousness on Disease Management

Millennials are extremely cost conscious, especially when it comes to their health care. According to a 2015 survey of more than 5000 adults aged 21 and older, more than half of millennials admit to delaying or avoiding medical treatment due to cost.[26] Millennials ranked being able to afford necessary care as the most important aspect of the health care system,[27] and are requesting estimates of out-of-pocket cost before agreeing to treatment options. Thirty-four percent of millennials reported their final health bill was higher than their initial estimate, thereby fueling the positive feedback loop that will discourage more and more millennials from seeking medical care.[26] Furthermore, 1 in 5 millennials cannot afford routine health care expenses.[27] Within the industry, it well known that MS is an expensive disease. Health care costs related to MS in the United States have been estimated to range from $8,500 to upwards of $52,000 per patient per year.[28] How will this frugal health care mentality impact a millennial who is newly diagnosed with MS? Millennials are more likely to skip a doctor's visit, laboratory test, or MRI scan to avoid costs, putting them at higher risk for disease progression. Thankfully, many of the disease-modifying therapies (DMTs) approved by the Food and Drug Administration for MS have patient assistance programs to help patients who do not have the financial means to pay for their MS treatments. In select cases, laboratory studies that are required for safety monitoring while on a given therapy may be provided at zero cost to the patient. However, these services are typically reserved for those who are commercially insured. Individuals with federal-funded or state-funded insurance plans must find supplemental funding through charitable organizations. Nonetheless, many patients have high deductible insurance plans or substantial coinsurance payments that result in financial strain and increased stress. MRI scans are another financial burden for patients; however, the data gained from the scans are essential to effective MS management. As MRI changes outnumber clinical relapses at a 10:1 ratio,[29] MRI is the most sensitive measure of MS disease progression available today. The increased likelihood of millennials omitting key components of disease management in an effort to reduce costs is a major concern. In general, millennials need to be better motivated to prioritize their health even if it means incurring additional costs.

Millennials' Need for Immediate Feedback

Growing up in the era of fast food, instant messaging, and the Internet, it is no surprise millennials have more than a preference for speed and efficiency; they demand it.[11] This coincides with their preferences for more frequent feedback,[30] whether that be from their teacher, boss, or the product they just bought online. In the education system, most grades are now posted online immediately after the assignment has been evaluated, leaving no need to wait until the next class session to receive the grade. When ordering a pizza from Domino's, its progress can be tracked step by step from when it was created, put in the oven, and sent out for delivery. In contrast, many aspects of the MS health care system are exceptionally slow and outdated. Some patients find it difficult to schedule their first appointment with an MS specialist in a timely manner due to physicians' heavily booked schedules. Routine chart reviews reveal countless examples of patients being diagnosed with MS months to years after their initial symptoms. Furthermore, once a patient is finally diagnosed with MS and a DMT is prescribed, it is not uncommon for patients to wait an additional 6 to 8 weeks before receiving their first dose. Millennials may experience both increased stress and frustration throughout the process, having expectations of more immediate gratification. On the most basic level, clear expectations surrounding the timeline of DMT initiation or the interpretation of diagnostic studies must be reinforced by the physician. Unique strategies may need to be implemented to better engage the millennial patient with MS as customary practices of disease management may be ineffective.

The Lack of Primary Care Physicians Among Millennials

Mainly due to inconvenience and cost, fewer and fewer millennials are establishing care with a primary care physician. Only approximately 60% of millennials visit their primary care physician compared with 80% of baby boomers.[26] Instead, millennials are trending toward retail clinics, acute care clinics, and telemedicine. Thirty-four percent of millennials prefer retail clinics to seeing a primary care physician compared with only 17% of baby boomers.[26] The number of retail clinics in the United States has skyrocketed, growing by nearly 900% between 2006 and 2014. In 2012, retail clinic visits totaled to 10.5 million, representing 2% of all primary care encounters in the country.[31] Possibly growing even faster than retail clinics is millennials' preferences for telemedicine, connecting with physicians via technology on a mobile device, tablet, or computer. Amwell, a popular telehealth app launched in 2013, gives users live video access to a US board-certified doctor 24/7 within 2 minutes on average. The app reached 1 million downloads within 1 year.[32] A 2015 survey found that 74% of millennials are interested in using telehealth.[33] Millennials are valuing cost and convenience over in-person examinations and continuity of care. In fact, nearly half of millennials do not have a personal relationship with their physician.[34] For a patient with MS, having one primary care physician, seen routinely throughout their lifetime, is imperative for effective care due to the complexity of the disease as well as the chronic nature of the disease. Common colds and other infections can cause an increase in MS symptoms and may even lead to a relapse if not treated. A primary care physician who is fully up to date on the medical history of a patient with MS can provide the best guidance compared with a doctor who has not been following the patient's care long term. Furthermore, preventive measures are especially critical for a patient with MS who may be immunosuppressed due to their DMT. These preventive checkups, like cancer and diabetes screenings, may be missed if a millennial is seeing a physician only to treat an acute infection, ultimately leaving the patient at greater risk for comorbid conditions. Currently, 93% of millennials do not schedule preventive physician visits,[35] and the numbers will most likely increase in accordance with current millennial health care trends. The value of a genuine, in-person, continuous relationship between a patient with MS and a primary care physician cannot be overemphasized and cannot be replicated using acute care clinics or today's telemedicine resources.

FUTURE STEPS TOWARD NEXT-GENERATION CARE

It is imperative to find innovative solutions to the challenges presented. Creating resources that are tailored specifically to millennial patients' preferences and unique needs is the future of MS care. Health care providers also should be mindful that not all individuals who fall into this generational category will align with all strata described, and heterogeneity regarding expectations and degree of technological engagement will exist. However, by incorporating technology into more aspects of patient management, emphasizing the power of prevention and the importance of patient-provider relationships through providing more educational resources within the first year of diagnosis, and integrating more financial resources and incentives into standardized care (**Fig. 1**), the delivery of health care and long-term outcomes of preventing disability will significantly improve among millennial patients with MS.

Incorporating Technology to Increase Patient Engagement

One of the best ways to engage millennials is undoubtedly through technology. In 2014, 85% of millennials owned a smartphone,[36] and the numbers are increasing

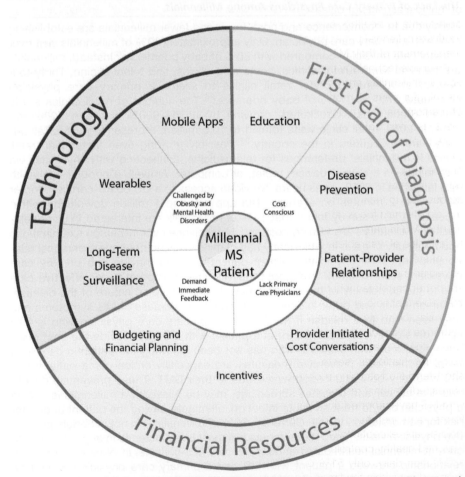

Fig. 1. Summary of the unique challenges presented by a millennial patient with MS and suggested innovative solutions to create millennial patient–specific care.

each year. When it comes to health care, most millennials want to see technology incorporated into multiple aspects of their health care experience. Seventy-one percent of millennials would like their doctor to use a mobile app, and 74% of millennials choose a doctor according to if they can book appointments and pay bills online.[34] To answer the millennial call, mobile resources and other technological devices specifically tailored for the patient with MS need to be developed. For example, incorporating nutrition and exercise with standard MS management tools into a mobile application could help fight the rising problem of obesity among millennial patients with MS. This has been done with success in the diabetes community among millennials. The use of smartphone-based glucose monitors and applications led to improved A1C levels and self-management in diabetes care.[37] Furthermore, 55% of millennials with diabetes reported they are connecting with their doctor more frequently because of health apps.[38] A plethora of diabetes smartphone applications are on the market that not only allow users to track glucose levels but also track exercise, glucose intake, help remind patients of their appointments, and even remind users of the meals they ate at restaurants and how their blood sugar levels were affected afterward.[39] Creating apps that offer more all-inclusive coordination of multiple aspects of disease management, from tracking medications and MRI appointments to healthy recipes and exercise routines, all in one place, could better motivate millennial patients with MS to engage in their general health while improving management of their MS.

Wearable technology that passively tracks individualized health data is also trending among millennials and in today's health care technology space in general. Finding meaningful ways to monitor the patient in-between face-to-face visits is the future of medicine, and to many, wearable technology is the solution. Particularly, patients feel these wearables will further motivate them to engage in a healthier lifestyle, but more importantly, patients feel the data gained from the technology would be useful to their doctor. Eighty percent of millennials feel that wearables would make transferring health care information to physicians more convenient.[40] Enamored with technology, millennials feel providing personal data points acquired through the latest gadget across time to their doctor will improve their care. However, the quality of data should remain the main focus rather than the quantity or ease of acquisition. For the management of MS in particular, one must think critically about the value of data provided by today's line of wearables to disease management or clinical outcomes. Will the number of steps a patient takes each day or a patient's heart rate, for example, impact a physician's recommended treatment plan? Finding more predictive data points that are better correlated with disease state and that can be passively monitored through wearable technology is essential to truly enhancing MS patient care.

Similar to the aims of wearables, efforts have been made to use mobile and online platforms to acquire personal, longitudinal data in hopes of determining more naturalistic outcome measures of patients with chronic diseases. On the surface, such technological platforms seem optimal for millennial engagement. In fact, multiple short-term studies using mobile phones and mobile applications to deliver questionnaires, educational resources, cognitive tests, and even exercise routines to patients with MS have reported success in terms of patient engagement, acceptance of platforms, and increased independence.[41–43] However, attrition rates for long-term studies are exceptionally high. In a 1-year study in which patients with MS and matched healthy controls were asked to complete a small task or survey on a mobile application daily, only 51% of enrolled participants completed the study, and 25% dropped out within the first 4 months.[44] Although these established platforms provide the opportunity to acquire specific data more relevant to an MS provider, long-term use of currently available platforms by patients is unrealistic. Possible causes for diminished usage are the absence of feedback or incentive given for completion of tasks or surveys, the amount of time it takes to complete recommended tasks, as well as the nonexistent end date in real-life application. Furthermore, there may be a lack of perceived value of such surveys or minor tests aimed at disease surveillance by patients. Overall, more innovative technological platforms that incorporate both short-term completion motivators as well as incentives emphasizing the possibilities of improving disease outcomes over the course of a patient's lifetime and increasing scientific knowledge about MS should be generated with authentic, longstanding patient usage as a primary indicator of effectiveness.

Emphasizing Prevention, Education, and Relationships Early On

The first year after diagnosis represents the most formative time for developing life-style changes in the patient; patients are most eager to learn more about MS and the best practices to help prevent disease progression immediately following their diagnosis. This presents an opportunity to form essential habits the patient will continue throughout their lifetime based on the resources provided to them during this crucial stage. Effectively capitalizing on this period will help reorient millennial trends of cutting health care corners. More educational resources that emphasize pre-vention should be afforded to millennial patients with MS soon after they receive their diagnosis. As a cure for MS has yet to be developed, preventing further demyelinating events within the central nervous system is key to preserving long-term function in a patient with MS. This key feature should be emphasized to young patients who can capitalize on their young age to make lifestyle changes that will have a significant impact on their long-term disease outcome, even if this means incurring additional costs initially. The form these educational resources should take is still up for debate. Perhaps answering the call of millennials for more immediate feedback and more health care technology is an electronic health advisor system specifically designed for the new patient with MS. An option to chat 24/7 with someone knowledgeable on MS would provide optimal support for the millennial patient during an often over-whelming and confusing time. The patient could connect with the same health advisor throughout the year, allowing the patient to form a connection with a health care pro-vider and encouraging the patient to create other long-term relationships with other health care providers, principally a primary care physician. Along with answering any questions the patient may have, the health advisor could give advice concerning lifestyle changes, like increasing exercise, eating a healthier diet, or seeking help for a mental health disorder. The health advisor could even evaluate a patient's medical data to provide more accurate and personalized advice. In general, resources pro-vided to millennials should be more technologically based, as well as interactive and visual, compared with lengthy texts, which have been the foundation of educa-tional materials until now. Most importantly, these resources must be provided within the first year of diagnosis to encourage millennial patients with MS to establish habits that will best benefit their long-term prognosis and to capitalize on this formative year.

Integrating Financial Resources and Incentives into Standardized Care

Resources specific to financial matters in connection with disease management should be provided in an effort to directly address millennials' cost-conscious ten-dencies. Using monetary incentives may help increase patient engagement across multiple aspects of MS care. For example, logging in personal health care data into a mobile app to be rewarded with points over time, which can ultimately be redeemed for monetary prizes, such as gym membership discounts, grocery credits, or even health insurance discounts, could help increase long-term engagement and improve disease surveillance. Compliance to a DMT regimen also can be incentivized with decreased costs of the therapies by pharmaceutical companies. Currently, patients are financially penalized by third-party payers if they engage in unhealthy behaviors like smoking. Inverting this system of financial penalties into financial rewards for active engagement in beneficial health habits would bode well with millennials who want to cut costs as much as possible. Furthermore, resources that provide financial education are also important to better support a millennial patient with MS. Mobile applications or online platforms that provide tips on budgeting for health care expenses, how to best schedule medical procedures throughout the year to coincide with insurance deductibles or work pay schedules, or the charities and nonprofit organizations with funds available for patients with MS should be developed and highlighted to millennial patients. Although some MS-specific charities offer a certain degree of personal finance counseling free of cost, this type of resource can be expanded to specifically target millennial patients with MS who are younger and are more likely to be navigating financial independence for the first time. On the most basic level, cost conversations should be regularly included in patient-provider discussions. Many times, patients will neglect bringing up concerns related to costs they may incur in an effort to not disappoint their doctor. Therefore, providers should initiate these types of conversations with their patients to help give patients a better financial forecast for the year. Providers can help patients balance expenses by prioritizing studies and distributing costs over multiple time points, scheduling more expensive measures like an MRI at a time most financially convenient for a patient or in line with a patient's pay schedule. These simpler planning efforts can tremendously help a patient financially but are often opportunities missed because the responsibility most commonly lies with the patient to voice concerns, whether financial or otherwise. Provider-initiated conversations about cost should be encouraged to best meet the needs of cost-conscious millennial patients with MS.

SUMMARY

The most effective treatment plan for a patient with MS is one that is specifically tailored to the patient's individual needs and preferences. This increases engagement, which in turn enhances prognostic outcomes. Most patients newly diagnosed with MS over the next 10 to 15 years will be from the millennial generation. Neurologists and MS specialists who care for patients with MS should recognize the unique characteristics, preferences, and trends shared by this generation as a whole and use this information to drive innovative solutions. If done effectively, the millennial patient with MS could have access to resources designed for their specific needs along with technology that will allow for better outcomes as a result of increased patient engagement and disease management when compared with any other generation before them.

REFERENCES

1. United States Census Bureau. Millennials outnumber baby boomers and are far more diverse, Census Bureau reports. 2015. Available at: https://www.census.gov/newsroom/press-releases/2015/cb15-113.html. Accessed March 22, 2017.
2. Howe N, Strauss W. The next 20 years: how customer and workforce attitudes will evolve. Harv Business Rev 2007;85(7–8):41–52, 191.
3. Keeter S, Taylor P. The millennials. Pew Research Center; 2009. Available at: http://www.pewresearch.org/2009/12/10/the-millennials/. Accessed March 15, 2017.

4. Pew Research Center. The whys and hows of generations research. 2013. http://www.people-press.org/2015/09/03/the-whys-and-hows-of-generations-research/. Accessed March 20, 2017.

5. Seppanen S. The millennial generation: research review. Washington, DC: National Chamber Foundation; 2012.

6. Strauss W, Howe N. Generations: the history of America's future, 1584 to 2069. New York: William Morrow and Company, Inc; 1991.

7. Howe N, Strauss W. Millennials go to college: strategies for a new generation on campus. Virginia: Lifecourse Associates; 2007.

8. Pew Research Center. Millennials. Confident. Connected. Open to Change. 2010. Available at: http://pewsocialtrends.org/pubs/751/millennials-confident-connected-open-tochange. Accessed March 22, 2017.

9. American Psychological Association. Stress in America 2017: technology and social media. 2017. Available at: http://www.apa.org/news/press/releases/stress/2017/technology-social-media.PDF. Accessed March 15, 2017.

10. Patten E. How millennials today compare with their grandparents 50 years ago. 2015. Available at: http://www.pewresearch.org/fact-tank/2015/03/19/how-millennials-compare-with-their-grandparents/-!14. Accessed March 22, 2017.

11. Kurup V. The new learners–millennials!! Int Anesthesiol Clin 2010;48(3):13–25.

12. Lucardie AT, Berkenbosch L, van den Berg J, et al. Flipping the classroom to teach millennial residents medical leadership: a proof of concept. Adv Med Educ Pract 2017;8:57–61.

13. Hennessy CM, Kirkpatrick E, Smith CF, et al. Social media and anatomy education: using twitter to enhance the student learning experience in anatomy. Anat Sci Educ 2016;9(6):505–15.

14. Berkowitz SJ, Kung JW, Eisenberg RL, et al. Resident iPad use: has it really changed the game? J Am Coll Radiol 2014;11(2):180–4.

15. Bahner DP, Adkins E, Patel N, et al. How we use social media to supplement a novel curriculum in medical education. Med Teach 2012;34(6):439–44.

16. Hunter SF. Overview and diagnosis of multiple sclerosis. Am J Manag Care 2016;22(6 Suppl):s141–50.

17. Ogden CL, Carroll MD, Curtin LR, et al. Prevalence of high body mass index in US children and adolescents, 2007-2008. JAMA 2010;303(3):242–9.

18. Eaton DK, Kann L, Kinchen S, et al. Youth risk behavior surveillance–United States, 2007. MMWR Surveill Summ 2008;57(4):1–131.

19. Ogden CL, Carroll MD, Fryar CD, et al. Prevalence of obesity among adults and youth: United States, 2011-2014. NCHS Data Brief 2015;(219):1–8.

20. Hedstrom AK, Olsson T, Alfredsson L. High body mass index before age 20 is associated with increased risk for multiple sclerosis in both men and women. Mult Scler 2012;18(9):1334–6.

21. Gianfrancesco MA, Acuna B, Shen L, et al. Obesity during childhood and adolescence increases susceptibility to multiple sclerosis after accounting for established genetic and environmental risk factors. Obes Res Clin Pract 2014;8(5):e435–47.

22. Munger KL, Chitnis T, Ascherio A. Body size and risk of MS in two cohorts of US women. Neurology 2009;73(19):1543–50.

23. Depression and work: the impact of depression on different generations of employees. Available at: http://www.bensingerdupont.com/eap-research-white-paper-development2014. Accessed March 15, 2017.

24. Brenner P, Piehl F. Fatigue and depression in multiple sclerosis: pharmacological and non-pharmacological interventions. Acta Neurol Scand 2016;134(Suppl 200):47–54.

25. Center for collegiate mental health (CCMH). 2016 annual report. Pennsylvania: Penn State University; 2016. Available at: https://sites.psu.edu/ccmh/files/2017/01/2016-Annual-Report-FINAL_2016_01_09-1gc2hj6.pdf. Accessed March 15, 2017.

26. PNC Healthcare. Five ways tech-savvy millennials alter health care landscapes. 2015. Available at: http://www.prnewswire.com/news-releases/five-ways-tech-savvy-millennials-alter-health-care-landscape-300054028.html. Accessed March 21, 2017.

27. Transamerica Center for Health Studies. Millennial Survey: Young adults' healthcare reality. Transamerica Institute; 2016. Available at: https://www. transamericacenterforhealthstudies.org/docs/default-source/research/tchs-2016-millennial-survey-embargoed.pdf. Accessed March 15, 2017.

28. Adelman G, Rane SG, Villa KF. The cost burden of multiple sclerosis in the United States: a systematic review of the literature. J Med Econ 2013;16(5): 639–47.

29. Lebrun C, Bensa C, Debouverie M, et al. Unexpected multiple sclerosis: follow-up of 30 patients with magnetic resonance imaging and clinical conversion profile. J Neurol Neurosurg Psychiatry 2008;79(2):195–8.

30. Lourenco AP, Cronan JJ. Teaching and working with millennial trainees: impact on radiological education and work performance. J Am Coll Radiol 2017;14(1):92–5.

31. Deborah Bachrach JF, Garcimonde A, Nevitt K. Building a culture of health: the value proposition of retail clinics. New York: Manatt Health; 2015. Available at: https://www.transamericacenterforhealthstudies.org/docs/default-source/research/tchs-2016-millennial-survey-embargoed.pdf. Accessed March 15, 2017.

32. Hyatt A. American well announces mobile milestone of 1 million downloads. 2014. Available at: https://www.americanwell.com/american-well-announces-mobile-milestone-of-1-million-downloads-2/. Accessed March 22, 2017.

33. Telehealth index: 2015 Consumer survey highlights. American well; 2015: Available at: http://go.americanwell.com/rs/335-QLG-882/images/American_Well_Telehealth_Index_2017_Consumer_Survey.pdf. Accessed March 15, 2017.

34. Salesforce. 2015 state of the connected patient: healthcare insights from more than 1,700 adults. San Francisco (CA): Salesforce; 2015. Available at: https://secure2. sfdcstatic.com/assets/pdf/industries/2015-State-of-the-Connected-Patient.pdf. Accessed March 15, 2017.

35. Barnet S. Preventative health visits in danger of extinction. 2015. Available at: http://www.beckershospitalreview.com/quality/preventative-health-visits-in-danger-of-extinction.html. Accessed March 15, 2017.

36. The Nielsen Company. Mobile millennials: over 85% of generation Y owns smartphones. 2014. Available at: http://www.nielsen.com/us/en/insights/news/2014/mobile-millennials-over-85-percent-of-generation-y-owns-smartphones.html. Accessed March 20, 2017.

37. Hunt CW. Technology and diabetes self-management: an integrative review. World J Diabetes 2015;6(2):225–33.

38. Pennic J. 55% of millennials would trust a health app over health professionals. 2015. Available at: http://hitconsultant.net/2015/06/10/55-millennials-trust-health-app-health-professionals/. Accessed March 15, 2017.

39. Tran J, Tran R Jr, White JR. Smartphone-based glucose monitors and applications in the management of diabetes: an overview of 10 salient "Apps" and a

novel smartphone-connected blood glucose monitor. Clin Diabetes 2012; 2012(4):173–8.

40. PricewaterhouseCoopers. The Wearable Future. PwC network; 2014. Available at: http://www.pwc.com/us/en/technology/publications/assets/pwc-wearable-tech-design-oct-8th.pdf. Accessed March 15, 2017.

41. Finkelstein J, Cha E, Wood J, et al. Predictors of successful acceptance of home telemanagement in veterans with multiple sclerosis. Conf Proc IEEE Eng Med Biol Soc 2013;2013:7314–7.

42. Tacchino A, Pedulla L, Bonzano L, et al. A new app for at-home cognitive training: description and pilot testing on patients with multiple sclerosis. JMIR Mhealth Uhealth 2015;3(3):e85.

43. Greiner P, Sawka A, Imison E. Patient and physician perspectives on msdialog, an electronic PRO diary in multiple sclerosis. Patient 2015;8(6):541–50.

44. Bove R, White CC, Giovannoni G, et al. Evaluating more naturalistic outcome measures: a 1-year smartphone study in multiple sclerosis. Neurol Neuroimmunol Neuroinflamm 2015;2(6):e162.

Moving?

Make sure your subscription moves with you!

To notify us of your new address, find your **Clinics Account Number** (located on your mailing label above your name), and contact customer service at:

Email: journalscustomerservice-usa@elsevier.com

800-654-2452 (subscribers in the U.S. & Canada)
314-447-8871 (subscribers outside of the U.S. & Canada)

Fax number: 314-447-8029

Elsevier Health Sciences Division
Subscription Customer Service
3251 Riverport Lane
Maryland Heights, MO 63043

*To ensure uninterrupted delivery of your subscription, please notify us at least 4 weeks in advance of move.